T0261057

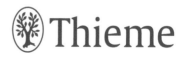

# Top 3 Differentials in Nuclear Medicine

A Case Review

**Ely A. Wolin, MD**
Lieutenant Colonel, United States Air Force
Program Director, Diagnostic Radiology Residency
Chief, Nuclear Medicine Services
David Grant USAF Medical Center
Assistant Professor of Radiology/Radiological Sciences
Uniformed Services University of the Health Sciences
Bethesda, Maryland

Series Editor:

**William T. O'Brien, Sr., DO, FAOCR**
Director, Pediatric Neuroradiology Fellowship
Cincinnati Children's Hospital Medical Center
Associate Professor of Radiology
University of Cincinnati College of Medicine
Cincinnati, Ohio

267 illustrations

Thieme
New York • Stuttgart • Delhi • Rio de Janeiro

Executive Editor: William Lamsback
Managing Editors: Apoorva Goel
Director, Editorial Services: Mary Jo Casey
Production Editor: Rohit Dev Bhardwaj
International Production Director: Andreas Schabert
Editorial Director: Sue Hodgson
International Marketing Director: Fiona Henderson
International Sales Director: Louisa Turrell
Director, Institutional Sales: Adam Bernacki
Senior Vice President and Chief Operating Officer:
   Sarah Vanderbilt
President: Brian D. Scanlan

**Library of Congress Cataloging-in-Publication Data**
is available from the publisher.

©2019 Thieme Medical Publishers, Inc.

Thieme Publishers New York
333 Seventh Avenue, New York, NY 10001 USA
+1 800 782 3488, customerservice@thieme.com

Thieme Publishers Stuttgart
Rüdigerstrasse 14, 70469 Stuttgart, Germany
+49 [0]711 8931 421, customerservice@thieme.de

Thieme Publishers Delhi
A-12, Second Floor, Sector-2, Noida-201301
Uttar Pradesh, India
+91 120 45 566 00, customerservice@thieme.in

Thieme Publishers Rio de Janeiro,
Thieme Publicações Ltda.
Edifício Rodolpho de Paoli, 25º andar
Av. Nilo Peçanha, 50 – Sala 2508,
Rio de Janeiro 20020-906 Brasil
+55 21 3172-2297

Cover design: Thieme Publishing Group
Typesetting by DiTech Process Solutions, India

Printed in USA by King Printing Company, Inc.          5 4 3 2 1

ISBN: 978-1-62623-344-7

Also available as an e-book:
eISBN: 978-1-62623-354-6

**Important note:** Medicine is an ever-changing science undergoing continual development. Research and clinical experience are continually expanding our knowledge, in particular our knowledge of proper treatment and drug therapy. Insofar as this book mentions any dosage or application, readers may rest assured that the authors, editors, and publishers have made every effort to ensure that such references are in accordance with **the state of knowledge at the time of production of the book.**

Nevertheless, this does not involve, imply, or express any guarantee or responsibility on the part of the publishers in respect to any dosage instructions and forms of applications stated in the book. **Every user is requested to examine carefully** the manufacturers' leaflets accompanying each drug and to check, if necessary in consultation with a physician or specialist, whether the dosage schedules mentioned therein or the contraindications stated by the manufacturers differ from the statements made in the present book. Such examination is particularly important with drugs that are either rarely used or have been newly released on the market. Every dosage schedule or every form of application used is entirely at the user's own risk and responsibility. The authors and publishers request every user to report to the publishers any discrepancies or inaccuracies noticed. If errors in this work are found after publication, errata will be posted at www.thieme.com on the product description page.

Some of the product names, patents, and registered designs referred to in this book are in fact registered trademarks or proprietary names even though specific reference to this fact is not always made in the text. Therefore, the appearance of a name without designation as proprietary is not to be construed as a representation by the publisher that it is in the public domain.

The views expressed in this book are those of the author and contributors, and do not reflect the official policy or position of the United States Government, the Department of Defense, Department of the Army or the Department of the Air Force

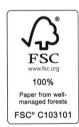

This book, including all parts thereof, is legally protected by copyright. Any use, exploitation, or commercialization outside the narrow limits set by copyright legislation, without the publisher's consent, is illegal and liable to prosecution. This applies in particular to photostat reproduction, copying, mimeographing, preparation of microfilms, and electronic data processing and storage.

*I dedicate this book to my amazing wife and children. You are my "why."*

# Contents

# Series Foreword

The original "Top 3" concept was something engrained in us during our residency training in the military. From day 1, our program emphasized the importance of having gamut-based differentials as part of our daily readout sessions, as well as during didactic and clinical case-based conferences. The bulk of residency training was then centered around learning the key clinical and imaging manifestations of each entity on the list of differentials to be able to distinguish one from another, when possible. To avoid providing clinicians with a laundry list of differentials that would be of little value, we were encouraged to consider the "Top 3" differentials and any other important considerations based on the specific clinical scenario or imaging finding(s) presented. I found this concept and approach to radiology so useful that I continue to utilize it to this day.

One thing I have learned throughout my radiology career, especially as a residency program director, is that not every individual learns or processes information in the same manner. Some individuals can read through a traditional textbook that is organized by pathology (i.e., developmental abnormalities, infectious processes, neoplasms, etc.) and readily recognize that the developmental abnormality in Chapter 1 is in the same differential for the infectious process in Chapter 2 and a few neoplasms in Chapter 3. Others, like me, best learn from gamut-based resources where content is organized based on the key imaging findings, similar to how we practice radiology. If you are part of the latter group, then the "Top 3" approach may be the right fit for you. The intent of the series is to provide a comprehensive case-based alternative to traditional subspecialty textbooks where the focus remains on differential diagnoses.

After all, when the dust settles and the core and certifying exams are nothing but distant (and hopefully pleasant) memories, this is what radiology is all about.

This Nuclear Medicine Top 3 book is edited by Dr. Ely Wolin, who is an academic radiologist and is also affiliated to the residency program at David Grant USAF Medical Center (DGMC), Travis AFB, CA. I first met Dr. Wolin when we were stationed together as faculty at DGMC and was immediately impressed by his style of lectures and at-the-monitor teaching. His emphasis on working through differentials was reminiscent of how I was trained and embraced by our residents. He was presented with our coveted teaching award in just his first year as faculty. After witnessing his work as the Nuclear Medicine editor for the second edition of the original Top 3 book, there was no question that he was the ideal candidate to author and edit the Nuclear Medicine subspecialty series edition.

*Top 3 Differentials in Nuclear Medicine* is organized into 12 parts, encompassing all body regions and radiopharmaceuticals. The initial parts are dedicated to specific body regions, while the latter parts discuss imaging of various inflammatory processes and neoplasms. The final part covers the important topic of quality control, which is essential both for board review and clinical practice. As with the original Top 3 book, the emphasis is on differential-based cases with the addition of Roentgen Classics where appropriate.

It is my sincere hope that you find this subspecialty Top 3 book both enjoyable and educational.

*William T. O'Brien Sr., DO, FAOCR*

# Preface

It is with humble excitement that I present *Top 3 Differentials in Nuclear Medicine: A Case Review*. I am hopeful that this subspecialty edition will help radiology residents, nuclear medicine residents and fellows, and staff radiologists prepare for their certification or continued certification testing, as well as provide a useful framework for all those who utilize nuclear medicine in their practice.

This book is organized primarily by body system, with additional sections for infection and inflammation, PET, and tumor imaging, as well as physics/QC. Sections follow the "Top 3" series format first used by William T. O'Brien in his 2010 publication and include unknown differential-based cases. The first page for each case provides a brief clinical history, an image, and an image legend. The images are intended to illustrate a key imaging finding which is expressly defined at the beginning of the second page. The key imaging finding is followed by a differential-based discussion for that finding that is broken down into Top 3 and additional diagnostic considerations, including a review of important imaging and clinical details for each differential. This is followed by imaging pearls to provide a quick review of key points. Altogether, this provides a high-yield differential-based

reference which is hopefully very useful for both board exam preparation and clinical practice. While the final diagnosis for each case is provided, when available, the focus of the book is on the differential discussion for the imaging finding and not on the final diagnosis itself.

Although I believe this book will prove to be useful to all those learning and practicing nuclear medicine, it is not meant to be a comprehensive reference book. Many new or novel radiopharmaceuticals are not included, as they are not yet ubiquitous in practice. The focus while creating this book was on providing key findings likely to be encountered in both clinical practice and the exam setting to initiate a gamut-based differential discussion.

I found the approach of the original Top 3 book to be incredibly helpful during radiology residency and beyond. I sincerely hope you will find this book helpful as well. Thank you for the honor of allowing me to contribute to the rewarding goal of lifelong learning!

*Ely A. Wolin, MD*

# Acknowledgments

This book would not have been possible without the efforts of many people. First, I would like to thank Dr. William T. O'Brien for paving the way with the original Top 3 book and leading me to this opportunity. Some cases from the nuclear medicine chapter of the second edition of the original work are included in this book. I would like to thank all those who trained me during my radiology residency at Penn State Health MS Hershey Medical Center and my nuclear medicine fellowship at the San Antonio Uniformed Services Health Education Consortium; it is because of you all that I am inspired to continue a career in academic radiology. Specific thanks to Dr. Don Fleming for taking a chance on me—I am forever in your debt.

Many people contributed directly to this book. I would like to thank Joe Fotos, Mickaila Johnston, and Kate Wagner who were kind enough to serve as chapter editors. Thanks to all the residents and colleagues who authored or contributed to cases. I truly cannot thank any of them enough for helping make this project a reality!

Most importantly, I would like to thank my loving family! My wife, Lisa, has provided continuous love and support through the ups and downs, and many moves of my career. I am in awe of her strength daily. My daughters, Kiley and Makenzie, bring more joy to my life than I could have ever imagined! I have much to be grateful for!

*Ely A. Wolin, MD*

*Note:* The views expressed in this material are those of the author and do not reflect the official policy or position of the U.S. Government, the Department of Defense, or the Department of the Air Force.

# Contributors

**Victoria A. Campbell, MD**
Lieutenant Commander, United States Navy
Department of Radiology
Naval Medical Center
San Diego, California

**Brady S. Davis, DO**
Captain, United States Air Force
Department of Diagnostic Imaging
David Grant USAF Medical Center
Travis Air Force Base, California

**John Dryden, MD**
Lieutenant Commander, United States Navy
Diagnostic Radiologist
Mammography and Diagnostic Divisional Officer
U.S. Naval Hospital
Okinawa, Japan

**David W. Erickson, MS**
Captain, United States Air Force
Department of Diagnostic Imaging, Medical Physics
Travis Air Force Base, California

**Cameron C. Foster, MD**
Associate Professor
Clinical Director of Nuclear Medicine and PET
Nuclear Medicine Residency Program Director
University of California Davis Health
Sacramento, California

**Joseph S. Fotos, MD**
Assistant Professor of Radiology
Division of Nuclear Medicine
Penn State Milton S. Hershey Medical Center
Hershey, Pennsylvania

**Britain A. Gailliot, MD**
Captain, United States Air Force
Department of Diagnostic Imaging
David Grant USAF Medical Center
Travis Air Force Base, California

**James J. Gullo, MD**
Captain, United States Air Force
Department of Diagnostic Imaging
David Grant USAF Medical Center
Travis Air Force Base, California

**Mickaila Johnston, MD, FACNM**
Commander, MC (UMO), United States Navy
Senior Medical Officer
USS Frank Cable
USS Frank Cole

**Brian J. Lewis, DO**
Major, United States Air Force
Department of Radiology
10th Medical Group
United States Air Force Academy
Colorado Springs, Colorado

**John P. Lichtenberger, MD**
Lieutenant Colonel, United States Air Force
Cardiothoracic Radiologist
Associate Professor
Radiology
Uniformed Services University of the Health Sciences (USU)
Bethesda, Maryland

**Jonathan Muldermans, MD**
Captain, United States Air Force
Department of Diagnostic Imaging
David Grant USAF Medical Center
Travis Air Force Base, California

**Vicki Nagano, MD**
Department of Nuclear Medicine
Kaiser Sacramento
Sacramento, California

**William T. O'Brien, Sr.**
Director, Pediatric Neuroradiology Fellowship
Cincinnati Children's Hospital Medical Center
Associate Professor of Radiology
University of Cincinnati College of Medicine
Cincinnati, Ohio

**Kamal D. Singh, MD**
Chief
Nuclear Medicine
Kaiser West Los Angeles
Los Angeles, California

**Trevor A. Thompson, MD**
Major, United States Air Force
Officer In-Charge
Nuclear Medicine Section
Mike O'Callaghan Military Medical Center
Nellis Air Force Base
Las Vegas, Nevada

**Kathryn R. Wagner, MS**
Assistant Radiation Safety Officer
Medical University of South Carolina
Charleston, South Carolina

**Ely A. Wolin**
Lieutenant Colonel, United States Air Force
Program Director, Diagnostic Radiology Residency
Chief, Nuclear Medicine Services
David Grant USAF Medical Center
Assistant Professor of Radiology/Radiological Sciences
Uniformed Services University of the Health Sciences
Bethesda, Maryland

**Joseph M. Yetto, Jr., MD**
Lieutenant Commander, United States Navy
Chief Resident
Diagnostic Radiology
Naval Medical Center
San Diego, California

**Cathy Zhou, MD**
Resident
Nuclear Medicine and Diagnostic Radiology
University of California, Davis
Sacramento, California

# Part 1

## Neuro

# Case 1

*Joseph S. Fotos*

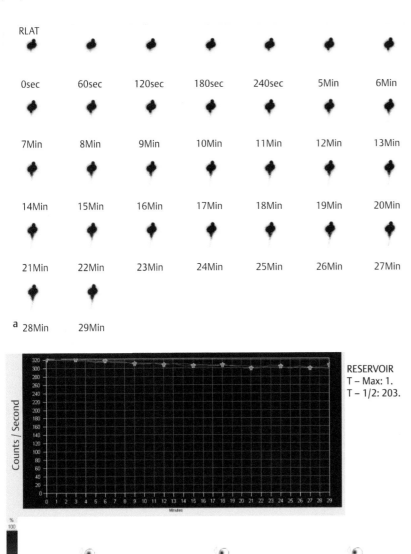

**Fig. 1.1** Cerebrospinal fluid (CSF) flow study with indium-111 (In-111) diethylenetriamine pentaacetic acid (DTPA). Dynamic imaging **(a)** demonstrates activity localization within the reservoir and backflow into the ventricles and remaining neuraxis. Calculated T ½ with a region of interest (ROI) at the reservoir **(b)** measures 203 minutes, markedly abnormal (normal is 5 minutes or less).

RESERVOIR
T – Max: 1.
T – 1/2: 203.

## ■ Clinical History

89-year-old male with history of idiopathic normal pressure hydrocephalus and worsening symptoms (▸ Fig. 1.1).

## ▪ Key Finding

Absent CSF flow through ventricular shunt tubing

## ▪ Top 2 Differential Diagnoses

• **Shunt obstruction.** Ventriculoperitoneal and ventriculoatrial shunts are commonly placed in patients with obstructive hydrocephalus. These shunts are placed percutaneously by neurosurgery. A reservoir, with an internal valve, is placed in the subcutaneous tissues superficial to the skull. Afferent tubing is then passed through the skull and into the ventricular system adjacent to the foramen of Monro. Efferent tubing is connected to the reservoir superficially and courses under the skin and down the neck and chest before terminating within the peritoneal cavity in the abdomen, or extending into the venous system and terminating in the right atrium. Worsening clinical symptoms or increasing ventricular size raises concern for obstruction of the shunt tubing. To evaluate the flow, the reservoir is accessed by the neurosurgical service and a small amount of the patient's CSF is removed. The dose of In-111 DTPA is then injected into the reservoir in sterile saline, followed by a flush with the previously removed autologous CSF. The efferent tubing can be blocked if evaluation of the afferent tubing is needed. Dynamic imaging is performed for 30 minutes to visualize the flow of CSF. Quantification can be performed by drawing an ROI around the reservoir and measuring the time to half activity, normally 5 minutes or less. Normal examinations should demonstrate flow of activity from the lateral ventricles through the afferent tubing to the reservoir, and then through the efferent tubing to either the peritoneal or venous system. Complete obstruction will show flow of activity into the ventricles and absence of flow into the tubing or reservoir with no terminal destination activity. Possible etiologies for shunt obstruction include injury to the choroid plexus, increasing cellular debris within the CSF, as well as red blood cell and platelet aggregates in patients with intracranial hemorrhage.

• **Peritoneal pseudocyst.** Normally, CSF that drains into the peritoneal cavity is absorbed over time. However, in rare cases a walled-off collection of the drained CSF can form within the peritoneal cavity. This collection is termed a peritoneal CSF pseudocyst which is formed by a wall of fibrous tissue and epithelium. As the cyst grows, backpressure through the peritoneal tubing increases leading to decreased and eventual absent forward flow. If the cyst is imaged early on in its development and growth, focal accumulation of activity within the abdomen is seen. If this diagnosis is suspected and no such accumulation is seen on CSF flow imaging, further imaging with abdominal ultrasound (US) or CT is essential for correct interpretation.

## ▪ Diagnosis

CSF ventriculoperitoneal shunt tubing obstruction.

## ✓ Pearls

• Normal exams demonstrate flow from the ventricles to either the peritoneal cavity or venous system.
• Shunt obstruction will present with absent or delayed antegrade flow.
• Peritoneal CSF pseudocyst formation is a rare complication of VP shunt tubing placement.

• Cross-sectional imaging is needed if CSF pseudocyst is suspected and flow imaging is negative.
• In-111 DTPA is an ideal CSF label. It is nonpyrogenic with a favorable half-life and photon energy.

## Suggested Readings

Khan F, Rehman A, Shamim MS, Bari ME. Factors affecting ventriculoperitoneal shunt survival in adult patients. Surg Neurol Int. 2015; 6:25
Mai DT, Vasinrapee P, Cook RE. Diagnosis of abdominal cerebrospinal fluid pseudocyst by scintigraphy. Clin Nucl Med. 1993; 18(3):237–238

Sigg D, Rich R, Ashby S, Jabour B, Glass E. Radionuclide shuntogram demonstrating migration of distal ventriculoperitoneal shunt tubing out of the peritoneal cavity. Clin Nucl Med. 2005; 30(8):552–554

# Case 2

*Kamal D. Singh*

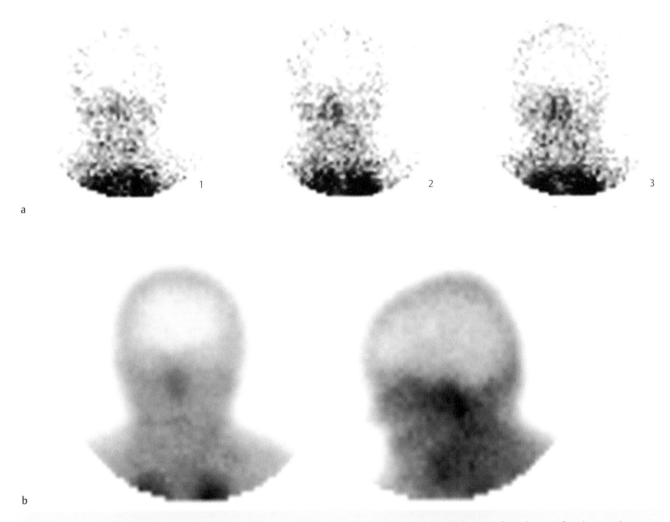

**Fig. 2.1** Brain death study with Technetium-99m (Tc-99m) hexamethylpropyleneamine (HMPAO). Selected images from dynamic flow (1 second per frame for 1 minute) **(a)** demonstrate absence of intracranial flow. Blood pool imaging in anterior and lateral projections **(b)** reveals absent cerebral or cerebellar uptake and physiologic faint scalp activity, along with increased activity in the nasopharyngeal region ("hot nose" sign). These findings were confirmed on delayed single-photon emission computed tomography (SPECT) imaging of the head (not included).

■ **Clinical History**
...........................................................................................................................

57-year-old male unresponsive after a motor vehicle accident
(▶Fig. 2.1).

## ■ Key Finding

Absent intracranial activity on a Tc-99m HMPAO scan

## ■ Top 3 Differential Diagnoses

- **Brain death.** Brain death is a clinical diagnosis utilizing a combination of physical examination, electroencephalography, and imaging findings. A brain death scan has high specificity as a confirmatory study for absent intracranial perfusion. Scintigraphic imaging can be performed at the patient's bedside with a portable gamma camera. Imaging may be performed with a nonspecific flow agent (Tc-99m diethylenetriamine pentaacetic acid [DTPA]), or with lipophilic brain perfusion agents (Tc-99m HMPAO or Tc-99m ethyl cysteinate dimer [ECD]) which cross the blood–brain barrier (BBB) and are extracted by viable brain tissue proportional to cerebral flow. A scalp band or tourniquet may be placed around the head to avoid interfering activity from extracranial vessels. The scalp band, however, is contraindicated in pediatric patients due to increased intracranial pressure. First-minute dynamic flow imaging is performed in an anterior projection, with subsequent static blood pool images in both anterior and lateral projections. Delayed SPECT imaging may improve sensitivity in cases where lipophilic agents are utilized. Normal imaging reveals symmetric flow within the anterior and middle cerebral arteries ("trident" sign) on the anterior view, with visualization of dural venous sinuses on blood pool imaging. In brain death, there is termination of carotid activity at the skull base due to increased intracranial pressure overcoming perfusion pressure, thereby shunting blood through the external carotid artery branches projecting over the nasopharyngeal region ("hot nose" sign).
- **Injection error.** Peripheral intravenous injection of the radiotracer is performed as a rapid/tight bolus. A proper bolus is confirmed by visualizing distinct activity within the proximal common carotid arteries. Dose infiltration, slow radiotracer injection, or missed bolus can result in false-positive studies, especially when flow agents (like Tc-99m DTPA, which do not cross the BBB) are used. Tc-99m DTPA is rapidly cleared through renal excretion which allows for reinjection and reimaging in the setting of equivocal or technically limited studies.
- **Poor radiopharmaceutical labeling/quality control.** Quality control is essential with lipophilic brain-specific agents. Poor labeling and instability can result in a false-positive exam. HMPAO should be labeled with fresh eluate within 2 hours of elution. If it is stabilized, it has a shelf life of 4 hours after labeling.

## ■ Diagnosis

Brain death.

## ✓ Pearls

- Besides brain death, Tc-99m HMPAO can image cerebral ischemia, seizure focus, and dementia.
- Absent intracranial flow and no cerebral/cerebellar uptake of Tc-99m HMPAO confirm brain death.
- Brain parenchymal uptake of radiotracer is not seen with flow agents like Tc-99m DTPA.
- Scintigraphic evaluation is unaffected by drug intoxication, hypothermia, or metabolic derangements.

## Suggested Readings

Conrad GR, Sinha P. Scintigraphy as a confirmatory test of brain death. Semin Nucl Med. 2003; 33(4):312–323

Donohoe KJ, Agrawal G, Frey KA, et al. SNM practice guideline for brain death scintigraphy 2.0. J Nucl Med Technol. 2012; 40(3):198–203

Sinha P, Conrad GR. Scintigraphic confirmation of brain death. Semin Nucl Med. 2012; 42(1):27–32

# Case 3

*Joseph S. Fotos*

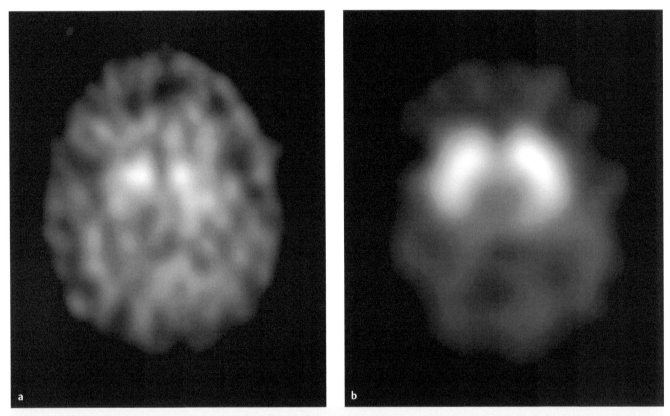

**Fig. 3.1** Abnormal Iodine-123 (I-123) Ioflupane scan **(a)**, with asymmetric bilateral decreased uptake within the striatum, most severe within the putamina. For comparison, a normal scan **(b)** demonstrates symmetric uptake bilaterally in a smooth comma-shaped distribution.

## ■ Clinical History

64-year-old male with history of postural tremor (▶ Fig. 3.1).

## ■ Key Finding

Asymmetric decreased uptake within the striatum on I-123 Ioflupane scan

## ■ Top 3 Differential Diagnoses

- **Parkinson's disease.** Parkinson's disease (PD) is a movement disorder that occurs due to loss of dopaminergic neurons within the substantia nigra. The disease presents after age 60 and includes resting tremor, bradykinesia, rigidity, and loss of balance and coordination. Differentiation between PD and essential tremor (ET) is often difficult. ET is a different tremor disorder of unknown cause that presents with intention or postural tremors, and many patients with ET are misdiagnosed with PD. Recent advances in imaging of the dopaminergic pathways have provided an elegant means of differentiating these two disorders. I-123 Ioflupane (DATscan, GE Healthcare, Chicago, IL) binds to the presynaptic dopamine transporters present at the end of axons of the nigrostriatal pathway that course from the substantia nigra to the striatum. Uptake of this radiopharmaceutical is seen within the striatum itself and not the substantia nigra where the neurons originate. Normal scans demonstrate symmetric uptake within the striata bilaterally, which appear as smooth comma–shaped structures.

Abnormal uptake consists of any decrease in uptake and is usually asymmetric.

- **Dementia with Lewy Bodies.** Dementia with Lewy Bodies (DLB) is the second most common neurodegenerative disorder in patients over the age of 65. In contrast to Alzheimer's disease (AD), memory deficits often present as a later finding, with initial loss of attention and visuospatial function. Still, when presenting with memory deficits, it is sometimes difficult to differentiate these two entities based on symptoms alone. Recent studies have demonstrated a progressive loss of dopaminergic neurons in patients with DLB, representing an important differentiating feature between DLB and AD.
- **Other parkinsonian syndromes.** Other parkinsonian syndromes, such as progressive supranuclear palsy (PSP) and multiple system atrophy (MSA), also involve loss of dopaminergic neurons and will demonstrate similar findings on I-123 Ioflupane scanning. Studies have shown this scan to improve physician confidence in their diagnosis of these syndromes.

## ■ Diagnosis

Presynaptic dopaminergic defect within the striatum, consistent with a parkinsonian syndrome in the appropriate clinical setting.

## ✓ Pearls

- I-123 Ioflupane binds to presynaptic dopaminergic transporters within the striatum.
- Abnormal scans show loss of comma–shaped striatal uptake with asymmetric decreased uptake.

- Abnormal DATscan suggests dopaminergic neurodegenerative disease (PD, PSP, or MSA).
- DLB also involves progressive loss of dopaminergic neurons, which differentiates it from AD.

## Suggested Readings

Benamer TS, Patterson J, Grosset DG, et al. Accurate differentiation of parkinsonism and essential tremor using visual assessment of [123I]-FP-CIT SPECT imaging: the [123I]-FP-CIT study group. Mov Disord. 2000; 15(3):503–510

Colloby SJ, Williams ED, Burn DJ, Lloyd JJ, McKeith IG, O'Brien JT. Progression of dopaminergic degeneration in dementia with Lewy bodies and Parkinson's disease with and without dementia assessed using 123I-FP-CIT SPECT. Eur J Nucl Med Mol Imaging. 2005; 32(10):1176–1185

Seifert KD, Wiener JI. The impact of DaTscan on the diagnosis and management of movement disorders: A retrospective study. Am J Neurodegener Dis. 2013; 2(1):29–34

# Case 4

*Joseph S. Fotos*

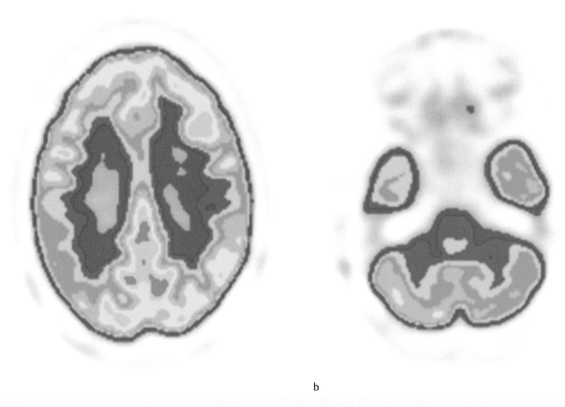

a                                               b

**Fig. 4.1** Axial fluorine-18 fluorodeoxyglucose positron-emission tomography (F-18 FDG PET) in patient with chronic intractable seizures. Axial slice of brain **(a)** demostrates marked hypometabolism within the right parietal lobe, localizing to areas on concurrent Electroencephalography (EEG) (not shown) indicating an area of seizure susceptibility. Note the relatively decreased metabolism seen within the left cerebellar lobe **(b)**.

## ■ Clinical History

48-year-old female patient with chronic intractable complex partial epilepsy (▶Fig. 4.1).

## ■ Key Finding

Unilateral decreased cerebellar perfusion or metabolism

## ■ Top 3 Differential Diagnoses

- **Crossed cerebellar diaschisis.** The term "diaschisis" was originally coined in 1914 by Constantin von Monakow, meaning "shocked throughout" in Greek. Crossed cerebellar diaschisis (CCD) refers to the loss of function within an undamaged part of the cerebellum that is distantly connected to a damaged part of the cerebrum via long axons. This leads to disruption of the corticopontocerebellar tracts, depressed metabolism and blood flow, and eventual cortical atrophy. Given the normal contralateral crossing pattern of cerebral neurons that occurs within the brainstem, connected areas within the cerebellum lose function when areas of the contralateral cerebral cortex are damaged (hence the term "crossed"). As the cerebellum serves the important function of providing coordination of motor impulses, this pattern is often seen following an insult to the motor cortex within the parietal lobe. Possible associated supratentorial pathologies include tumor, seizure focus, and stroke. Similar findings of decreased uptake will be seen on both F-18 FDG PET metabolism imaging and brain perfusion single-photon emission computed tomography (SPECT).
- **Stroke.** Infarcted brain will show little to no metabolism on F-18 FDG positron emission tomography/computed tomography (PET/CT) and decreased perfusion on SPECT imaging, depending on the extent of damage. In these cases, the CT images of the brain are essential for correct interpretation. As with all studies, ensure that all available comparison studies are used as part of the current study interpretation.
- **Prior surgery.** As one would expect, following surgical resection of a portion of the cerebellum (often for tumor), decreased metabolism and perfusion will be seen within the location of the absent cerebellar tissue. It is essential to compare findings with correlative anatomic imaging, available previous studies, as well as the patient's medical and surgical history.

## ■ Diagnosis

Crossed cerebellar diaschisis secondary to intractable right temporoparietal seizures.

## ✓ Pearls

- CCD is the loss of cerebellar function from damage to the contralateral supratentorial brain.
- Other etiologies for decreased cerebellar uptake include infarct or surgical resection.
- Correlation with prior studies and the patient's surgical and medical history is essential.
- CCD on standard "eyes to thighs" PET scan indicates the need to image the supratentorial brain.

## Suggested Readings

Al-Faham Z, Zein RK, Wong CY. 18F-FDG PET assessment of Lewy body dementia with cerebellar diaschisis. J Nucl Med Technol. 2014; 42(4):306–307

Mewasingh LD, Christiaens F, Aeby A, Christophe C, Dan B. Crossed cerebellar diaschisis secondary to refractory frontal seizures in childhood. Seizure. 2002; 11(8):489–493

Shih WJ, Huang WS, Milan PP. F-18 FDG PET demonstrates crossed cerebellar diaschisis 20 years after stroke. Clin Nucl Med. 2006; 31(5):259–261

Tien RD, Ashdown BC. Crossed cerebellar diaschisis and crossed cerebellar atrophy: correlation of MR findings, clinical symptoms, and supratentorial diseases in 26 patients. AJR Am J Roentgenol. 1992; 158(5):1155–1159

# Case 5

*Joseph S. Fotos*

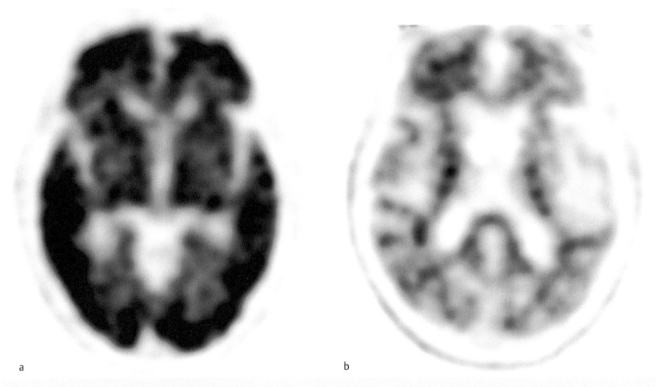

a                                                                b

**Fig. 5.1** Beta-amyloid scan using the fluorine-18 (F-18) based PET tracer florbetapir (Amyvid, Eli Lilly, Indianapolis, IN). Intense and diffuse cortical binding of the radiotracer **(a)** with complete loss of the normal gray-white matter differentiation. For comparison, the normal binding pattern is shown **(b)** throughout the white matter tracts, with little binding seen in the cortical gray matter.

## ■ Clinical History

75-year-old male with progressive cognitive decline (▶ Fig. 5.1).

## ■ Key Finding

Diffuse cortical binding of F-18 florbetapir, loss of normal gray-white differentiation

## ■ Top 3 Differential Diagnoses

- **Alzheimer's disease (AD).** AD is a progressive neurologic disorder, usually presenting after 60 years of age. It is characterized by progressive loss of memory and cognitive skills. While no cure currently exists, there has been some success in managing symptoms with medication and behavioral management. The pathophysiology remains poorly understood. However, pathologic postmortem analysis on brain tissue in patients diagnosed with AD reveals an association with increased accumulation of neurofibrillary tangles and beta-amyloid plaques. Beta-amyloid accumulation has been studied as an imaging target for novel radiotracers, including ongoing trials using F-18 based PET tracers. A normal scan with F-18 florbetapir will show activity distributed within the white matter tracts much greater than within the cortical gray matter, providing a clear gray-white differentiation. Abnormal scans demonstrate loss of this differentiation with increased cortical binding. Results of these scans can be used as part of an overall assessment for AD. Cortical uptake is highly suggestive but not diagnostic of AD, as other neurologic disorders and even patients with normal cognition may present with a similar pattern. A positive study has, however, been shown to identify patients at risk of a progressive cognitive decline. When negative, the likelihood that the patient's neurological symptoms are due to AD are reduced.
- **Dementia with Lewy bodies.** Dementia with Lewy bodies (DLB) is the second most common neurodegenerative disorder in patients over the age of 65 years. In contrast to AD, memory deficits often present as a later finding, with initial loss of attention and visuospatial function. Beta-amyloid deposition has also been seen in patients with DLB, though it is not present in all patients and is therefore not useful in the diagnosis of DLB. Studies have demonstrated an association with increased beta-amyloid deposition and an increased severity of overall cognitive impairment in these patients, and may help predict future cognitive decline in these patients.
- **Amyloid angiopathy.** Deposition of beta-amyloid within the walls of the cortical blood vessels is a common age-related process, termed cerebral amyloid angiopathy (CAA), and may play a role in increasing the risk for spontaneous intracerebral hemorrhage. Multiple beta-amyloid imaging agents have been shown to bind to this type of vascular deposition as well.

## ■ Diagnosis

Positive F-18 florbetapir scan, supportive of a diagnosis of AD.

## ✓ Pearls

- Increased beta-amyloid deposition within the cortical gray matter is associated with AD.
- Multiple F-18 based PET tracers are currently under investigation to assist in the diagnosis of AD.
- Beta-amyloid can also be seen in DLB, especially in patients with severe cognitive impairment.
- Beta-amyloid binding agents also have been shown to bind the vascular deposition seen in CAA.

## Suggested Readings

Clark CM, Pontecorvo MJ, Beach TG, et al. AV-45-A16 Study Group. Cerebral PET with florbetapir compared with neuropathology at autopsy for detection of neuritic amyloid-β plaques: a prospective cohort study. Lancet Neurol. 2012; 11(8):669–678

Donaghy P, Thomas AJ, O'Brien JT. Amyloid PET imaging in Lewy body disorders. Am J Geriatr Psychiatry. 2015; 23(1):23–37

Doraiswamy PM, Sperling RA, Coleman RE, et al. AV45-A11 Study Group. Amyloid-β assessed by florbetapir F 18 PET and 18-month cognitive decline: a multicenter study. Neurology. 2012; 79(16):1636–1644

Gurol ME, Becker JA, Fotiadis P, et al. Florbetapir-PET to diagnose cerebral amyloid angiopathy: A prospective study. Neurology. 2016; 87(19):2043–2049

# Case 6

*Cameron C. Foster*

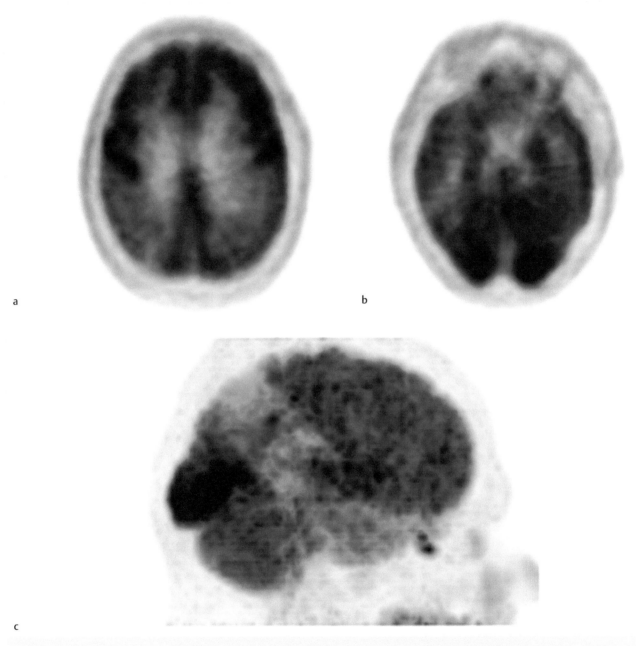

**Fig. 6.1** Attenuation corrected axial FDG PET images of the brain demonstrate decreased activity within the bilateral parietal **(a)** and temporal **(b)** lobes with intact normal activity within the bilateral frontal and occipital lobes. Attenuation corrected FDG PET maximum intensity projection (MIP) image in sagittal projection **(c)** demonstrates decreased activity in both the parietal and temporal lobes with intact normal activity within the cerebellum, frontal and occipital lobes.

■ Clinical History

62-year-old male with 6-year history of cognitive decline (▶Fig. 6.1).

## ■ Key Finding

Decreased cortical FDG activity in the setting of dementia

## ■ Top 3 Differential Diagnoses

- **Alzheimer's disease.** It is the most common dementing disorder affecting adults. Presentation is usually after 65 years of age and prevalence increases with age. Initial imaging findings are of decreased metabolism (FDG PET) and blood flow (single-photon emission computed tomography [SPECT]) in the bilateral temporoparietal areas with relative sparing of the primary motor, somatosensory, and visual cortices. One of the earliest findings include hypometabolic posterior cingulate gyri. Early stage Alzheimer's disease (AD) may show hemispheric asymmetry. Later stage AD will also begin to show metabolic decline in the frontal lobes at a faster rate than normal aging dementia. In general, the amount of decreased metabolism directly correlates with the degree of symptoms.
- **Pick's disease.** It is a classic, although rare member of the frontotemporal dementia (FTD) family. It is characterized by decreased metabolism in the bilateral frontal lobes and anterior temporal lobes on FDG PET imaging. Differentiation from other disorders such as AD are based on symptoms, such as Pick's disease has memory impairment as a secondary or absent feature rather than a primary symptom as is seen in AD. Differential considerations for isolated decreased metabolism in the frontotemporal regions include such entities as depression, cocaine abuse, and amyotrophic lateral sclerosis (ALS). This distribution is rarely seen in AD.
- **Multi-infarct dementia (MID).** It is the most common cause of vascular dementia and is the second most common cause of all dementias for adults over 65 years of age (after AD). While MID is usually identified via CT or MRI, FDG PET and SPECT imaging show similar patterns of decreased activity in a diffuse or multifocal distribution that progress over time. Frontotemporal distribution can be seen in MID and can be difficult to differentiate from other FTDs; diffuse distribution of MID can also be difficult to differentiate from severe AD.

## ■ Additional Diagnostic Consideration

- **Parkinson's disease (PD):** PD is largely a clinical diagnosis that has normal appearance on FDG PET in the early stages (striatum may be mildly increased). In later stages, decreased activity will be seen in the cortices and will progress along with the disease. Use of serial FDOPA PET scans in patients with PD will initially show decreased activity within the posterior putamen with sparing of the caudate that, over time, will involve more of the putamen and eventually include the posterior aspect of the caudate.

## ■ Diagnosis

Alzheimer's disease.

## ✓ Pearls

- AD shows bilateral temporoparietal hypometabolism with sparing of the occipital lobes (visual cortices).
- Frontal lobe hypometabolism can be seen in FTD (e.g., Pick's disease), depression, and schizophrenia.
- MID presents as multifocal regions of decreased activity.
- Dementia with Lew Bodies (DLB) has similar appearance to AD with less sparing of occipital lobe.

## Suggested Readings

Herholz K, Herscovitch P, Heiss WD. NeuroPET. Berlin, Germany: Springer-Verlag, 2004

Hoffman JM, Welsh-Bohmer KA, Hanson M, et al. FDG PET imaging in patients with pathologically verified dementia. J Nucl Med. 2000; 41(11):1920–1928

Van Heertum RL, Tikofsky RS. Positron emission tomography and single-photon emission computed tomography brain imaging in the evaluation of dementia. Semin Nucl Med. 2003; 33(1):77–85

# Case 7

*Joseph S. Fotos*

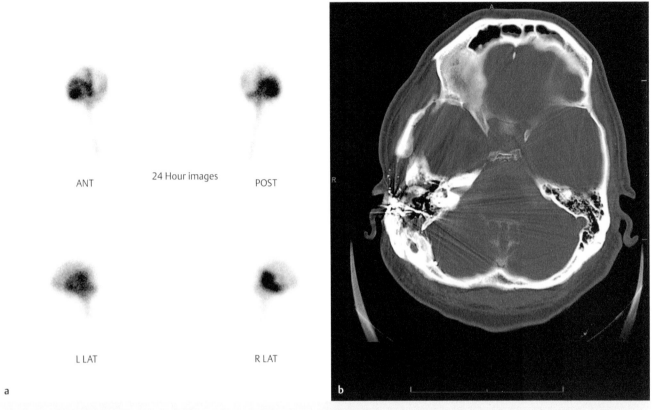

Fig. 7.1 Extra-axial accumulation of radiotracer is noted in the region of the right ear on 24-hour cerebrospinal fluid (CSF) flow study images (a). This correlates with findings of significant trauma to the right mastoid, external and internal auditory structures on CT (b). Note the scattered hyperdense material at the right ear, representing bullet fragments.

■ Clinical History

34-year-old male with otorrhea following gunshot wound to the right ear (▶ Fig. 7.1).

## ■ Key Finding

Extra-axial CSF on CSF flow study

## ■ Top 3 Differential Diagnoses

• **Posttraumatic CSF leak.** In cases of facial trauma, the cribriform plate may become disrupted, leading to dural tears and leakage of CSF from the anterior cranial fossa. Temporal bone trauma may lead to disruption of the inner and middle ear structures, causing similar dural tears that communicate with the middle ear (which then may drain via the Eustachian tubes and present as rhinorrhea), mastoid air cells, and even the external auditory canal. CSF otorrhea and rhinorrhea can be investigated with the use of Indium (In-111) diethylenetriamine pentaacetic acid (DTPA). A lumber puncture is performed with injection of the radiopharmaceutical into the thecal sac. Static images of the head and spine are then obtained at 2 and 24 hours. Extrathecal localization of radiotracer is then visualized on planar imaging. Slow CSF rhinorrhea that is not visualized on planar images can be identified by measuring activity within nasal pledgets that are placed prior to the initial lumbar puncture. The nasal pledgets are removed after planar imaging, weighed and placed in a well counter for quantitative count analysis. The patient's plasma is obtained at the same time and also placed in the well counter. A ratio of the pledget/plasma counts is then calculated for each pledget, taking care to label the location that each pledget was placed within the nasal cavity.

A single pledget/plasma ratio of 1.3 or more is considered abnormal and concerning for a CSF leak.

• **Lumbar CSF leak.** A traumatic tap resulting in a persistent lumbar CSF leak should be considered if there are clinical concerns for intracranial hypotension after a recent lumbar puncture. Care should be taken to perform the lumbar puncture for these studies at a different level than the previous procedure, occasionally performed at the skull base if needed. A CSF leak will appear as a collection of activity outside the neuraxis, particularly on lateral images. Repair is usually performed using a "blood patch," in which a small amount of autologous blood is injected at the location of the leak, which then clots and seals the leak. CSF leaks within the lumbar spine may also be suspected following spinal surgery or significant trauma.

• **Dural ectasia.** Marfan's syndrome is a connective tissue disease caused by a mutation in the fibrillin gene on the long arm of chromosome 15. Multiple neurologic complications have been described, including dural ectasia and meningocele formation. The dura becomes lax and dilated leading to areas of weakness and bulging. This increased thecal capacity can lead to postural headaches and other symptoms of intracranial hypotension, even without a frank tear and leak into the soft tissues. CSF flow study images will show a dilated and ectatic thecal sac.

## ■ Diagnosis

CSF leak at the right mastoid secondary to trauma from a gunshot wound.

## ✓ Pearls

• Any localization of activity outside the neuraxis on CSF imaging is abnormal.
• CSF rhinorrhea is often diagnosed using nasal pledgets placed in the nasal cavity.

• At 24 hours, a ratio of counts within nasal pledgets to the patient's plasma > 1.3 is abnormal.
• Dural ectasia in Marfan's syndrome appears as areas of bulging or frank ectasia of spinal activity.

## Suggested Readings

Davenport RJ, Chataway SJ, Warlow CP. Spontaneous intracranial hypotension from a CSF leak in a patient with Marfan's syndrome. J Neurol Neurosurg Psychiatry. 1995; 59(5):516–519

Grantham VV, Blakley B, Winn J. Technical review and considerations for a cerebrospinal fluid leakage study. J Nucl Med Technol. 2006; 34(1):48–51

Khan SH, Mahone T, Logic JR. CSF otorrhea. Clin Nucl Med. 1994; 19(3):236–237

# Case 8

*Joseph S. Fotos*

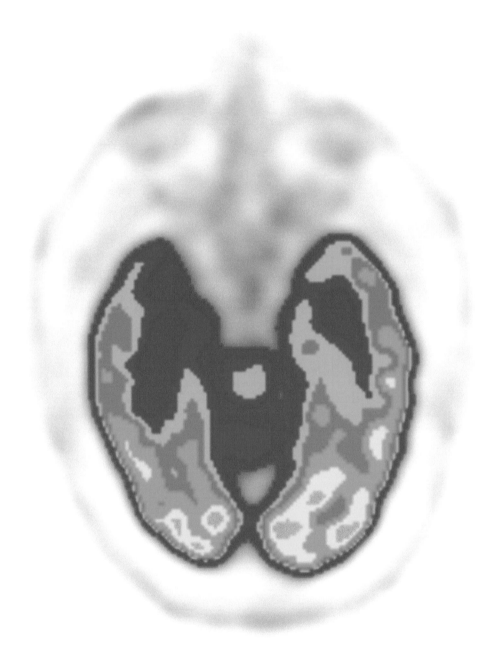

**Fig. 8.1** Interictal positron emission tomography/computed tomography (PET/CT) examination demonstrating asymmetrically decreased uptake within the right anterior temporal horn. This focus correlated with electroencephalography (EEG) results in localization of the patient's epileptogenic seizure focus.

■ **Clinical History**

63-year-old male with history of refractory seizures (▶ Fig. 8.1).

## ■ Key Finding

Focal defect in FDG avidity on PET/CT of the brain

## ■ Top 3 Differential Diagnoses

- **Seizure focus.** PET/CT of the brain has shown to be very helpful in the localization of a seizure focus in patients with refractory epilepsy and otherwise equivocal imaging findings on routine seizure work-up. Due to the relatively short half-life of fluorine-18 (F-18) (~110 minutes), PET/CT for this purpose is performed between seizures, or "interictal." When imaging the metabolism of the interictal brain, seizure foci will appear as areas of decreased metabolism relative to the remaining brain tissue. Mechanisms for this hypometabolism include atrophy and neuron loss, as well as neuronal deactivation and abnormal synaptogenesis. As with most nuclear medicine examinations, it is important to use symmetry in this examination to evaluate for an abnormality, as any look up table used to display the uptake data will be based on the highest activity and then scaled accordingly. Patients will often be imaged with a concurrent EEG for comparison. Often, patients with complex partial seizures may have additional areas of subtly decreased adjacent hypometabolism that may represent areas of subsequent seizure spread.
- **Stroke.** Not surprisingly, areas of infarcted brain will show little to no metabolism on F-18 FDG PET/CT, depending on the extent of damage. In these cases, the CT images of the brain are essential for correct interpretation. In addition, these patients often present for this examination after a brain MRI. Information from available comparison studies can aid in current study interpretation.
- **Hemorrhage.** Similarly, hemorrhagic stroke will show little to no metabolism on F-18 FDG PET/CT, making the CT images an essential part of the study interpretation. Depending on the severity of the insult, displacement of the surrounding brain tissue is common.

## ■ Additional Diagnostic Consideration

- **Tumor/treated tumor:** Successful radiation treatment to a brain tumor will also result in a photopenic defect on subsequent PET brain imaging, allowing F-18 FDG imaging to help differentiate between radiation necrosis and tumor recurrence. Some tumors may also be hypometabolic themselves, with increased uptake on follow up imaging suggesting anaplastic transformation.

## ■ Diagnosis

Right temporal seizure focus.

## ✓ Pearls

- Seizure foci on interictal PET/CT appear as areas of relative hypometabolism.
- F-18 FDG PET can help differentiate between radiation necrosis and tumor recurrence.
- Interval increase in F-18 FDG uptake in a brain tumor suggests anaplastic transformation.

## Suggested Readings

Chen W. Clinical applications of PET in brain tumors. J Nucl Med. 2007; 48(9):1468–1481

Kuhl DE, Phelps ME, Kowell AP, Metter EJ, Selin C, Winter J. Effects of stroke on local cerebral metabolism and perfusion: mapping by emission computed tomography of 18FDG and 13NH3. Ann Neurol. 1980; 8(1):47–60

Menon RN, Radhakrishnan A, Parameswaran R, et al. Does F-18 FDG-PET substantially alter the surgical decision-making in drug-resistant partial epilepsy? Epilepsy Behav. 2015; 51:133–139

# Case 9

*Joseph S. Fotos*

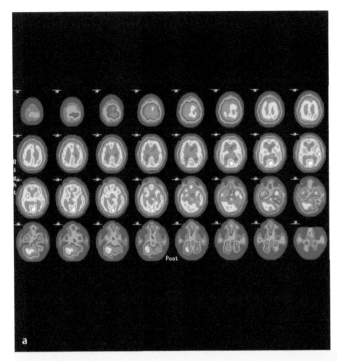 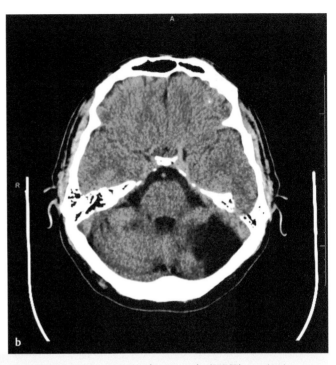

**Fig. 9.1** Axial slices from Tc-99m hexamethylpropyleneamine oxime (HMPAO) single-photon emission computed tomography (SPECT) examination (**a**) show asymmetrically decreased radiotracer localization within the left lobe of the cerebellum which localizes to an area of encephalomalacia on correlative CT scan (**b**).

## ■ Clinical History

50-year-old male with history of gait instability (▶ Fig. 9.1).

## ■ Key Finding

Focal decreased activity on brain perfusion SPECT

## ■ Top 3 Differential Diagnoses

- **Stroke.** As per the American Stroke Association 2016 data, stroke causes 1 out of 20 deaths in the United States, and is the leading cause of preventable disability. Tc-99m HMPAO is a lipophilic compound that can cross the blood-brain barrier (BBB) to gain access to the cerebral parenchyma. Once there, the compound passes into the neuronal cell body where it is trapped, likely via a combination of conversion to a hydrophilic compound and binding to intracellular components. Cerebral ischemia is, by definition, a decrease in blood flow to a portion of cerebral parenchyma, and uncorrected leads to infarction. This results in decreased delivery of the radiotracer to the affected area and relative photopenia.
- **Tumor.** Although Tc-99m HMPAO SPECT is no longer used as a primary investigation in a patient with a brain tumor, it is important to keep tumor on the differential diagnosis as it may be encountered incidentally. Previous studies have reported wide variability in uptake within brain tumors. As the mechanism of localization within neuronal cells is not dependent on a specific receptor, these differences are likely due to differences in perfusion in different brain tumors, which vary widely in their vascularity and ability to incite neovascularity to support continued tumor growth. Therefore, tumor, including metastasis, could be in the differential for a photopenic defect.
- **Abscess.** Similar to the discussions above, localization of the radiotracer within abscesses will depend on the overall blood flow distribution and the viability of the cells to which the radiotracer is delivered. Typically, an abscess will show decreased perfusion centrally as the internal core is a combination of the infective organism and immune cells. Cerebral abscesses are uncommon but are serious and life threatening, presenting with classic symptoms of fever, headache, and focal neurologic defects (though a recent meta-analysis notes that this triad is only apparent in approximately 20% of patients). It is important to remember this discussion concerns Tc-99m HMPAO distribution, and not Tc-99m HMPAO-labeled leukocytes that will have a higher degree of localization in areas of infection.

## ■ Additional Consideration

- **Seizure focus:** Brain perfusion imaging is frequently utilized to help localize a seizure focus. A seizure focus will show focally decreased perfusion if imaging is performed in the interictal state.

## ■ Diagnosis

Left cerebellar encephalomalacia.

## ✓ Pearls

- On Tc-99m HMPAO SPECT, stroke appears as a photopenic defect secondary to decreased perfusion.
- Damaged parenchyma shows decreased uptake since an intact cell membrane is needed for localization.
- Tumors show varying degrees of uptake, from decreased to focally increased.
- Cerebral abscesses are uncommon but remain an important consideration in the right clinical setting.

## Suggested Readings

Abumiya T, Katoh M, Moriwaki T, et al. Utility of early post-treatment single-photon emission computed tomography imaging to predict outcome in stroke patients treated with intravenous tissue plasminogen activator. J Stroke Cerebrovasc Dis. 2014; 23(5):896–901

Babich JW, Keeling F, Flower MA, et al. Initial experience with Tc-99m-HM-PAO in the study of brain tumors. Eur J Nucl Med. 1988; 14(1):39–44

Berger JD, Witte RJ, Holdeman KP, et al. Neuroradiologic applications of central nervous system SPECT. Radiographics. 1996; 16(4):777–785

# Case 10

*Joseph S. Fotos*

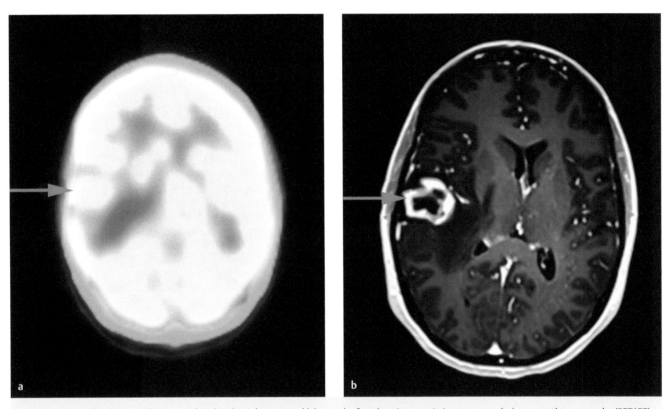

**Fig. 10.1** Intense focal FDG avidity is noted within the right temporal lobe on the fused positron emission tomography/computed tomography (PET/CT) image **(a)**. This correlates with a peripherally enhancing lesion on post contrast magnetization prepared rapid acquisition GRE (MPRAGE) MRI **(b)**.

■ **Clinical History**

41-year-old female with history of metastatic breast cancer (▶Fig. 10.1).

## ■ Key Finding

Focal increased uptake in FDG avidity on PET/CT of the brain

## ■ Top 3 Differential Diagnoses

- **Tumor.** While the resolution of PET/CT imaging often limits its evaluation in areas of complex anatomy, such as the brain, larger brain metastases are occasionally seen, especially in studies performed in patients with lung cancer, breast cancer, and malignant melanoma. This increased uptake of fluorine-18 fluorodeoxyglucose (F-18 FDG) relies on the Warburg effect wherein cancer cells tend to produce energy through a high rate of glycolysis. Once phosphorylated by hexokinase, FDG is unable to proceed through glycolysis or leave the cell. This causes a proportional accumulation of FDG, which is often very intense and similar to the high metabolic demands of the obligate glycolytic tissue of the brain. Due to the intense avidity of the brain, it is critical to change the window width and level of the brain images. Tumor may appear as a focus of intense confluent uptake or an area of peripheral uptake and central necrosis. New amino acid-based PET tracers are also being used to image brain tumors, including F-18 fluoro-ethyl-tyrosine (F18-FET), C-11 methionine (C11-MET), and nucleoside tracers such as F-18 fluorothymidine (F-18 FLT).

- **Abscess.** Similar high metabolic demands are present within inflammatory tissue, leading to increased uptake around abscesses. Clinical context is essential, as patients with brain abscesses tend to be very ill. Abscesses will tend to appear as a rim of intense FDG uptake with a central area of photopenia. Recent studies have shown the potential for other PET tracer use in differentiating tumor from an abscess including N-13 ammonia. MRI provides better soft-tissue characterization and should be employed following identification of suspicious uptake on PET/CT brain imaging, if not already performed.

- **Seizure focus.** It is generally impractical to use fluorine-18 fluorodeoxyglucose positron-emission tomography (F-18 FDG PET)/CT for imaging a seizure focus at the time of the seizure, known as "intraictal" imaging, as the half-life of F-18 is only 110 minutes. While grand mal seizures would be obvious due to patient motion, more subtle complex partial seizures may not and may occur during imaging. An active seizure focus will appear as a focus of increased uptake. This contrasts with the focal decreased uptake found in the commonly used "interictal" PET/CT imaging strategy (see Case 8 for further details).

## ■ Diagnosis

Breast cancer metastatic to the brain.

## ✓ Pearls

- Images should only be reviewed after changing the window width/level to reveal subtle abnormalities.
- Brain metastases are not uncommon, especially in lung cancer, breast cancer, and malignant melanoma.

- Both brain tumors and abscesses may demonstrate peripheral avidity with central photopenia.
- "Intraictal" PET/CT is impractical for most services; seizure foci would appear as focal intense uptake.

## Suggested Readings

Chen W. Clinical applications of PET in brain tumors. J Nucl Med. 2007; 48(9):1468–1481

Heiss WD, Raab P, Lanfermann H. Multimodality assessment of brain tumors and tumor recurrence. J Nucl Med. 2011; 52(10):1585–1600

Van den Broeck B, Jansen K, Goffin K. Delineation of seizure onset zone using ictal PET in epilepsia partialis continua. Eur J Nucl Med Mol Imaging. 2014; 41(12):2360

# Case 11

*Joseph S. Fotos*

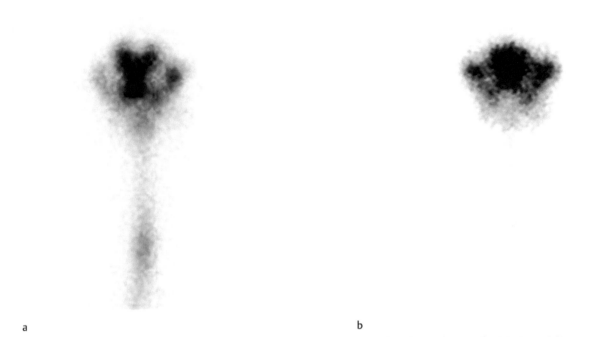

a                                                b

**Fig. 11.1** Cerebrospinal fluid (CSF) flow study shows reflux of activity within the lateral ventricles at 4 hours **(a)**, with persistent activity at 24 hours **(b)**. No activity is seen over the cerebral convexities.

## ■ Clinical History

80-year-old male with dementia (▶Fig. 11.1).

## ■ Key Finding

Lateral ventricle activity and delayed activity ascent on CSF flow study

## ■ Top 2 Differential Diagnoses

- **Normal pressure hydrocephalus (NPH).** A CSF flow study begins with a lumbar puncture. Once access to the subarachnoid space is gained, In-111 diethylenetriamine pentaacetic acid (DTPA) is then introduced into the CSF. Commonly, opening pressure is measured at the same time, and a small amount of CSF is sent for laboratory testing. Images are then obtained at 4 hours of the head and entire spine, followed by delayed images of the head and superior spinal cord at 24, 48, and sometimes 72 hours. Over this time the radiotracer follows the course of the patient's CSF flow patterns. The normal CSF flow pattern begins with formation by the choroid plexus primarily within the lateral ventricles. Flow then proceeds inferiorly along the central canal and then superiorly to return to the basal cisterns before traveling to the cerebral convexities where it is reabsorbed by the arachnoid granulations and dura. Normal imaging shows this flow pattern, with ascent of activity over the cerebral convexities by 24 hours. This pattern is abnormal in NPH, as characteristic reflux of activity into the lateral ventricles is seen on early imaging, with delayed ascent of radiotracer over the cerebral convexities (if at all, in some cases). These findings should be put into the context of the patient presentation, often correlating with clinical symptoms of urinary incontinence, dementia, and abnormal gait. Cross-sectional imaging may demonstrate dilation of the lateral and third ventricles out of proportion to the convexity sulci.
- **Decreased CSF reabsorption.** Subarachnoid hemorrhage is known to cause obstruction of CSF reabsorption at the arachnoid granulations. This causes abnormal CSF flow that may cause a similar pattern of tracer distribution as seen in NPH. In cases where this is suspected, correlation with patient history and cross-sectional imaging (CT or MRI) is essential for accurate interpretation.

## ■ Diagnosis

Normal pressure hydrocephalus.

## ✓ Pearls

- Normal CSF flow begins in the lateral ventricles, descends to the sacrum, ascends to the skull vertex.
- Reflux of activity into the lateral ventricles is abnormal and a classic early finding in NPH.
- Delayed ascent over the cerebral convexities beyond 24 hours is a classic late finding in NPH.
- Subarachnoid hemorrhage can cause a similar flow pattern due to obstruction of CSF flow reabsorption.

## Suggested Readings

Kazumata K, Kamiyama H, Ishikawa T, et al. Clinical study of cerebrospinal fluid dynamics using 111In-DTPA SPECT in patients with subarachnoid hemorrhage. Neurol Med Chir (Tokyo). 2006; 46(1):11–17, discussion 17–18

Thut DP, Kreychman A, Obando JA. (1)(1)(1)In-DTPA cisternography with SPECT/CT for the evaluation of normal pressure hydrocephalus. J Nucl Med Technol. 2014; 42(1):70–74

# Part 2

## Thyroid and Parathyroid

# Case 12

*Brian J. Lewis*

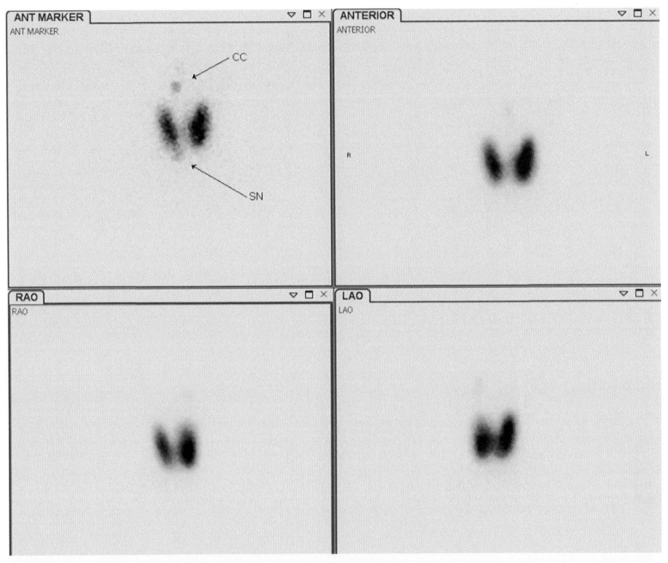

**Fig. 12.1** 24-hour images from I-123 thyroid scan show diffuse homogeneous uptake throughout the thyroid gland with no focal areas of decreased or increased activity. 4-hour uptake was 49%, 24-hour uptake was 67%.

## ■ Clinical History

62-year-old male with hyperthyroidism. Laboratory values at time of exam: thyroid stimulating hormone (TSH) < 0.005 µIU/mL (normal 0.270–4.20), free T4 > 5.18 (normal range 0.93–1.7 ng/dL) (▶ Fig. 12.1).

## ■ Key Finding

Increased thyroid radioiodine uptake in the setting of hyperthyroidism

## ■ Top 3 Differential Diagnoses

- **Graves' Disease.** Graves occurs secondary to thyroid-stimulating antibodies that bind to thyroid-stimulating hormone (TSH) receptors, stimulating the gland to create hormone independent of the central axis. Radioiodine (I-123) scan will show diffuse homogeneous thyroid uptake, possibly a pyramidal lobe, and increased uptake at both 4 and 24 hours. Uptake may be normal at 24 hours in cases of rapid iodine turnover. Normal uptake values are for a euthyroid patient, so "normal" values in a patient with suppressed TSH are not normal and indicate subclinical Graves. I-131 ablation can be used for treatment with dosages generally calculated taking thyroid gland size and 24-hour iodine uptake percentage in account, typically around 12–15 mCi.
- **Toxic multinodular goiter (TMNG).** TMNG occurs when a multinodular goiter develops some autonomous function.

Imaging shows an enlarged gland with multiple cold, warm, and hot nodules. Uptake values may be normal or elevated. I-131 ablation is used for treatment, often with 30 mCi.
- **Hyperfunctioning adenoma.** A hyperfunctioning thyroid adenoma may result in hyperthyroidism. Imaging usually demonstrates a single hot nodule with suppression of the rest of the gland. Uptake values may be normal or increased. A hot nodule on Tc-99m pertechnetate should be followed with an I-123 scan to rule out a discordant nodule, as thyroid carcinoma will be hot on a pertechnetate scan. Adenomas may be more resistant to I-131 and are typically ablated with around 30 mCi. Patients may return to a euthyroid state after ablation as the remainder of the thyroid gland is suppressed and may not take up I-131.

## ■ Additional Diagnostic Considerations

- **Hashimoto's thyroiditis:** Radioiodine uptake may be increased early in the disease as the body responds to a drop in thyroid function by increasing TSH production. Patients are rarely imaged in this stage, and hyperthyroidism (Hashitoxicosis) would have been present prior to imaging.
- **Gestational trophoblastic disease (GTD):** Human chorionic gonadotropin (HCG)-secreting GTD can result in hyperthyroidism as HCG is structurally similar to TSH, typically occurs with HCG over 300 IU/mL.

## ■ Diagnosis

Graves' disease.

## ✓ Pearls

- Normal uptake on a thyroid scan is 6–18% at 4–6 hours and 10–30% at 24 hours, in a euthyroid patient.
- In Graves' disease, uptake can be normal at 24 hours in cases of rapid iodine turnover or subclinical disease.

- Typical I-131 ablation doses are 15 mCi for Graves and 30 mCi for TMNG and hyperfunctioning adenoma.
- It is important to remember that "normal" uptake values are abnormal in the setting of a suppressed TSH.

## Suggested Readings

Day TA, Chu A, Hoang KG. Multinodular goiter. Otolaryngol Clin North Am. 2003; 36(1):35–54

Nachiappan AC, Metwalli ZA, Hailey BS, Patel RA, Ostrowski ML, Wynne DM. The thyroid: review of imaging features and biopsy techniques with radiologic-pathologic correlation. Radiographics. 2014; 34(2):276–293

Nayak B, Hodak SP. Hyperthyroidism. Endocrinol Metab Clin North Am. 2007; 36(3):617–656, v

# Case 13

*James J. Gullo*

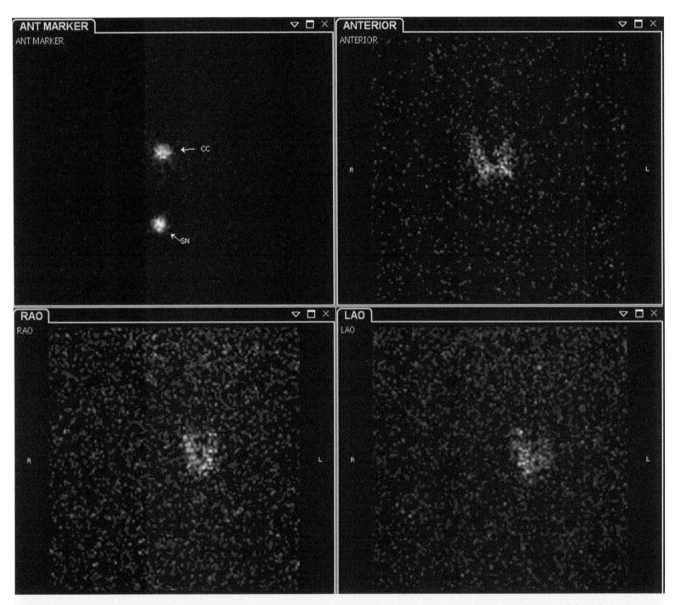

**Fig. 13.1** Planar images of the thyroid obtained 24 hours after the administration of I-123 demonstrate global diminished uptake of the radiotracer. Uptake at 4 hours was 1.5% (normal 6–18%) and uptake at 24 hours was 1.1% (normal 10–30%).

■ **Clinical History**

37-year-old woman with symptomatic and laboratory evidence of thyrotoxicosis (▶Fig. 13.1).

## ■ Key Finding

Decreased thyroid uptake in the setting of hyperthyroidism

## ■ Top 3 Differential Diagnoses

- **Subacute thyroiditis.** It results from an inflammatory response following a viral illness leading to giant cell infiltration of thyroid follicles. The follicles swell and eventually rupture leading to release of thyroid hormone and thyrotoxicosis. The swelling of the follicles results in the clinical symptoms of a painful and tender thyroid gland. Free thyroid hormone levels are elevated resulting in suppression of thyroid stimulating hormone (TSH) and decreased iodine uptake, also in part due to disruption of the follicular membrane. Treatment is anti-inflammatory medications and, in severe cases, steroids.
- **Induced thyrotoxicosis.** It results when an individual is exposed to excessive amounts of iodine either via medication such as amiodarone or radiographic contrast agents. Normally the *Wolff–Chaikoff effect* prevents excessive thyroid hormone synthesis during exposure to excessive amounts of iodine. *Jod-Basedow phenomenon* results when there are autonomous areas within the thyroid gland that produce excessive thyroid hormone with exposure to excessive amounts of iodine

resulting in TSH suppression and reduced radioiodine uptake. A recent large iodine load could have a similar effect via competitive inhibition, possibly masking an underlying productive cause of hyperthyroidism, such as Graves' disease or multinodular goiter.

- **Struma ovarii.** It is a rare ovarian teratoma that contains functioning thyroid tissue. While most cases do not produce a significant amount of thyroid hormone, on rare occasions the exogenous thyroid hormone production can be symptomatic. T3 and T4 levels will be elevated and TSH levels will be suppressed. There will be decreased uptake in the thyroid gland on thyroid scintigraphy due to the production of the ectopic thyroid hormone with increased uptake in the ovarian tumor. The ectopic thyroid tissue is better demonstrated with I-123 than with pertechnetate since urinary excretion of the pertechnetate could obscure the ovarian mass. It is important to image the pelvis in a female patient sent for hyperthyroid evaluation with decreased iodine uptake in the neck to exclude this diagnosis.

## ■ Additional Differential Diagnoses

- **Thyrotoxicosis factitia:** It is thyrotoxicosis caused by exogenous thyroid hormone administration, either knowingly or unknowingly. There will be elevation of serum T3 and T4 levels, often with a higher serum T4/T3 ratio than in endogenous

thyrotoxicosis, since the exogenous hormone is often pure T4, and there will be decreased uptake on scintigraphy due to suppressed TSH. Serum thyroglobulin (Tg) level will be very low or undetectable with thyrotoxicosis factitia.

## ■ Diagnosis

Subacute thyroiditis.

## ✓ Pearls

- Subacute thyroiditis will have a history of recent viral illness and a tender, enlarged thyroid.
- There will be a history of recent exposure to iodine (contrast, medications) with induced thyrotoxicosis.

- Suspect struma ovarii with a pelvic mass and decreased thyroid uptake in the setting of hyperthyroidism.
- Serum Tg levels will be very low/undetectable with thyrotoxicosis factitia.

## Suggested Readings

Dujardin MI, Sekhri P, Turnbull LW. Struma ovarii: role of imaging? Insights Imaging. 2014; 5(1):41–51

Intenzo CM, dePapp AE, Jabbour S, Miller JL, Kim SM, Capuzzi DM. Scintigraphic manifestations of thyrotoxicosis. Radiographics. 2003; 23(4):857–869

Mittra ES, Niederkohr RD, Rodriguez C, El-Maghraby T, McDougall IR. Uncommon causes of thyrotoxicosis. J Nucl Med. 2008; 49(2):265–278

# Case 14

*Kamal D. Singh*

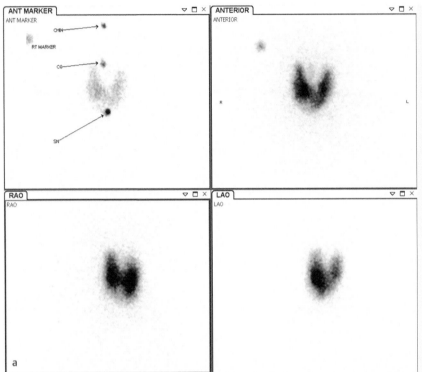

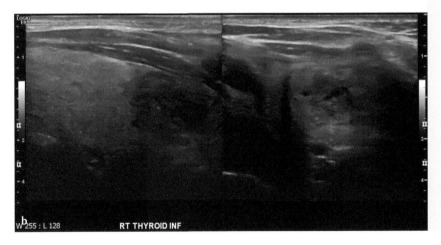

Fig. 14.1 Planar imaging of the thyroid with I-123 performed at 24 hours after oral radioiodine administration (a) demonstrates photopenia in the inferior right thyroid lobe. Both 4-hour and 24-hour uptake measurements were normal, and thyroid stimulating hormone (TSH) was normal at the time of the exam. Sonographic images (b) show a correlative nodule.

## ■ Clinical History

63-year-old male with solitary 2-cm right thyroid nodule and long history of labs consistent with subclinical hyperthyroidism (▶Fig. 14.1).

## ■ Key Finding

Cold nodule on I-123 thyroid scan

## ■ Top 3 Differential Diagnoses

- **Thyroid carcinoma.** Ultrasound and fine needle aspiration (FNA) are the primary diagnostic procedures for thyroid nodule in a euthyroid patient. Nuclear medicine thyroid imaging for nodule characterization should be reserved for patients with hyperthyroidism (suppressed TSH), or an indeterminate biopsy. Cold or nonfunctioning nodules on I-123 thyroid scans are nonspecific and may represent colloid cyst (40%), nonfunctioning adenoma (40%), or thyroid carcinoma (15–20%). The incidence of cancer is lower (< 5%) in the setting of multinodular goiter. Hot or hyperfunctioning nodules on I-123 scan, defined as uptake in the nodule suppressing the rest of the thyroid gland, are essentially always benign. However, a hot nodule on pertechnetate scan requires further evaluation with I-123 scan to exclude a discordant nodule, which requires FNA to exclude thyroid carcinoma. Risk factors for thyroid malignancy include age < 20 or > 60 years, male patient, family history, prior radiation therapy to the head/neck, and/or a dominant nodule with concerning ultrasound features (solid, hypoechoic, hypervascular nodule with microcalcifications). Papillary carcinoma is the most common subtype, followed by follicular. Medullary and anaplastic carcinomas are less common and highly aggressive. Treatment of localized thyroid carcinoma typically consists of total thyroidectomy followed by I-131 ablation therapy. Patients are followed with thyroglobulin (Tg) levels, as well as whole-body I-131 imaging, for at least 2 years after radioiodine ablation (RIA).
- **Colloid cyst.** These are benign localized follicles filled with gelatinous colloid. They usually originate from cystic degeneration of thyroid adenomas and are hyperintense on T1-weighted MRI due to high protein content. Ultrasound characteristics include a cystic lesion with inspissated colloid, which is hyperechoic and demonstrates ring-down or comet tail artifact.
- **Nonfunctioning adenoma.** Thyroid adenomas are benign lesions that may be functioning (hot nodule) or nonfunctioning (cold nodule). They can be multiple in the setting of multinodular goiter. On ultrasound, benign adenomas are typically well encapsulated with a hypoechoic halo. Interval growth is not unusual. A dominant hyperfunctioning adenoma with suppression of the remainder of the gland in the setting of hyperthyroidism is called an autonomous nodule (produces thyroid hormones independent of TSH). Multinodular goiter and autonomous nodules are generally more resistant to ablation therapy than Graves' disease; hence, these patients are treated with higher doses of I-131 (about 30 mCi).

## ■ Diagnosis

Nonfunctioning adenoma.

## ✓ Pearls

- I-123 thyroid scan is indicated in hyperthyroidism or nodule evaluation after an indeterminate biopsy.
- A cold nodule may be a colloid cyst (40%), nonfunctioning adenoma (40%), or thyroid cancer (15–20%).
- A hot nodule on Tc pertechnetate may be cold or "discordant" on I-123 (trapping without organification).
- Papillary and follicular cancers are amenable to I-131 ablation, medullary and anaplastic carcinomas are not.

## Suggested Readings

Intenzo CM, Dam HQ, Manzone TA, Kim SM. Imaging of the thyroid in benign and malignant disease. Semin Nucl Med. 2012; 42(1):49–61

Nachiappan AC, Metwalli ZA, Hailey BS, Patel RA, Ostrowski ML, Wynne DM. The thyroid: review of imaging features and biopsy techniques with radiologic-pathologic correlation. Radiographics. 2014; 34(2):276–293

Yeung MJ, Serpell JW. Management of the solitary thyroid nodule. Oncologist. 2008; 13(2):105–112

# Case 15

*Ely A. Wolin*

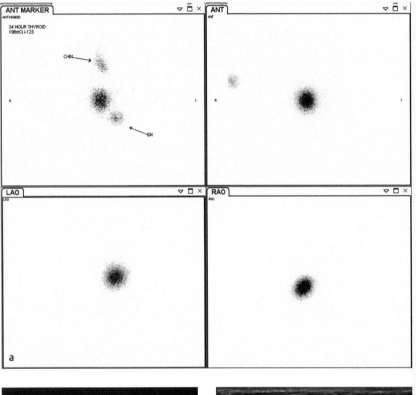

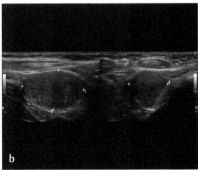

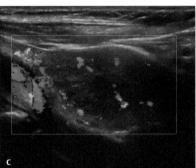

Fig. 15.1 24-hour images from I-123 thyroid scan (a) show a focal area of radiotracer uptake in the region of the inferior right thyroid lobe with no uptake in the remainder of the thyroid gland. Correlative ultrasound images show a nodule in the inferior right thyroid lobe (b) with internal vascularity (c).

■ **Clinical History**

82-year-old woman with suppressed thyroid stimulating hormone (TSH) (▶Fig. 15.1).

■ **Key Finding**

Focal area of increased uptake on radioiodine thyroid scan with washout of the rest of the thyroid gland

■ **Top 2 Differential Diagnoses**

- **Toxic adenoma.** Radioiodine thyroid uptake and scan is most frequently performed for the evaluation of hyperthyroidism. However, the study can also be useful for the evaluation of a thyroid nodule, particularly in the setting of an indeterminate biopsy with concerning imaging features. A "hot" nodule on thyroid scintigraphy will appear as a focal area of increased radioiodine uptake with washout of the remaining thyroid gland. This is reassuring of benignity as this appearance is nearly pathognomic for a hyperfunctioning, or toxic, thyroid adenoma. A true hot nodule has a very low chance of being malignant as even well-differentiated carcinomas are rarely hyperfunctioning. The washout of the remaining thyroid gland is an important feature because it proves that the nodule is producing thyroid hormone independently while the remaining gland is responding appropriately to the central axis. The autonomous nature of toxic adenomas is thought to be due to the mutation of the TSH receptors resulting in continuous activation. Toxic adenomas can be treated with I-131 ablation, usually utilizing a 30-mCi dose. Patients who receive radioiodine ablation (RIA) may end up euthyroid and without the need for thyroid hormone replacement as the appropriately suppressed iodine uptake of the remaining thyroid gland can be protective.

- **Thyroid carcinoma.** It most commonly presents as a cold nodule on thyroid scintigraphy performed with radioiodine. However, while it is rare, thyroid carcinoma can present with the ability to trap and organify iodine independent of the central axis. This occurs in well-differentiated cancers, and even when present they are rarely hyperfunctioning to the point of resulting in clinical hyperthyroidism. However, as a "hot" nodule is not definitively benign, a nodule that has imaging characteristics which meet criteria for biopsy per standard guidelines should be biopsied regardless of radioiodine thyroid scan findings.

■ **Diagnosis**

Hyperfunctioning thyroid adenoma.

✓ **Pearls**

- A "hot" nodule on radioiodine thyroid scintigraphy is almost always a benign toxic thyroid adenoma.
- Suppression of the remaining thyroid gland on scintigraphy makes a benign toxic adenoma more likely.
- Thyroid scan findings should not negate biopsy of a nodule with concerning imaging features.
- Thyroid carcinoma can rarely present as a functioning nodule, mimicking a benign toxic adenoma.

**Suggested Readings**

Intenzo CM, dePapp AE, Jabbour S, Miller JL, Kim SM, Capuzzi DM. Scintigraphic manifestations of thyrotoxicosis. Radiographics. 2003; 23(4):857–869

Lee ES, Kim JH, Na DG, et al. Hyperfunction thyroid nodules: their risk for becoming or being associated with thyroid cancers. Korean J Radiol. 2013; 14(4):643–652

Mirfakhraee S, Mathews D, Peng L, Woodruff S, Zigman JM. A solitary hyperfunctioning thyroid nodule harboring thyroid carcinoma: review of the literature. Thyroid Res. 2013; 6(1):7

# Case 16

*Trevor A. Thompson*

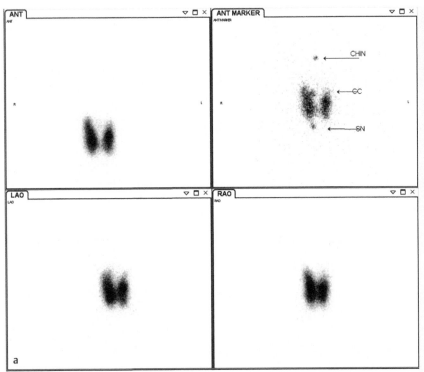

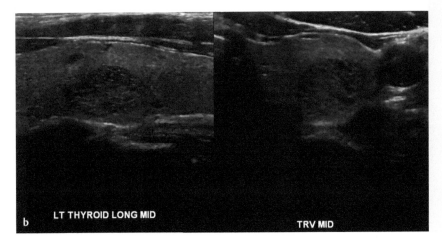

**Fig. 16.1** I-123 scan (a) shows diffuse uptake throughout the thyroid gland with no areas of focal increased or decreased activity. Specifically, there is no abnormal uptake noted in the region of the dominant nodule in the mid left lobe of the thyroid gland seen on correlative ultrasound images (b).

■ **Clinical History**

60-year-old female with presumptive Graves' disease in the past with recent reports of suppressed thyroid stimulating hormone (TSH) and palpitations and nodules noted on thyroid ultrasound (▶ Fig. 16.1).

## ■ Key Finding

"Warm" thyroid nodule

## ■ Top 3 Differential Diagnoses

• **Thyroid adenoma.** "Warm" thyroid nodules on planar radio-iodine scintigraphy may represent isofunctioning thyroid tissue or a nonfunctioning "cold" nodule surrounded by normally functioning unsuppressed thyroid tissue. The large majority (80–85%) of thyroid nodules are "cold" with 15–20% of these representing malignancy. In comparison, "hot" nodules are uncommon (~5%) with a less than 1% chance of malignancy. Thyroid (follicular) adenoma represents a benign proliferation of thyroid follicles surrounded by a complete capsule. Adenomas typically manifest as a solitary lesion within an otherwise normal-appearing thyroid gland. While adenomas account for nearly all "hot" thyroid nodules, only 1% of these create sufficient thyroid hormone to produce clinical hyperthyroidism ("toxic adenomas"). The majority of adenomas demonstrate low uptake on thyroid scintigraphy when compared to the remainder of the gland. As nontoxic adenomas may be autonomous (TSH-independent), semiautonomous or nonautonomous (TSH-responsive), these may appear as either "warm" or "cold" nodules without associated suppression of the background thyroid tissues. As adenomas enlarge, they frequently undergo necrosis that could be perceived as a central "warm" or even "cold" region on thyroid scintigraphy.

• **Thyroid hyperplasia.** Nodular hyperplasia (goiter) represents the development of hyperplastic nodules within the thyroid gland as a response to intrinsic abnormalities of thyroid hormone production or an iodine-deficient diet (rare in the developed world). Additional causes of hyperplasia include compensatory hyperplasia (secondary to gland fibrosis most commonly due to Hashimoto's thyroiditis) and physiologic hyperplasia (secondary to congenital thyroid lobar agenesis or partial thyroidectomy). Patient history and laboratory testing may help to distinguish between these entities as hyperplasic nodules demonstrate nonspecific heterogeneous radioiodine uptake ranging from "cold" to "hot" on thyroid scintigraphy.

• **Differentiated thyroid carcinoma.** It is divided into papillary and follicular subtypes. Papillary carcinoma is the most common primary thyroid malignancy (80% of cases) followed by follicular carcinoma (~10%). Due to alterations in iodine uptake and organification, secondary to changes in function of the sodium-iodide symporter (NIS) and decreased expression of thyroperoxidase, thyroglobulin (Tg), and pendrin, these malignancies show significantly decreased radioiodine activity when compared to the native gland and classically appear as a "cold" nodule. A degree of preserved function and continued responsiveness of these tissues to TSH, however, can rarely result in detectable activity and present as either a "warm" or even "hot" nodule. Continued expression of TSH receptors also makes these malignancies responsive to TSH stimulation and allows radioiodine ablation (RIA) as well as scintigraphic evaluation for disease recurrence following thyroidectomy and RIA.

## ■ Diagnosis

Isofunctioning thyroid nodule.

## ✓ Pearls

• "Warm" thyroid nodules may be isofunctioning or nonfunctioning but surrounded by normal thyroid tissue.
• Thyroid adenomas can range from "hot" to "cold" based on TSH responsiveness and presence of necrosis.

• Thyroid hyperplasia can result from a variety of intrinsic and extrinsic causes.
• Nodules should be considered as "hot" or "not hot" as a "warm" nodule may be cancerous and needs biopsy.

## Suggested Readings

McHenry CR, Phitayakorn R. Follicular adenoma and carcinoma of the thyroid gland. Oncologist. 2011; 16(5):585–593

Nachiappan AC, Metwalli ZA, Hailey BS, Patel RA, Ostrowski ML, Wynne DM. The thyroid: review of imaging features and biopsy techniques with radiologic-pathologic correlation. Radiographics. 2014; 34(2):276–293

Robbins RJ, Schlumberger MJ. The evolving role of (131)I for the treatment of differentiated thyroid carcinoma. J Nucl Med. 2005; 46(Suppl 1):28S–37S

# Case 17

*Ely A. Wolin*

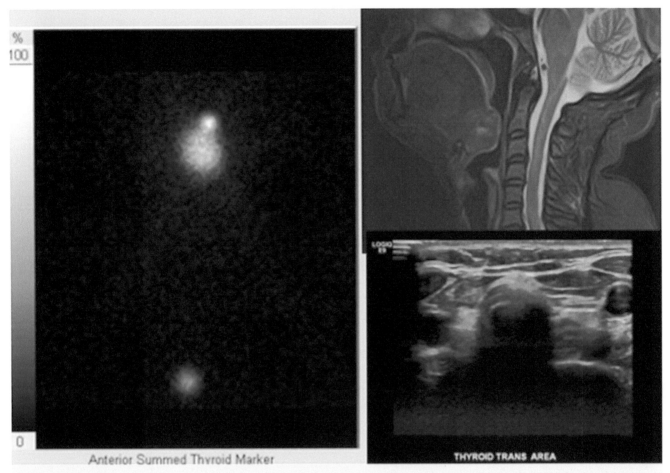

**Fig. 17.1** Anterior view from I-123 scan shows focal uptake just inferior to the chin marker with no uptake in the expected region of the thyroid gland. Uptake correlates with a heterogeneous mass at the base of the tongue shown on sagittal T2-weighted MRI. Image from thyroid ultrasound which was performed before the I-123 scan shows no definite thyroid tissue in the thyroid bed.

## ■ Clinical History

40-year-old female presenting with heat intolerance and neck swelling (▶ Fig. 17.1).

(Case courtesy of Brian F. McQuillan, MD, and Michael S. McLaughlin, MD, Mike O'Callaghan Military Medical Center, Nellis AFB, NV.)

## ◼ Key Finding

Focal uptake localizing to the tongue on nuclear medicine thyroid scan

## ◼ Diagnosis

- **Lingual thyroid.** Thyroid embryogenesis begins in the primitive pharynx around the 6th week of gestation. Normally, the thyroid then descends with the heart and major vessels along the thyroglossal duct to reach its final position at the infrahyoid base of the neck. The thyroglossal duct then usually involutes between the 8th and 10th weeks of gestation. Failure in complete migration of the thyroid gland results in thyroid ectopia. The base of the tongue, the location of the foramen cecum which is the point of origin of the thyroglossal tract, is the most common site for ectopic thyroid tissue (around 90%). Remaining sites of ectopia can occur anywhere along the thyroglossal duct tract, some more lateral than expected. Other sites include sublingual region, prelaryngeal area, lateral neck, and mediastinum. There are rare reports of ectopic thyroid tissue in more remote locations such as the adrenal glands. Although unlikely, it is also possible to have multiple foci of ectopic thyroid tissue.

  Ectopic lingual thyroid may be the patient's only functioning thyroid tissue. However, around one-fifth of the time thyroid tissue will also be found in the thyroid bed. Evaluation for orthotopic thyroid tissue is important prior to therapy for lingual thyroid ectopia for prediction of the post therapy thyroid state.

  Ectopic lingual thyroid tissue can be symptomatic. Symptoms can arise from resultant oropharyngeal obstruction leading to dysphonia, dysphagia, glomus sensation, snoring, and occasional bleeding. Symptoms can also be secondary to hypothyroidism, which occurs in around 60% of cases, as the ectopic tissue may not be able to produce enough thyroid hormone. The ectopic tissue is also susceptible to all disease that can affect a normally positioned thyroid gland.

  Treatment can include exogenous thyroid hormone administration, usually with levothyroxine, to both treat associated hypothyroidism as well as to decrease the size of the ectopic gland through hormone suppression. However, surgery is necessary if medical therapy fails, or in the case of acute obstructive symptoms and other complications including bleeding and malignancy. Radioiodine ablation (RIA) has also been used as an alternative therapy, usually in patients who are not good surgical candidates.

## ◼ Diagnosis

Lingual thyroid ectopia.

## ✓ Pearls

- Ectopic thyroid tissue is the only thyroid tissue present in approximately 80% of the cases.
- Ectopic tissue cannot always make enough hormone to meet demand resulting in hypothyroidism.
- Surgical excision is necessary in the setting of acute obstructive symptoms and other complications.
- The base of the tongue is the most common location for thyroid ectopia.

## Suggested Readings

Gandhi A, Wong KK, Gross MD, Avram AM. Lingual thyroid ectopisL diagnostic SPECT/CT imaging and radioactive iodine treatment. Thyroid. 2016; 26(4):573–579

Kumar LK, Kurien NM, Jacob MM, Menon PV, Khalam SA. Lingual thyroid. Ann Maxillofac Surg. 2015; 5(1):104–107

Zander DA, Smoker WRK. Imaging of ectopic thyroid tissue and thyroglossal duct cysts. Radiographics. 2014; 34(1):37–50

# Case 18

*Trevor A. Thompson*

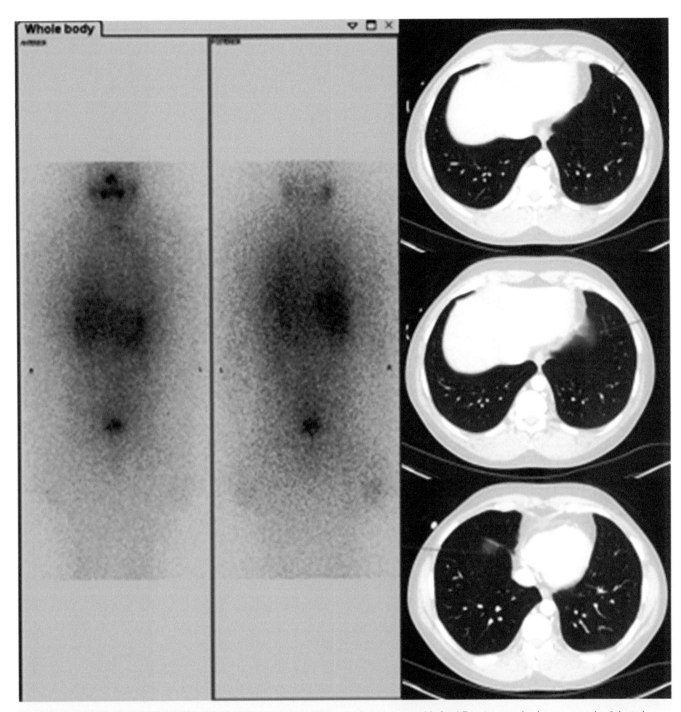

**Fig. 18.1** Whole body images obtained 8 days after administration of 220 mCi of I-131 are notable for diffuse increased pulmonary uptake. Selected axial slices from correlative CT imaging of the lungs show scattered pulmonary nodules which were new since prior imaging.

## ■ Clinical History

45-year-old male imaged 8 days after ablation with 220 mCi of I-131 for differentiated papillary thyroid carcinoma with nodal metastases (▶Fig. 18.1).

## ■ Key Finding

Pulmonary uptake on post therapy I-131 imaging

## ■ Top 3 Differential Diagnoses

- **Lung metastases.** Around 1–9% of differentiated thyroid cancer (DTC) patients have distant metastatic disease at the time of diagnosis. Approximately half will have isolated involvement of the lungs; the follicular subtype has a higher propensity for pulmonary spread. Miliary DTC pulmonary metastatic disease can result in diffuse lung uptake on I-131 whole-body scan (WBS). Metastatic thyroid cancer following thyroidectomy and radioiodine ablation (RIA) is typically heralded by a newly detectable or increasing serum thyroglobulin (Tg) level; however, pulmonary metastatic disease has been reported in the setting of undetectable Tg levels. As such, undetectable serum Tg does not exclude metastatic disease as a cause of increased pulmonary uptake.
- **Inflammation/infection.** Both acute and chronic infectious and inflammatory pathologies can be associated with increased radioiodine uptake. The uptake mechanism is not definitively known, but likely is secondary to associated hyperemia and increased capillary permeability, along with possible leukocyte radioiodine accumulation. Infectious uptake is more typically focal or nodular in appearance, but may be diffuse mimicking metastatic disease. Both focal and diffuse uptake has been described in the setting of bronchiectasis, and nodular uptake can be seen with rheumatoid lung disease. Cross-sectional imaging can frequently help distinguish between infectious/inflammatory causes of abnormal uptake and metastatic disease.
- **Pleural effusion.** Hypothyroidism related to thyroidectomy and RIA for DTC contributes to the development of pleural effusions through increased vascular permeability as well as osmotic interstitial changes. As there is normally low-level expression of the sodium-iodide symporter (NIS) within the lung parenchyma, I-131 can collect within these pleural fluid collections and present as diffuse lung uptake due to patient positioning at the time of imaging. Prominence of lung uptake on the posterior planar images can suggest this diagnosis due to layering of the fluid on typical supine imaging.

## ■ Additional Diagnostic Considerations

- **Nonthyroidal tumor:** Benign and malignant nonthyroidal tumors can result in increased I-131 pulmonary uptake and include mesothelioma, primary lung malignancy, and metastatic spread of breast or cervical cancer to the lung. Benign and malignant primary breast lesions, including breast cancer and fibroadenoma, can also overlie the lungs on planar imaging and appear as focally increased I-131 uptake.

## ■ Diagnosis

Presumed pulmonary metastases from differentiated papillary thyroid carcinoma.

## ✓ Pearls

- Pulmonary I-131 uptake suggests metastatic thyroid cancer even in the absence of detectable Tg.
- Infectious/inflammatory pulmonary I-131 uptake can be either focal or diffuse, and may mimic metastases.
- Prominent pulmonary I-131 uptake on posterior planar images suggests layering pleural effusion.
- With lung mets, I-131 dosage is adjusted so < 75–80 mCi goes to the lungs to avoid pulmonary fibrosis.

## Suggested Readings

Choi HS, Kim SH, Park SY, Park HL, Seo YY, Choi WH. Clinical significance of diffuse intrathoracic uptake on post-therapy I-131 scans in thyroid cancer patients. Nucl Med Mol Imaging. 2014; 48(1):63–71

Jang S, Chung JK, Kang KW, et al. Assessment of pulmonary uptake in post-therapy I-131 whole body scan in well-differentiated thyroid cancer patients. J Nucl Med. 2009; 50(Suppl. 2):389

Oh JR, Ahn BC. False-positive uptake on radioiodine whole-body scintigraphy: physiologic and pathologic variants unrelated to thyroid cancer. Am J Nucl Med Mol Imaging. 2012; 2(3):362–385

Triggiani V, Moschetta M, Giagulli VA, Licchelli B, Guastamacchia E. Diffuse 131I lung uptake in bronchiectasis: a potential pitfall in the follow-up of differentiated thyroid carcinoma. Thyroid. 2012; 22(12):1287–1290

# Case 19

*Kamal D. Singh*

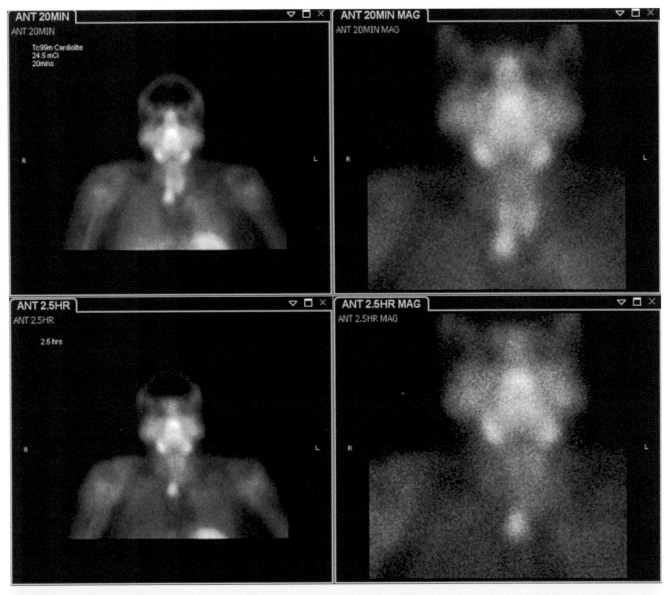

**Fig. 19.1** Dual-phase parathyroid scan with Technetium-99m (Tc-99m) Sestamibi. Early imaging 20 minute post injection demonstrates radiotracer uptake within the thyroid gland, along with a focus of moderately intense uptake inferior to right lobe of the thyroid gland. Delayed imaging 2 hours post injection reveals appropriate washout of thyroid activity with persistent focal uptake inferior to the right thyroid pole. Physiologic activity is seen within salivary glands and myocardium on both early and delayed imaging.

## ■ Clinical History

56-year-old female with labs consistent with primary hyper-parathyroidism (▶ Fig. 19.1).

## ■ Key Finding

Persistent focal cervical uptake on delayed Sestamibi imaging

## ■ Top 3 Differential Diagnoses

• **Parathyroid adenoma.** Etiologies of primary hyperparathyroidism include parathyroid adenoma (90–94%), hyperplasia (6%), and much less common parathyroid carcinoma (<1%). Clinically, patients have manifestations of serum hypercalcemia and hypophosphatasia due to elevated parathyroid hormone (PTH), although more than half may be asymptomatic. Tc-99m sestamibi initially localizes within both the thyroid gland and hyperfunctioning parathyroid adenoma with normal washout of thyroid activity on delayed scan. Dual phase (early and delayed) parathyroid scan utilizes this differential washout between thyroid gland and hyperfunctioning parathyroid tissue to localize an adenoma. While the majority of parathyroid adenomas are solitary and located adjacent to the thyroid tissue, they can be multiple in number and/or ectopic in location (10–15%); hence, the mediastinum is included in the field of view. Single-photon emission computed tomography (SPECT) imaging can improve contrast resolution for detection and localization of adenomas. Frequently, parathyroid adenomas may demonstrate rapid washout of radiotracer (similar to thyroid tissue), resulting in a false negative study since no discrete focus persists on delayed imaging. In such cases, either I-123 (oral) or Tc-99m pertechnetate (IV) scan can be performed to outline normal thyroid tissue, and this image may be subtracted from the early Tc-99m sestamibi image making the parathyroid adenoma more conspicuous.

• **Thyroid adenoma or carcinoma.** Tc-99m sestamibi demonstrates nonspecific localization in tumors via passive transport across cell membranes and active transport into mitochondria. False positive studies include thyroid adenoma (most common), thyroid carcinoma, and parathyroid carcinoma. Dual isotope imaging (Tc-99m sestamibi plus either I-123 or Tc-99m pertechnetate) with or without subtraction can improve sensitivity and avoid some of these pitfalls. Moreover, correlation with ultrasound or any cross-sectional imaging can be helpful.

• **Metastatic lymphadenopathy.** Tc-99m sestamibi is a nonspecific tumor localization agent. Focal cervical activity may be seen within metastatic lymph nodes from any primary malignancy (including thyroid, head/neck, and breast cancers). Correlation with clinical history and any cross-sectional imaging is helpful in these cases.

## ■ Diagnosis

Parathyroid adenoma.

## ✓ Pearls

• Parathyroid scan is performed as a localizing, not diagnostic, procedure prior to surgical exploration.
• Parathyroid adenoma is seen as focal persistent activity on delayed Tc-99m sestamibi scan.

• False positives include thyroid adenoma, thyroid carcinoma, and parathyroid carcinoma.
• Thyroid imaging with either I-123 or Tc-99m pertechnetate can be used for problem solving.

## Suggested Readings

Eslamy HK, Ziessman HA. Parathyroid scintigraphy in patients with primary hyperparathyroidism: 99mTc sestamibi SPECT and SPECT/CT. Radiographics. 2008; 28(5):1461–1476

Johnson NA, Tublin ME, Ogilvie JB. Parathyroid imaging: technique and role in the preoperative evaluation of primary hyperparathyroidism. AJR Am J Roentgenol. 2007; 188(6):1706–1715

Lavely WC, Goetze S, Friedman KP, et al. Comparison of SPECT/CT, SPECT, and planar imaging with single- and dual-phase (99m)Tc-sestamibi parathyroid scintigraphy. J Nucl Med. 2007; 48(7):1084–1089

# Case 20

*Ely A. Wolin*

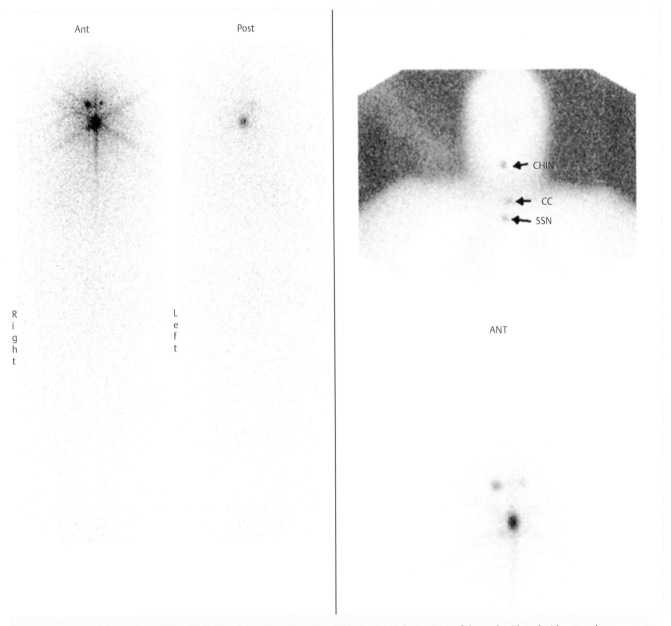

**Fig. 20.1** Postablation I-131 whole body scan. Anterior and posterior whole body images and spot views of the neck with and without markers demonstrate midline cervical uptake in the expected region of the thyroid bed with "star artifact."

## ■ Clinical History

37-year-old female with history of papillary thyroid carcinoma post total thyroidectomy and 107mCi I-131 therapy (▶ Fig. 20.1).

## ■ Key Finding

Focal neck uptake on I-131 postablation scan

## ■ Top 3 Differential Diagnoses

- **Residual thyroid tissue.** Patients with differentiated thyroid carcinoma are typically treated surgically with postoperative radioiodine (I-131) ablation. The goals of postoperative radioiodine therapy are: to ablate residual thyroid tissue to facilitate surveillance, provide adjuvant therapy for microscopic iodine avid disease, and further evaluation for metastases with post-treatment scan. The I-131 dose is determined by risk of recurrence, typically falling between 75 and 200 mCi. Limiting factors generally include no more than 200 R to bone marrow and a 1Ci lifetime limit. Limiting dose to the lungs with known pulmonary metastases is also important to avoid pulmonary fibrosis. There has been a push to decrease to a 30-mCi remnant ablation dose in low-risk patients, or not ablate at all, but that approach has not been completely validated as preablation staging is markedly limited. In preparation for ablation, the patient should discontinue thyroid hormone replacement therapy (6 weeks for T4, 2 weeks for T3) and should be on a low iodine diet for at least 10–14 days. Recombinant thyroid stimulating hormone (TSH) may be administered 48 and 24 hours prior to dose administration alternatively to hormone withdrawal. If there is concern for a significant thyroid remnant, a preablation scan can be performed with 1–2 mCi I-123 or < 5 mCi I-131, although with I-131 specifically there is a concern for thyroid stunning which might limit effectiveness of the therapy dose. Postablation imaging is usually performed 7–10 days after therapy as a baseline for future surveillance scans and to provide more accurate staging information. On any I-131 imaging study, a high degree of functional thyroid tissue (residual thyroid tissue or metastatic disease) may result in septal penetration due to the high energy of the I-131 photons (364 keV), causing the "star artifact."

- **Cervical nodal metastases.** Thyroid carcinoma may have local (cervical nodes) or distant (mediastinal, pulmonary, or osseous) metastases, which require a larger I-131 ablation dose than does ablation of a normal thyroid gland remnant. Papillary carcinoma typically spreads via lymphatics to local cervical lymph nodes, whereas follicular carcinoma spreads hematogenously to distant sites. After initial radioiodine therapy, surveillance includes serum thyroglobulin (Tg) levels and I-131 or I-123 whole-body metascans. I-131 ablation may be repeated in the event of recurrent disease with generally a 6 month to 1 year interval between ablation doses.

- **Physiologic pharyngeal/esophageal activity.** On all I-131 or I-123 scans, physiologic uptake is expected within the salivary glands, stomach, intestines, and urinary bladder. Nonfocal hepatic uptake is also seen in cases where there is residual functioning thyroid tissue, since thyroid hormone is metabolized by the liver. Focal increased activity, however, is more suggestive of metastases. In addition to primary renal excretion, radioiodine is excreted in saliva. Therefore, transient swallowed activity within the pharynx or esophagus may mimic cervical or mediastinal metastases; this can be confirmed by reimaging after the patient drinks water.

## ■ Diagnosis

Residual or remnant thyroid bed activity.

## ✓ Pearls

- Pretherapy I-123 or I-131 diagnostic metascan can identify residual thyroid and detect metastases.
- Using I-131 for pretherapy scan comes with risk of thyroid "stunning" prior to therapy.
- Postablation I-131 whole body scan (WBS) provides additional staging information and establishes a baseline.

- fluorine-18 fluorodeoxyglucose (F-18 FDG) positron emission tomography/computed tomography (PET/CT) is recommended if follow-up Tg is elevated and radioiodine scan is negative.

## Suggested Readings

Blumhardt R, Wolin EA, Phillips WT, et al. Current controversies in the initial post-surgical radioactive iodine therapy for thyroid cancer: a narrative review. Endocr Relat Cancer. 2014; 21(6):R473–R484

Haugen BR, Alexander EK, Bible KC, et al. 2015. American Thyroid Association management guidelines for adult patients with thyroid nodules and differentiated thyroid cancer: The American Thyroid Association Guidelines Task Force on Thyroid Nodules and Differentiated Thyroid Cancer. Thyroid. 2016; 26(1):1–133

Mazzaferri EL. Managing thyroid microcarcinomas. Yonsei Med J. 2012; 53(1):1–14

# Case 21

*Ely A. Wolin*

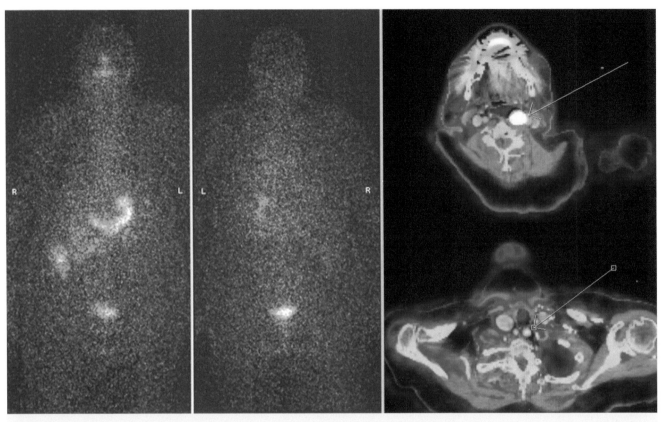

**Fig. 21.1** Anterior and posterior images from a whole-body scan obtained 24 hours after the oral administration of approximately 2 mCi of I-123 show physiologic uptake in the nasopharynx, bowel, and bladder, with no other areas of uptake to suggest recurrent iodine avid disease. Representative axial fused images from subsequent fluorine-18 fluorodeoxyglucose positron-emission tomography (F-18 FDG PET)/CT show hypermetabolic nodes in the left neck and paraesophageal region.

## ■ Clinical History

80-year-old female with metastatic papillary thyroid carcinoma, 14 months post thyroidectomy and 12 months post ablation with 204 mCi I-131, with new elevation in thyroglobulin (Tg) level (▶Fig. 21.1).

## Key Finding

Negative radioiodine scan in the setting of positive serum Tg levels after initial therapy for differentiated thyroid cancer

## Top 3 Differential Diagnoses

- **Dedifferentiated cancer.** Initial therapy for differentiated (i.e., papillary or follicular) thyroid cancer usually involves total thyroidectomy with subsequent I-131 therapy. The main goals for initial postoperative radioiodine ablation (RIA) are to destroy any remaining thyroid tissue, removing beds for possible recurrence, and allowing for biochemical follow up with serum Tg levels, as adjuvant therapy to destroy any residual iodine-avid disease, and for improved staging with a posttherapy whole body scan (WBS). Follow up after initial therapy usually involves monitoring thyroid stimulating hormone (TSH)-stimulated serum Tg levels and WBS. An elevation of stimulated Tg levels is concerning, with Tg greater than 10 ng/mL after thyroid withdrawal, or 5 ng/mL after recombinant human TSH (rhTSH) stimulation, carrying a high predictive value for recurrence. A stimulated WBS should be obtained in this setting, usually using 3–5 mCi of I-131 or 1–2 mCi of I-123, to localize recurrent or metastatic disease. A negative WBS in this setting is concerning for dedifferentiated cancer which is no longer iodine avid. Both medullary and anaplastic thyroid carcinoma are known to result in a false negative WBS. F-18 FDG PET/CT can be useful in this setting, as noniodine avid disease frequently has increased F-18 FDG avidity.
- **Small metastases.** While a negative WBS in the setting of positive Tg is concerning for dedifferentiated cancer, it is possible that the Tg is being produced by metastatic foci that are below the size threshold for resolution on the WBS. Because of this possibility, patients that have a positive Tg, negative WBS, and subsequent negative F-18 FDG PET/CT are commonly empirically treated with additional high dose I-131 ablation, with the hope of treating small foci of avid disease as well as possibly visualizing the disease on the posttherapy scan due to the increased dosage.
- **False positive thyroglobulin**. It is routine to check for Tg antibodies (anti-Tg) during the initial laboratory assessment of thyroid cancer patients. The presence of anti-Tg makes serum Tg measurements less reliable, and sometimes falsely high.

## Additional Diagnostic Consideration

- **Poor prep for radioiodine scan:** Appropriate exam preparation is necessary to maximize the sensitivity of a WBS. This includes adherence to a low-iodine diet and appropriate TSH stimulation.

## Diagnosis

Dedifferentiated, noniodine avid, recurrent metastatic thyroid carcinoma.

## ✓ Pearls

- High serum Tg levels on follow up for thyroid cancer after initial therapy is concerning for recurrence.
- A negative radioiodine WBS in setting of high serum Tg levels may indicate dedifferentiated cancer.
- It is important to ensure appropriate exam preparations have been followed prior to WBS.
- The presence of anti-Tg makes Tg measurements less reliable.

## Suggested Readings

Blumhardt R, Wolin EA, Phillips WT, et al. Current controversies in the initial post-surgical radioactive iodine therapy for thyroid cancer: a narrative review. Endocr Relat Cancer. 2014; 21(6):R473–R484

Chao M. Management of differentiated thyroid cancer with rising thyroglobulin and negative diagnostic radioiodine whole body scan. Clin Oncol (R Coll Radiol). 2010; 22(6):438–447

Kloos RT. Approach to the patient with a positive serum thyroglobulin and a negative radioiodine scan after initial therapy for differentiated thyroid cancer. J Clin Endocrinol Metab. 2008; 93(5):1519–1525

# Part 3

## Cardiac

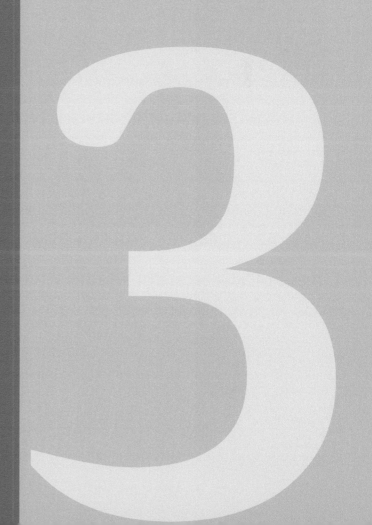

# Case 22

*Ely A. Wolin*

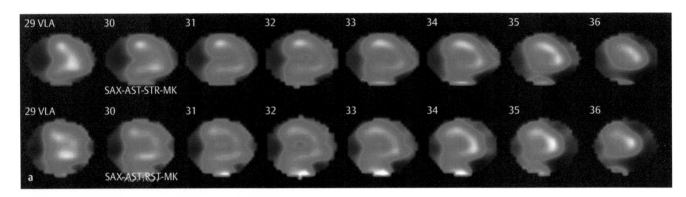

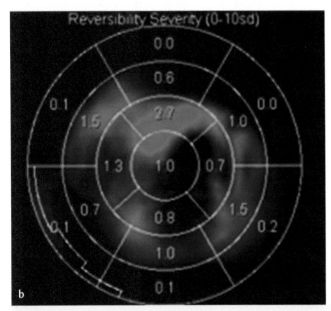

**Fig. 22.1** **(a)** Vertical long axis images and **(b)** reversibility polar map from a 1-day protocol myocardial perfusion scan using technetium-99m (Tc-99m) tetrofosmin show a primarily reversible distal anterior/apical defect.

## ■ Clinical History

55-year-old male with known coronary artery disease post pacemaker placement (▸ Fig. 22.1).

## ■ Key Finding

Myocardial perfusion defect which is worse on stress than rest images (reversible defect)

## ■ Top 2 Differential Diagnoses

- **Ischemia.** Single-photon emission computed tomography (SPECT) myocardial perfusion imaging (MPI) remains the most common exam performed in the majority of Nuclear Medicine departments. MPI is generally performed for risk stratification for possible coronary artery disease, to help determine which patients need cardiac catheterization, and possible reperfusion. Most commonly used radiopharmaceuticals are the mitochondrial imaging agents, Tc-99m sestamibi, and Tc-99m tetrofosmin, having mostly replace thallium-201 (Tl-201) due to more advantageous imaging and dose characteristics. For the Tc-99m-based mitochondrial agents a 1-day protocol is frequently used for patient and scheduling convenience. SPECT imaging is obtained at rest first after administration of around 8–11 mCi of the radiotracer. Either pharmacologic or exercise stress is then performed, and a stress dose of around 25–30 mCi is injected at the appropriate time with subsequent repeat SPECT imaging. A perfusion defect present only on the poststress images, or a "reversible" defect, is concerning for stress-induced ischemia and suggests the presence of coronary artery disease (CAD) while providing prognostic value for risk of a major cardiac event. Other stress-induced findings associated with CAD include increased pulmonary or right ventricular (RV) uptake, increased poststress left ventricular volumes (transient ischemic dilation), and decreased poststress ejection fraction.

MPI has good sensitivity for identifying CAD that results in greater than 50% luminal narrowing.

- **Shifting attenuation.** Attenuation is always a concern when reviewing MPI. The photons emitted from the injected radiopharmaceutical can be attenuated by the patient, as well as by anything overlying the patient, resulting in an apparent perfusion defect. Common causes for attenuation defects include the breasts, chest wall, diaphragm, implanted pacemaker/defibrillator, electrocardiography (EKG) leads, and implanted medication ports. Attenuation most frequently results in a defect that is worse on the rest images than the stress images, when using the 1-day protocol, since approximately one-third of the amount of radioactivity is used for the rest exam. Breast attenuation usually results in an anteroseptal defect, and diaphragm in an inferolateral defect. A defect can confidently be attributed to attenuation when it is in a common location, is worse on rest than stress, does not have a corresponding wall motion abnormality, and attenuation is seen on the rotating raw images. Attenuation can result in an apparent reversible defect when the cause of attenuation shifts in location between the rest and stress images. If this is considered, repeat stress images obtained in the prone position, or SPECT/CT with attenuation correction, can be used for problem solving, as long as the patient is still available for imaging.

## ■ Diagnosis

Myocardial ischemia. Subsequent cardiac catheterization revealed diffuse plaque in the proximal to mid left anterior descending coronary artery resulting in over 50% stenosis.

## ✓ Pearls

- A reversible myocardial perfusion defect, seen on stress but not rest images, is concerning for ischemia.
- Shifting attenuation can result in an apparent reversible defect.
- Prone imaging and attenuation correction with SPECT/CT are possible problem-solving techniques.

- Attenuation will usually result in a defect that is worse on rest than stress and without abnormal motion, when using a 1-day protocol.

## Suggested Readings

Hage FG, Ghimire G, Lester D, et al. The prognostic value of regadenoson myocardial perfusion imaging. J Nucl Cardiol. 2015; 22(6):1214–1221

Higgins JP, Higgins JA, Williams G. Stress-induced abnormalities in myocardial perfusion imaging that are not related to perfusion but are of diagnostic and prognostic importance. Eur J Nucl Med Mol Imaging. 2007; 34(4):584–595

Holder L, Lewis S, Abrames E, Wolin EA. Review of SPECT myocardial perfusion imaging. J Am Osteopath Coll Radiol. 2016; 5(3):5–13

# Case 23

*Ely A. Wolin*

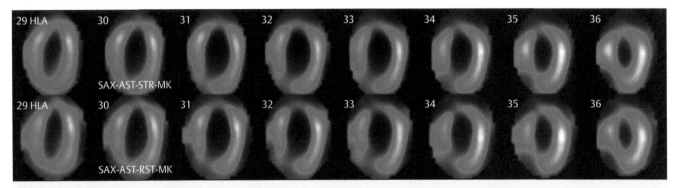

**Fig. 23.1** Horizontal long axis images from a myocardial perfusion scan show a large sized, severe to complete, fixed apical defect, with wall divergence. Gated images showed apical dyskinesia (not shown).

## ■ Clinical History

71-year-old male with ischemic cardiomyopathy and worsening exertional fatigue and dyspnea (▶ Fig. 23.1).

## ■ Key Finding

Myocardial perfusion defect present on both rest and stress images (fixed defect)

## ■ Top 3 Differential Diagnoses

- **Infarct.** A perfusion defect on single-photon emission computed tomography (SPECT) myocardial perfusion imaging (MPI) is generally described in terms of size, severity, location, and reversibility. A defect that is present on both the rest and stress images, or a "fixed" defect, is concerning for infarct. A true infarct should be associated with a wall motion abnormality on gated images. No differential is necessary if there is dyskinesia in the region of the fixed perfusion defect as that suggests the presence of a transmural infarct with aneurysm formation. There is some suggestion that the severity of a perfusion defect on SPECT MPI, particularly with Thallium-201 (Tl-201), can help predict the amount of infarcted tissue within the perfusion defect.

- **Hibernating myocardium.** Coronary artery occlusion can lead to a spectrum of results depending on severity and duration of occlusion. Short-duration ischemia can lead to myocardial stunning which presents as an area with normal perfusion but abnormal motion. This will spontaneously resolve. Long-term repetitive episodes of ischemia can lead to functional downregulation to promote myocyte survival by decreasing oxygen demand, known as hibernating myocardium. This is often indistinguishable from infarct on SPECT MPI, with possible distinction by the defect severity. However, differentiation may be important as hibernating myocardium is viable and will likely respond to revascularization. If determining the extent of hibernating versus infarcted myocardium is clinically warranted, most frequently needed in the setting of a reduced ejection fraction (EF) with a fixed defect, further evaluation can be done with Tl-201, fluorine-18 fluorodeoxyglucose (F-18 FDG), and cardiac MRI. Hibernating myocardium will show redistribution on 24-hour Tl-201 images, and uptake (occasionally increased relative to the remaining myocardium) on F-18 FDG images. Subendocardial delayed enhancement on cardiac MRI that involves less than 50% of the wall thickness is considered a marker for viability.

- **Attenuation.** Soft-tissue attenuation that remains in a fixed position can result in a fixed perfusion defect. This is commonly seen secondary to breast attenuation in the anterior/anteroseptal wall, and due to diaphragm attenuation in the inferior/inferolateral wall. Characteristics that suggest a perfusion defect is secondary to attenuation include location (often a nonvascular distribution), frequently worse on rest than stress with a 1-day protocol due to the lower administered dosage at rest, and wall motion and thickness are preserved.

## ■ Diagnosis

Apical infarct with aneurysm.

## ✓ Pearls

- Hibernating myocardium is dysfunctional with reduced perfusion but will respond to revascularization.
- Differentiating between viable and nonviable myocardium may be needed in the setting of reduced EF.
- F-18 FDG, Tl-201, and MR imaging can all be used to asses for myocardial viability.
- A fixed defect that has normal wall motion and thickening is likely secondary to attenuation.

## Suggested Readings

Dvorak RA, Brown RK, Corbett JR. Interpretation of SPECT/CT myocardial perfusion images: common artifacts and quality control techniques. Radiographics. 2011; 31(7):2041–2057

Mc Ardle BA, Beanlands RS. Myocardial viability: whom, what, why, which, and how? Can J Cardiol. 2013; 29(3):399–402

# Case 24

*Ely A. Wolin*

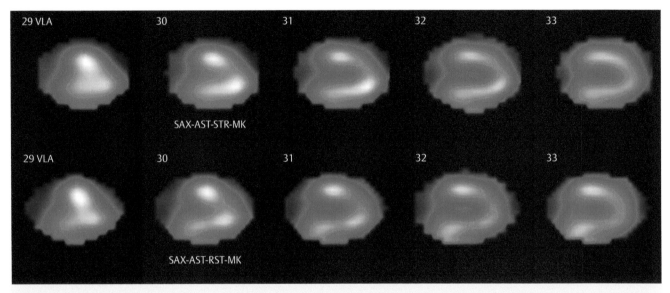

**Fig. 24.1** Representative vertical long axis from 1-day protocol Technetium-99m (Tc-99m) tetrofosmin myocardial perfusion imaging shows a defect in the distal anterior wall which appears worse on rest than stress.

## ■ Clinical History

73-year-old female referred for myocardial perfusion imaging (MPI) because of nonsustained supraventricular tachycardia on mobile telemetry (▶Fig. 24.1).

■ **Key Finding**

Resting myocardial perfusion defect that improves after stress ("reverse redistribution/perfusion")

■ **Top 3 Differential Diagnoses**

- **Attenuation/shifting attenuation.** Myocardial perfusion is most frequently performed for risk stratification of patients with suspected or known coronary artery disease (CAD). Stress images are the most important in this setting, as recognition of a stress-induced perfusion defect raises the concern for ischemia, possibly requiring coronary angiography and revascularization. While most facilities use a 1-day protocol, performing reduced dose rest imaging prior to either exercise or pharmacologic stress the same day, the 2-day protocol includes stress imaging first. If the stress images are normal, rest of the images are likely not necessary as they are primarily used to provide specificity to a stress defect. However, occasionally a perfusion defect will be seen at rest that improves after stress, termed "reverse redistribution" or "reverse perfusion." A possible cause is shifting attenuation. If an attenuating structure changes position between the rest and stress images, then the resulting defects will not be matched. Evaluation of the rotating raw images can help to visualize shifting attenuation. Attenuation on its own, that does not shift, can cause a defect that appears worse on rest than stress with 1-day protocol imaging due to the reduced dosage used for rest images.

- **Prior revascularization.** A rest perfusion defect that improves with stress can be seen in patients post revascularization. The etiology for this phenomenon is not completely clear. It may be secondary to slow flow through the revascularized vessel, stent, or graft. Theoretically, stress-induced vasodilation distal to the revascularization results in a greater pressure differential leading to sufficient flow through a conduit that is otherwise insufficient. Reverse perfusion may also be due to more rapid washout of radiotracer from hibernating or stunned myocardium. This finding was originally thought to represent effective reperfusion; however, some studies have shown patients with postreperfusion reverse redistribution have a higher risk for cardiac events even in the setting of proven myocardial viability.

- **Cardiac sarcoid.** Sarcoidosis is a multisystem disease of unknown etiology resulting in formation of noncaseating granulomas. Around 1 in 20 patients with sarcoidosis will have cardiac involvement, which may be asymptomatic or lead to sudden death. Reverse redistribution with cardiac sarcoid is thought to be secondary to constriction of coronary arterioles around granulomas. Fluorine-18 fluorodeoxyglucose (F-18 FDG) and cardiac MRI (cMRI) are better imaging agents for cardiac sarcoid and more frequently used.

■ **Diagnosis**

Attenuation (the defect resolved with attenuation correction, not shown).

✓ **Pearls**

- If a reverse perfusion pattern is seen, raw data should be evaluated for attenuation/shifting attenuation.
- Reverse perfusion post reperfusion may be due to slow flow requiring distal dilation to normalize.

- Reverse perfusion can be seen with cardiac sarcoid, better evaluated with F-18 FDG positron emission tomography (PET) and cMRI.

**Suggested Readings**

Schatka I, Bengel FM. Advanced imaging of cardiac sarcoidosis. J Nucl Med. 2014; 55(1):99–106

Schillaci O, Tavolozza M, Di Biagio D, et al. Reverse perfusion pattern in myocardial spect with 99mTc-sestaMIBI. J Med Life. 2013; 6(3):349–354

Swinkels BM, Hooghoudt TE, Schoenmakers EA, Zinder CG, de Boo TM, Verheugt FW. Clinical significance of reverse redistribution on technetium-99m tetrofosmin single-photon emission computed tomography: an 18-month follow-up study. Neth Heart J. 2003; 11(3):113–117

Tanaka R, Nakamura T, Chiba S, et al. Clinical implication of reverse redistribution on 99mTc-sestamibi images for evaluating ischemic heart disease. Ann Nucl Med. 2006; 20(5):349–356

# Case 25

*Ely A. Wolin*

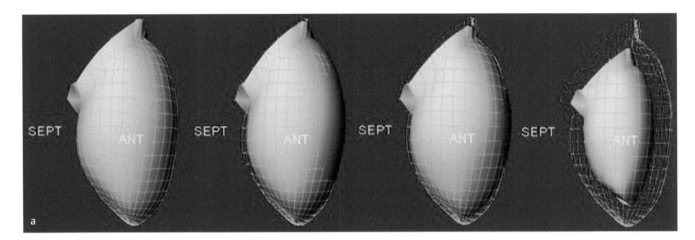

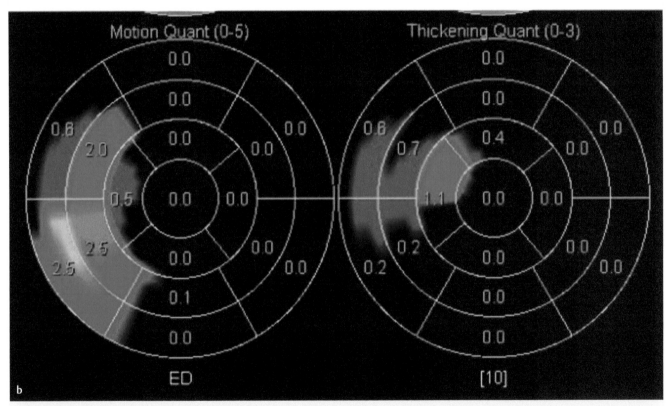

Fig. 25.1 (a) Representative volume rendered images from a gated myocardial perfusion scan show paradoxical inward motion of the septum during diastole. (b) Quantitative polar maps show that while the septum has abnormal motion it is thickening.

## ■ Clinical History

82-year-old female with new onset left bundle branch block (LBBB) and shortness of breath referred to evaluate for ischemia (▶Fig. 25.1).

## ■ Key Finding

Paradoxical bouncing motion of the interventricular septum during diastole, or "septal bounce"

## ■ Top 3 Differential Diagnoses

- **Ventricular interdependence.** Septal bounce is a wall motion abnormality that may be seen on gated single-photon emission computed tomography (SPECT) myocardial perfusion imaging (MPI) along with other imaging modalities that allow evaluation of cardiac wall motion to include echocardiography, cardiac CT and cardiac MRI (cMRI). During early diastole, the septum will show a paradoxical bouncing motion, initially moving toward and then away from the left ventricle (LV). This motion abnormality suggests restricted ventricular filling which results in a relatively fixed volume for the heart. This equates to ventricular interdependence, i.e., changes in volume and pressure of one ventricle are propagated through the septum into the other ventricle. This is most commonly seen with constrictive pericarditis, but can also be associated with cardiac tamponade.

- **Left bundle branch block.** Delayed conduction from a LBBB results in delayed LV activation. This alone can be associated with decreased LV function, even with normal myocyte contractility. Several septal wall motion abnormalities have been associated with LBBB, one of which is the septal bounce. Correlation with EKG obtained during performance of MPI can confirm the diagnosis.

- **Pulmonary hypertension.** Chronic pulmonary hypertension can result in paradoxical motion of the interventricular septum due to elevated right ventricle (RV) pressure. Pressure in the LV drops to near zero in early diastole allowing the greater RV pressure to push the septum toward the LV center.

## ■ Diagnosis

Left bundle branch block.

## ✓ Pearls

- Paradoxical bouncing of the septum toward the LV during diastole is known as a septal bounce.
- Ventricular interdependence due to constrictive pericarditis or tamponade can cause a septal bounce.
- Septal bounce can be due to delayed electrical activation of the LV in LBBB.
- Exercise or dobutamine stress should be avoided with LBBB due to a possible false septal defect.

## Suggested Readings

Breithardt G, Breithardt OA. Left bundle branch block, an old-new entity. J Cardiovasc Transl Res. 2012; 5(2):107–116

Dvorak RA, Brown RK, Corbett JR. Interpretation of SPECT/CT myocardial perfusion images: common artifacts and quality control techniques. Radiographics. 2011; 31(7):2041–2057

Walker CM, Chung JH, Reddy GP. "Septal bounce." J Thorac Imaging. 2012; 27(1):W1

# Case 26

*Ely A. Wolin*

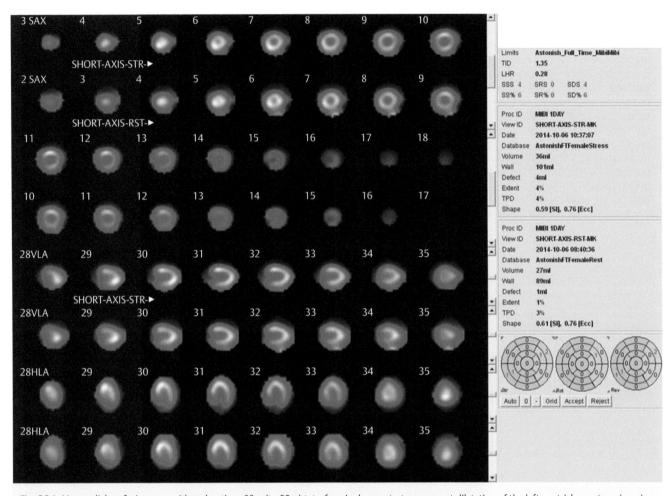

**Fig. 26.1** Myocardial perfusion scan with technetium-99m (tc-99m) tetrofosmin demonstrates apparent dilatation of the left ventricle on stress imaging, transient ischemic dilation (TID) ratio of 1.35, without apparent perfusion defect. TID, transient ischemic dilation.

## ■ Clinical History

80-year-old female with history of chronic obstructive pulmonary disease and atrial fibrillation presenting with chest pain (▶Fig. 26.1).

## ■ Key Finding

Transient ischemic dilation

## ■ Top 3 Differential Diagnoses

- **Multivessel coronary artery disease.** Myocardial perfusion imaging (MPI) is designed to detect areas of ischemia which may benefit from reperfusion. Ischemia is diagnosed by noting a reversible defect, decreased activity in a portion of the myocardium on post-stress imaging (exercise or chemical stress) in comparison to rest imaging. With multivessel balanced ischemia, however, focal regions of decreased activity may not be apparent as the images are normalized to the "hottest" pixels. In these situations, diffuse subendocardial ischemia may cause apparent dilation of the left ventricle (LV) cavity on post-stress imaging. This is an important finding to make as it may be the only sign of ischemia and can be associated with high-grade stenosis.

- **Hypertensive heart disease.** Global subendocardial ischemia, resulting in apparent dilation of the LV cavity on poststress imaging, may also be caused by severe hypertensive heart disease. This is likely a multifactorial process, but elevated end diastolic pressures in the LV are contributory as this leads to an increase in the required filling pressure of the epicardial coronary vessels. This can cause TID without any associated coronary artery stenosis.

- **Dilated cardiomyopathy.** TID can again be seen in the absence of coronary artery disease (CAD) rarely in patients with dilated cardiomyopathy. The subendocardial hypoperfusion in this case is likely due to decreased coronary flow reserve.

## ■ Additional Diagnostic Consideration

- **Misaligned single-photon emission computed tomography (SPECT) images:** Misaligned stress and rest images from SPECT analysis may result in apparent post-stress dilation of the LV cavity. A careful inspection of overall SPECT image alignment at rest and stress, as well as utilization of quantitative analysis, should be made to avoid this post processing pitfall.

## ■ Diagnosis

Multivessel coronary artery disease.

## ✓ Pearls

- Global subendocardial ischemia may result in apparent ventricular cavity dilation, TID.
- TID suggests diffuse subendocardial ischemia from balanced multivessel disease.

- In the setting of multivessel balanced ischemia, TID may be the only clue to underlying pathology.
- Be sure stress and rest SPECT images are appropriately aligned prior to visual interpretation.

## Suggested Readings

Abidov A, Bax JJ, Hayes SW, et al. Transient ischemic dilation ratio of the left ventricle is a significant predictor of future cardiac events in patients with otherwise normal myocardial perfusion SPECT. J Am Coll Cardiol. 2003; 42(10):1818–1825

McLaughlin MG, Danias PG. Transient ischemic dilation: a powerful diagnostic and prognostic finding of stress myocardial perfusion imaging. J Nucl Cardiol. 2002; 9(6):663–667

Robinson VJB, Corley JH, Marks DS, et al. Causes of transient dilatation of the left ventricle during myocardial perfusion imaging. AJR Am J Roentgenol. 2000; 174(5):1349–1352

# Case 27

*Ely A. Wolin*

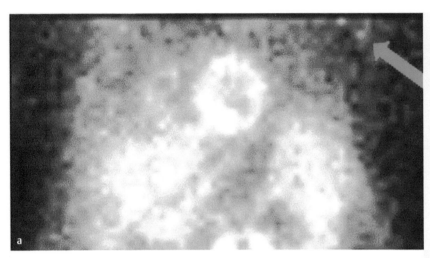

**Fig. 27.1** (a) Raw image from a myocardial perfusion scan shows foci of uptake in the left axilla (*red arrow*). (b) Images of the left arm injection site, before and after removal of the intravenous catheter, show local extravasation.

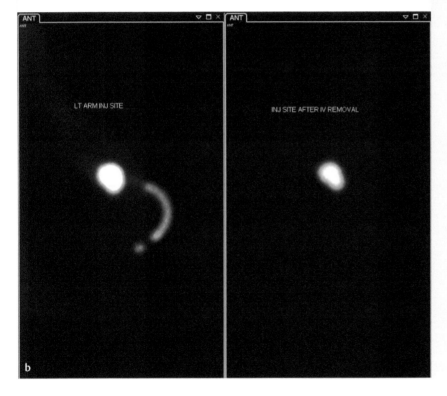

## ■ Clinical History

63-year-old male with coronary artery disease (CAD), hypertension, diabetes, and hyperlipidemia with ongoing substernal chest pain (▶ Fig. 27.1).

## ■ Key Finding

Axillary uptake on Tc-99m sestamibi or tetrofosmin myocardial perfusion imaging (MPI)

## ■ Top 2 Differential Diagnoses

- **Extravasation.** Extravasated radiopharmaceutical will be taken up by the lymphatic system and transported to the nearest nodal bed. As upper extremity injections are most common, this is usually the axillary lymph nodes. Axillary uptake noted on the raw data on the same side as the injection is most likely due to extravasation. This can be confirmed by obtaining a static image of the injection site. This is not specific to the myocardial imaging agents and is occasionally seen with bone scintigraphy as well.
- **Malignant lymphadenopathy.** The Tc-99m-based imaging agents used for MPI are mitochondrial imaging agents which were originally used as nonspecific tumor imaging agents.

Tc-99m sestamibi is currently the radiopharmaceutical used for breast-specific gamma imaging because of its tumor uptake characteristics. Axillary uptake can indicate nodal metastatic disease. Careful examination of the raw data for additional areas of nontarget uptake may show additional contributory findings, such as focal breast uptake. If axillary uptake is seen, and cannot be explained, correlation should be recommended with mammography and axillary ultrasound, when appropriate. Metastatic nodal uptake has been seen with malignancies other than breast primary, which is why mammography alone may not be sufficient for further work up.

## ■ Diagnosis

Radiopharmaceutical extravasation.

## ✓ Pearls

- Axillary uptake on MPI is likely due to lymphatic uptake of extravasated radiopharmaceutical.
- Extravasation can be confirmed if on the same side of injection with an image of the injection site.

- Mitochondrial imaging agents are tumor agents and axillary uptake may indicate nodal metastases.

## Suggested Readings

Bestetti A, Posterli R, Chiapparino R, Pedrazzini L, Tarolo GL. Tc-99m tetrofosmin lymph node uptake in myocardial perfusion imaging. Clin Nucl Med. 1996; 21(6):486–487

Burrell S, MacDonald A. Artifacts and pitfalls in myocardial perfusion imaging. J Nucl Med Technol. 2006; 34(4):193–211, quiz 212–214

Maharaj M, Korowlay NA. The role of routine whole volume SPECT reconstruction in comparison to cine raw data in the detection of extracardiac uptake on myocardiak perfusion scan. World J Nucl Med. 2011; 10(1):9–13

# Case 28

*Ely A. Wolin*

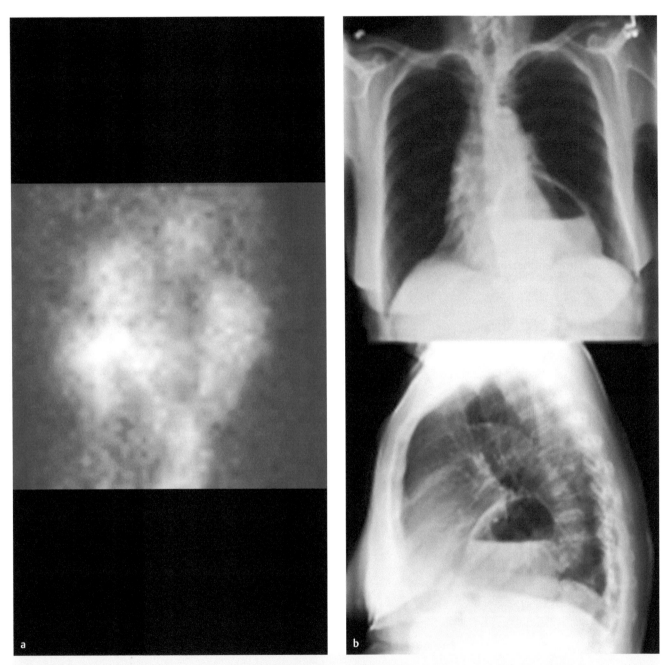

**Fig. 28.1** (a) Left anterior oblique projection from the raw data of a myocardial perfusion scan shows abnormal uptake posterior to the heart. (b) Correlative PA and lateral chest radiographs show a large hiatal hernia.

■ **Clinical History**

84-year-old female with hypertension, hyperlipidemia, and angina (▶Fig. 28.1).

## ■ Key Finding

Abnormal extracardiac uptake on myocardial perfusion imaging (MPI) other than axillary uptake

## ■ Top 3 Differential Diagnoses

- **Breast uptake.** The mitochondrial imaging agents and thallium-201 (Tl-201) are also nonspecific tumor imaging agents, with Tc-99m sestamibi used for breast-specific gamma imaging. Normal physiologic uptake in the breast will appear as mild diffuse uptake in both breasts, dependent on the amount of glandular tissue and hormonal status of the patient; this includes breast tissue uptake in male gynecomastia. Uptake will increase with lactation. Any focal increased uptake in the breasts, particularly if unilateral, is concerning for malignancy, primary or metastatic, and requires further evaluation. Focal breast uptake is not specific for malignancy, however, and has been seen with cystic disease, postsurgical scarring, benign microcalcifications, and fibroadenoma, among other benign processes.
- **Lung uptake.** Mild diffuse pulmonary uptake may also be seen normally on MPI. Increased diffuse pulmonary uptake is seen with increased pulmonary capillary wedge pressure, better appreciated with Tl-201 than the Tc-99m agents, and like transient ischemic dilation (TID) may suggest multivessel disease. Focal uptake of cardiac tracers in the lungs is concerning for malignancy. Uptake can also be seen in infectious and inflammatory conditions, such as pneumonia and granulomatous disease. Correlation with recent chest radiographs may be all that is necessary for added specificity.
- **Mediastinal uptake.** Mediastinal uptake of cardiac tracers can be seen with metastatic adenopathy, sarcoidosis, and primary neoplasms such as thymoma, esophageal carcinoma, and sarcoma. Activity can also be seen within a hiatal hernia from swallowed salivary secretions.

## ■ Additional Diagnostic Consideration

- **Thyroid/parathyroid:** Low level thyroid uptake may be present, normally. Abnormal thyroid uptake can be seen with multinodular goiter, thyroiditis, and carcinoma. Focal parathyroid uptake can be seen with adenoma, carcinoma, and hyperplasia; Tc-99m sestamibi is the radiopharmaceutical used for parathyroid imaging.

## ■ Diagnosis

Large hiatal hernia.

## ✓ Pearls

- Evaluation of the raw images is paramount to evaluate for clinically relevant extracardiac uptake.
- Focal uptake in the breast or lung on a myocardial perfusion scan requires evaluation for malignancy.
- Diffuse pulmonary uptake suggests high capillary wedge pressure, and may indicate multivessel disease.
- Abnormal uptake in the neck may indicate either thyroid or parathyroid pathology, including cancer.

## Suggested Readings

Gedik GK, Ergün EL, Aslan M, Caner B. Unusual extracardiac findings detected on myocardial perfusion single photon emission computed tomography studies with Tc-99m sestamibi. Clin Nucl Med. 2007; 32(12):920–926

Vijayakumar V, Gupta R, Rahman A. Pathologic extracardiac uptake of Tc-99m tetrofosmin identified in the chest during myocardial perfusion imaging. J Nucl Cardiol. 2005; 12(4):473–475

Williams KA, Hill KA, Sheridan CM. Noncardiac findings on dual-isotope myocardial perfusion SPECT. J Nucl Cardiol. 2003; 10(4):395–402

# Case 29

*Ely A. Wolin*

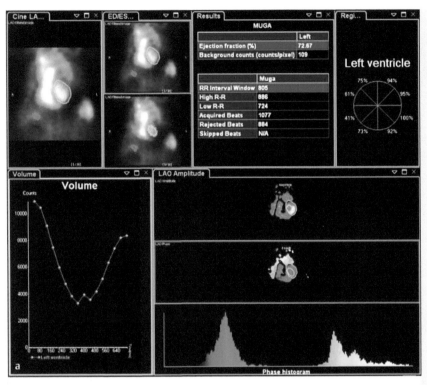

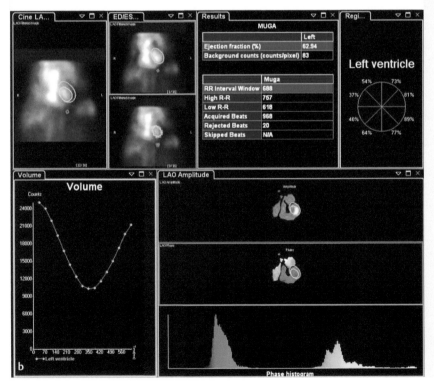

Fig. 29.1 (a) Gated ventriculography obtained after the administration of Technetium-99m (Tc-99m) RBCs shows a calculated ejection fraction of 73%. (b) After correction of the background region of interest (ROI) placement calculated ejection fraction is 63%.

## ■ Clinical History

71-year-old female on Herceptin (▶ Fig. 29.1).

## ■ Key Finding

Increased left ventricular ejection fraction (LVEF) on tagged red blood cell ventriculography

## ■ Top 2 Differential Diagnoses

• **Hyperdynamic left ventricle (LV).** Cardiac gated ventriculography performed with Tc-99m tagged red blood cells, frequently called a multi-gated acquisition (MUGA) scan, remains an accurate, noninvasive tool for LVEF determination. After injection of the radiopharmaceutical, cardiac gated dynamic images are obtained in the anterior, left lateral, and left anterior oblique views. The left anterior oblique imaging plane should be the angle that provides the best separation between the LV and right ventricle (RV) or the "best septal view." Some caudal tilt is usually helpful, depending on the cardiac axis. Using the best septal images, a region of interest (ROI) is drawn around the LV at both end diastole and end systole, along with a background ROI, to provide LVEF quantification. The anterior and lateral images provide additional information for qualitative assessment of wall motion, as well as to ensure the calculated LVEF appears accurate. This exam is most commonly used in patients who are about to start or are currently receiving cardiotoxic drugs such as Herceptin.

It can also be used for verification of ejection fraction (EF) when other anatomic modalities have provided conflicting data. A normal range for LVEF is generally considered to be around 50–80%, at rest. An LVEF below 50% may preclude initiating cardiotoxic therapy; and a drop in LVEF by more than 10% on follow-up exams may require discontinuing the therapy. An elevated LVEF, if calculated correctly, suggests a hyperdynamic LV which has multiple etiologies.

• **Poorly placed background ROI.** LVEF is determined on tagged red blood cell ventriculography by comparing background (BKG) corrected end systolic volume (ESV) to background corrected end diastolic volume (EDV). LVEF is calculated using the following calculation: $((EDV-BKG) - (ESV-BKG))/(EDV-BKG)$. Because the two BKG in the numerator cancel each other out, BKG ends up only affecting the denominator. If the BKG ROI is accidentally placed somewhere with too many counts, such as over the spleen or descending aorta, it will decrease the denominator and therefore falsely elevate the calculated LVEF.

## ■ Diagnosis

Background ROI placed over the liver resulting in an artificially elevated LVEF.

## ✓ Pearls

• Appropriate background ROI placement is essential for accurate LVEF determination on a MUGA scan.
• Placing the background ROI over the spleen or aorta will artificially increase the calculated LVEF.

• Tagged red blood cell ventriculography is a useful noninvasive tool to monitor cardiotoxic therapies.

## Suggested Readings

Corbett JR, Akinboboye OO, Bacharach SL, et al; Quality Assurance Committee of the American Society of Nuclear Cardiology. Equilibrium radionuclide angiocardiography. J Nucl Cardiol. 2006; 13(6):e56–e79

Robinson VJB, Corley JH, Marks DS, et al. Causes of transient dilatation of the left ventricle during myocardial perfusion imaging. AJR Am J Roentgenol. 2000; 174(5):1349–1352

# Case 30

*Ely A. Wolin*

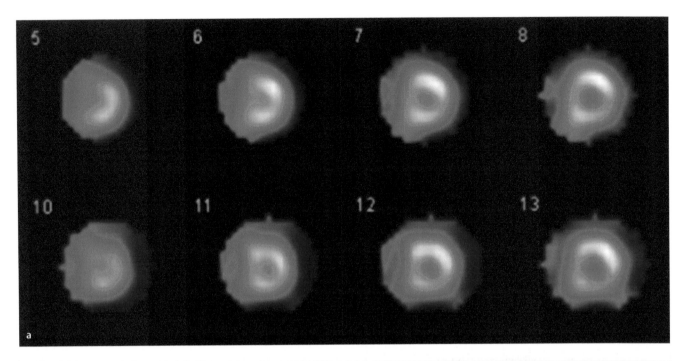

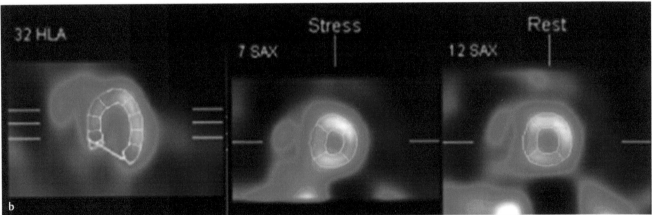

**Fig. 30.1** Representative images from a myocardial perfusion scan show right ventricular uptake present at both rest and stress. Also note the associated flattening of the interventricular septum and subtle increased activity at the right ventricle insertion point on the anteroseptal left ventricle, in this case.

■ Clinical History

80-year-old female with diabetes and hypertension and newly reduced left ventricular ejection fraction (LVEF) referred for myocardial perfusion imaging (MPI) (▶ Fig. 30.1).

## ■ Key Finding

Increased right ventricle (RV) uptake on myocardial perfusion imaging

## ■ Top 2 Differential Diagnoses

- **Right ventricular strain.** As the left ventricle (LV) myocardium is thicker than the RV, RV uptake is not usually seen on single-photon emission computed tomography (SPECT) myocardial perfusion imaging (MPI) with the exception of some low-level RV uptake with exercise testing. If RV uptake approaches the intensity of LV uptake, or is present at both rest and stress, it may indicate RV strain. This is commonly seen in the setting of heart failure and pulmonary arterial hypertension (PAH). With chronic PAH, SPECT MPI images may also show focal increased uptake in the anteroseptal LV wall at the RV insertion point.

- **Multivessel coronary artery disease.** Balanced multivessel ischemia can be difficult to identify with SPECT MPI since relative, not absolute, perfusion is presented. If perfusion is decreased throughout the heart, the entire heart will look normal. Increased RV uptake, particularly if seen at stress, may indicated multivessel or left main coronary artery disease. Transient ischemic dilation (TID) and increased pulmonary uptake (particularly with thallium-201 [Tl-201]) are other findings associated with balanced multivessel disease.

## ■ Diagnosis

RV strain. Correlative echocardiogram showed a dilated RV with increased wall thickness, reduced RV systolic function, and moderate pulmonary hypertension.

## ✓ Pearls

- Increased RV uptake on stress imaging may indicate multivessel or left main coronary artery disease.
- Increased RV uptake can also be seen with RV strain and PAH.

- Chronic PAH can cause focal increased uptake at the RV insertion point in the anteroseptal LV.

## Suggested Readings

Fang W, Zhao L, Xiong CM, et al. Comparison of 18F-FDG uptake by right ventricular myocardium in idiopathic pulmonary arterial hypertension and pulmonary arterial hypertension associated with congenital heart disease. Pulm Circ. 2012; 2(3):365–372

Williams KA, Schneider CM. Increased stress right ventricular activity on dual isotope perfusion SPECT: a sign of multivessel and/or left main coronary artery disease. J Am Coll Cardiol. 1999; 34(2):420–427

# Case 31

*Ely A. Wolin*

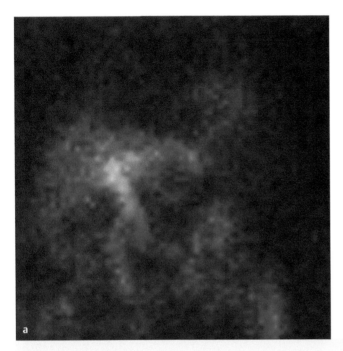 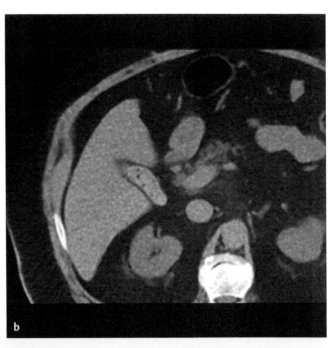

**Fig. 31.1** Raw image from a Technetium-99m (Tc-99m) tetrofosmin myocardial perfusion scan shows no uptake within the gallbladder. Cholelithiasis was seen on follow up ultrasound (not shown) and CT scan, without evidence of cholecystitis.

## ▪ Clinical History

69-year-old female referred for myocardial perfusion imaging (MPI) due to elevated BNP and dyspnea on exertion (▶ Fig. 31.1).

## ■ Key Finding

Nonvisualization of the gallbladder on myocardial perfusion imaging (MPI) using Tc-99m tagged sestamibi or tetrofosmin

## ■ Top 2 Differential Diagnoses

• **Cholecystectomy.** The Tc-99m imaging agents used for MPI are primarily cleared through the hepatobiliary system. Because of this, it is important to evaluate the imaged portions of the hepatobiliary system on the rotating raw data. The extent of hepatic uptake will depend on multiple factors including imaging agent used (sestamibi has more hepatic uptake and slower hepatic clearance), time between radiopharmaceutical injection and imaging, and type of stress performed (exercise stress should result in diversion from splanchnic blood flow resulting in less hepatic uptake). Any focal defects in the liver parenchyma require further evaluation to exclude a mass. If gallbladder activity is not visualized it is most likely secondary to cholecystectomy, easily confirmed through correlation with patient history.

• **Cholecystitis/cholelithiasis.** Nonvisualization of the gallbladder with Tc-99m-based MPI radiotracers without a history of cholecystectomy requires further evaluation. This may be secondary to cholecystitis, as complete or partial cystic duct obstruction will prevent hepatobiliary cleared radiotracer from entering the gallbladder due to the same physiology imaged with hepatobiliary imaging. Patients with nonvisualization of the gallbladder on MPI have been found to have acute cholecystitis, chronic cholecystitis, and cholelithiasis. Right upper quadrant ultrasound should be recommended if a history of cholecystectomy cannot be confirmed.

## ■ Diagnosis

Cholelithiasis.

## ✓ Pearls

• Tc-99m-based MPI agents have primarily hepatobiliary clearance.
• Nonvisualization of the gallbladder on MPI may be due to cholecystectomy or cholecystitis.

• Patients who have not had cholecystectomy, but their gallbladder is not visualized, require further evaluation.
• Focal defects in hepatic activity require further evaluation to exclude a mass.

## Suggested Readings

Chamarthy M, Travin MI. Altered biodistribution and incidental findings on myocardial perfusion imaging. Semin Nucl Med. 2010; 40(4):257–270

Gedik GK, Ergün EL, Aslan M, Caner B. Unusual extracardiac findings detected on myocardial perfusion single photon emission computed tomography studies with Tc-99m sestamibi. Clin Nucl Med. 2007; 32(12):920–926

Seo S, Angelina-Rivera A. Evaluation of gallbladder status on myocardial perfusion scan. J Nucl Med. 2016; 57:1669

# Case 32

*Ely A. Wolin*

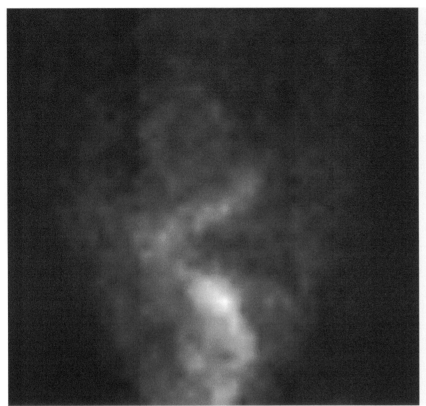

**Fig. 32.1** Left anterior oblique raw data projection from a Technetium-99m (Tc-99m) tetrofosmin myocardial perfusion scan shows absence of left renal activity.

## ■ Clinical History

87-year-old male with a history of prior myocardial infarct and a demand pacemaker undergoing preoperative assessment prior to resection of recurrent bladder cancer found to have inverted T waves in V2–V4 and two clinical risk factors for perioperative cardiovascular complications. Referred for myocardial perfusion imaging (MPI) for preoperative risk stratification (▶ Fig. 32.1).

## ▪ Key Finding

Absent renal uptake on MPI

## ▪ Top 3 Differential Diagnoses

• **Renal failure.** While the most commonly used MPI agents are primarily cleared through the hepatobiliary system, there is also some renal clearance. Depending on the field of view, the kidneys may be visible on the rotating raw images. The right kidney is often more difficult to ascertain than the left due to hepatic uptake as well as the usual 180 degrees of rotation around the left chest used to best image the heart. Nonvisualization of either kidney, if the visualization would be expected in the field of view, warrants further attention. Lack of renal radiotracer activity can be secondary to renal failure which on rare occasion may be unknown to the ordering clinical provider.

• **Nephrectomy.** Review of the medical record of a patient undergoing radionuclide MPI with no renal activity might show a history of nephrectomy.

• **Renal ectopia.** In the absence of renal failure or nephrectomy, absent renal activity on MPI may be secondary to renal ectopia. While renal ectopia is rare, common locations for ectopic kidney include the pelvis, intrathoracic, and cross-fused ectopia.

## ▪ Additional Diagnostic Consideration

• **Renal mass/space-occupying lesion:** The top 3 considerations discussed above are for general, or whole kidney, absent counts. However, it is important to thoroughly review renal uptake on the rotating raw data as a focal area of decreased activity suggests a renal mass. While most commonly a focal area of reduced renal counts is caused by a renal cyst or pelvicalyceal dilation, neoplasms such as renal cell carcinoma and oncocytoma will result in similar findings. If prior cross-sectional imaging is not available or prior imaging does not show a correlative finding, further evaluation should be recommended initially with renal ultrasound.

## ▪ Diagnosis

Unknown, as no follow up is available, but likely renal failure from obstructive uropathy.

## ✓ Pearls

• The kidneys should be seen on MPI, if in the field of view, due to some renal clearance of radiotracers.
• Absent renal activity suggests renal failure (which may be unknown), nephrectomy, or ectopia.

• Focal area of decreased renal activity is concerning for a mass and requires anatomic correlation.

## Suggested Readings

Jones SE, Aziz K, Yasuda T, Gewirtz H, Scott JA. Importance of systematic review of rotating projection images from Tc99m-sestamibi cardiac perfusion imaging for noncardiac findings. Nucl Med Commun. 2008; 29(7):607–613

Shih WJ, Kiefer V, Gross K, et al. Intrathoracic and intra-abdominal Tl-201 abnormalities seen on rotating raw cine data on dual radionuclide myocardial perfusion and gated SPECT. Clin Nucl Med. 2002; 27(1):40–44

Williams KA, Hill KA, Sheridan CM. Noncardiac findings on dual-isotope myocardial perfusion SPECT. J Nucl Cardiol. 2003; 10(4):395–402

# Case 33

*Ely A. Wolin*

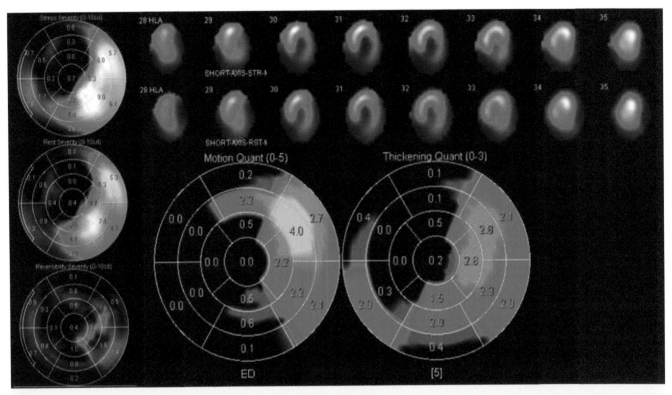

**Fig. 33.1** Select images from a Technetium-99m (Tc-99m) tetrofosmin myocardial perfusion scan show a large fixed lateral wall defect with associated decreased wall motion and thickening, qualitatively was noted as severe hypokinesis.

## ■ Clinical History

71-year-old male with dyspnea on exertion and chest pressure for 2 weeks, negative initial troponins, referred for myocardial perfusion imaging (MPI) for risk stratification (▶Fig. 33.1).

## ■ Key Finding

Focal wall motion abnormality on gated MPI

## ■ Top 3 Differential Diagnoses

- **Hypokinesia.** Electrographically gated myocardial perfusion single-photon emission computed tomography (GSPECT) allows for the simultaneous evaluation of myocardial perfusion and left ventricle (LV) function. During gated acquisition, the R-to-R interval is divided into equal segments, usually 8–16, and dynamically acquired information during each segment is used to create an image corresponding to that phase of the cardiac cycle. The endo- and epicardial borders are then used to define the myocardium. Regional wall motion (RWM) is determined by movement of the endocardial margin and systolic wall thickening (SWT) is measured by the change in counts between the end diastolic and end systolic images. The LV cavity is extrapolated from the endocardial contour. Functional analysis is generally not as accurate as radionuclide ventriculography during which the LV cavity is imaged directly. GSPECT can be performed with both rest and stress images, but this may be redundant as the stress images are obtained after the patient has already returned to resting physiology. A true wall motion abnormality will generally have both abnormal RWM and SWT, versus a post coronary artery bypass grafting septal rock, for example, which will have abnormal RWM but normal SWT. A focal area of hypokinesia suggests myocyte contractility dysfunction, and when associated with a fixed perfusion defect eliminates attenuation as a differential, limiting the possibilities to hibernating myocardium and infarct. Hypokinesia may be seen with ischemia on stress images if the patient has not fully recovered from stress.
- **Akinesia.** Continued progression of loss of myocyte contractility will lead to a complete lack of RWM and SWT, and again may be associated with hibernating myocardium or infarct.
- **Dyskinesia.** It is RWM opposite of the expected direction, or an area of the LV which appears to dilate during systole. This suggests the presence of a full thickness infarct with associated aneurysm formation. True LV aneurysm after myocardial infarct is more likely to occur along the anterior wall whereas pseudoaneurysm occurs along the inferior wall.

## ■ Diagnosis

Infarct versus less likely hibernating myocardium.

## ✓ Pearls

- GSPECT MPI allows for simultaneous evaluation of myocardial perfusion and LV function.
- GSPECT at stress only may be all that is necessary as the patient has returned to resting physiology.
- A fixed perfusion defect with abnormal RWM and SWT suggests infarct or hibernating myocardium.
- Dyskinesia suggests full thickness infarct with aneurysm formation.

## Suggested Readings

Chatziioannou SN, Moore WH, Dhekne RD, Ford PV. Gating of myocardial perfusion imaging for the identification of artifacts: is it useful for experienced physicians? Tex Heart Inst J. 2000; 27(1):14–18

Paul AK, Nabi HA. Gated myocardial perfusion SPECT: basic principles, technical aspects, and clinical applications. J Nucl Med Technol. 2004; 32(4):179–187, quiz 188–189

Schinkel AF, Bax JJ, van Domburg R, et al. Dobutamine-induced contractile reserve in stunned, hibernating, and scarred myocardium in patients with ischemic cardiomyopathy. J Nucl Med. 2003; 44(2):127–133

# Case 34

*Cathy Zhou*

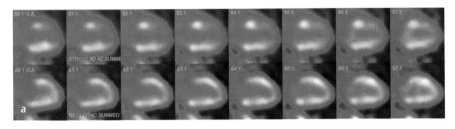
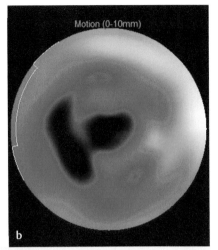
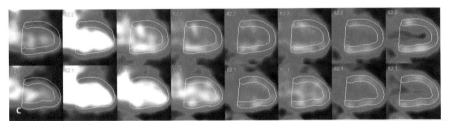

**Fig. 34.1** For the resting images, rubidium-82 infusion was performed over 20–30 seconds, and after 90–120 seconds an EKG-gated cardiac PET was acquired. For the stress images, Lexiscan was infused over 10 seconds, and after 40 seconds a second rubidium-82 infusion was performed. The poststress EKG-gated cardiac PET was then acquired. Rows of stress (*top*) and rest (*bottom*) attenuation-corrected PET perfusion images of the left ventricle in the vertical long axis demonstrate a perfusion defect of the anteroseptum, distal anterior wall and apex which completely reverses on rest images (**a**). A polar map of cardiac motion at stress demonstrates severe hypokinesis of the apex and anteroseptum, and milder hypokinesis of the distal anterior wall (**b**). Dynamic images of a selected frame in the vertical long axis at stress (*top row*) and rest (*bottom*) track flow of blood into and out of the left ventricle, followed by perfusion images (**c**).

■ **Clinical History**

82-year-old female with a history of hypertension, orthopnea, and chest pain on exertion evaluated with PET myocardial perfusion (▶ Fig. 34.1).

## ■ Key Finding

Reduced coronary flow reserve (CFR)

## ■ Top 3 Differential Diagnoses

- **Coronary artery disease.** Chronic atherosclerotic plaque formation in the coronary vessels leads to arterial stiffening and narrowing. Decreased myocardial perfusion, particularly with stress, can present symptomatically as angina pectoris, classically improving with rest. On myocardial perfusion imaging (MPI) regional perfusion deficits with or without associated motion and CFR deficits can be appreciated. EKG may also demonstrate inducible ST segment changes. Alternatively, patients with relatively balanced multivessel disease may present with uniform perfusion but global hypokinesis with stress and overall reduced CFR.
- **Hypertension.** Blood pressure elevation induces acute vasoconstriction and chronic remodeling and rarefaction of the microcirculation, leading to reduced tissue perfusion and vasodilator capacity. Hypertensive patients also exhibit increased resting coronary flow, which is likely secondary to the increased myocardial workload. Left ventricle (LV) hypertrophy may also result. In someone with hypertension and no known coronary artery stenosis, MPI may only demonstrate a blunted CFR. Hypertension is also a risk factor for coronary artery disease (CAD) and diabetes.
- **Diabetes mellitus.** Chronic hyperglycemia as a result of increased insulin resistance can lead to diabetic angiopathy and cardiomyopathy with autonomic neuropathy. Endothelial dysfunction affects the microvasculature and myocardial blood flow is reduced, while increased fatty acid oxidation raises baseline oxygen requirements and resting coronary flow. In otherwise anatomically normal patients, impaired blood flow can be reflected by a reduced CFR. Diabetes is also a risk factor for CAD and hypertension.

## ■ Additional Differential Diagnoses

- **Chronic kidney disease:** Kidney dysfunction can affect cardiovascular function in a number of ways, from the increase in toxins and metabolic end products prompting microvascular dysfunction, to secondary hyperparathyroidism and hyperphosphatemia leading to vascular calcification. Risk factors include hypertension and diabetes (most common). As with the above, on imaging one would appreciate a reduced CFR. Hemodialysis can also result in regional wall abnormalities, driven by repeated episodes of demand ischemia. These would be seen on imaging as regional perfusion defects.

## ■ Diagnosis

Coronary artery disease.

## ✓ Pearls

- PET MPI allows for coronary flow analysis.
- PET MPI also allows for real-time function evaluation, possibly showing ischemic changes in LV function.
- Decreased CFR is inversely associated with cardiac mortality in patients with CAD.

## Suggested Readings

Chade AR, Brosh D, Higano ST, Lennon RJ, Lerman LO, Lerman A. Mild renal insufficiency is associated with reduced coronary flow in patients with non-obstructive coronary artery disease. Kidney Int. 2006; 69(2):266–271

Levy BI, Schiffrin EL, Mourad JJ, et al. Impaired tissue perfusion: a pathology common to hypertension, obesity, and diabetes mellitus. Circulation. 2008; 118(9):968–976

Yokoyama I, Yonekura K, Ohtake T, et al. Coronary microangiopathy in type 2 diabetic patients: relation to glycemic control, sex, and microvascular angina rather than to coronary artery disease. J Nucl Med. 2000; 41(6):978–985

Ziadi MC, Dekemp RA, Williams K, et al. Does quantification of myocardial flow reserve using rubidium-82 positron emission tomography facilitate detection of multivessel coronary artery disease? J Nucl Cardiol. 2012; 19(4):670–680

# Case 35

*Ely A. Wolin*

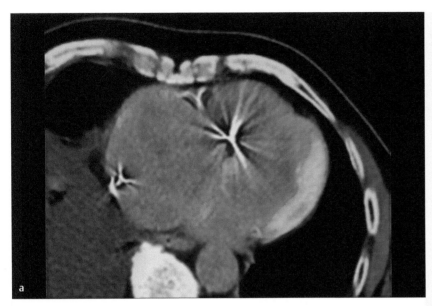

**Fig. 35.1** **(a)** Coned down image from oncologic fluorine-18 fluorodeoxyglucose (F-18 FDG) positron emission tomography/computed tomography (PET/CT) shows uptake in the left ventricular myocardium excluding an area involving the mid to distal septum and apex. **(b)** Myocardial perfusion scan performed 10 days prior shows normal myocardial perfusion.

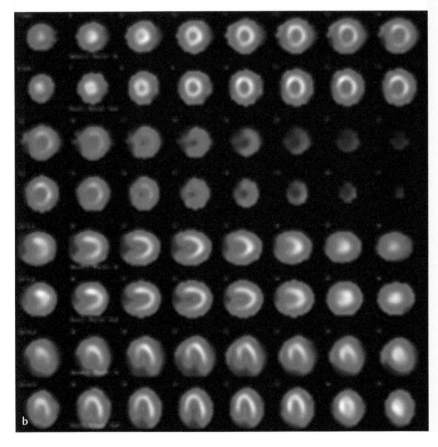

## ■ Clinical History

87-year-old male referred for PET scan for stage IIIA gastric gastrointestinal stromal tumor (▶ Fig. 35.1).

## ■ Key Finding

Regional decreased myocardial uptake on F-18 FDG PET/CT performed for a noncardiac indication

## ■ Top 2 Differential Diagnoses

• **Suboptimal patient preparation.** F-18 FDG PET/CT is most frequently used for oncologic imaging, primarily for staging and restaging exam. Appropriate patient preparation is important for exam quality. Part of the preparation includes a short fast, usually at least 4 hours, and at some institutions a low-carbohydrate diet for a period prior to the fast. This is in order to prevent large spikes in blood glucose. Elevated blood glucose affects systemic FDG uptake in two main ways: first, the elevated glucose leads to increased insulin levels which forces both glucose and FDG into skeletal muscles, and second there is some competitive inhibition for uptake on the glucose transporters between glucose and FDG. Another benefit of appropriate patient preparation, particularly when mediastinal evaluation is important, is decreased physiologic cardiac uptake. Myocardium will use the most efficient available metabolic fuel, preferring fatty acid metabolism in the fasting state. If the patient follows preparation appropriately, the myocardium will switch to fatty acid metabolism and not take up F-18 FDG. Incomplete transition will result in some areas of the heart taking up F-18 FDG, and others not. This heterogeneous myocardial uptake has been shown to occur despite persistent low glucose levels, in some patients, with spatial and temporal heterogeneity due to unknown causes. Some studies have shown the transition to fatty acid metabolism occurs from apex to base, suggesting incomplete preparation may result in an apparent distal defect.

• **Infarct.** F-18 FDG is used for cardiac viability assessment. With appropriate preparation, uptake of F-18 FDG, often increased compared to the remaining myocardium, in an area of a known myocardial perfusion defect indicates viability and thus a likely response to revascularization. Conversely, lack of F-18 FDG uptake indicates the lack of viable myocardium, or an infarct. When performing dedicated F-18 FDG cardiac metabolism imaging for evaluation of viability, patient preparation usually involves a fasting period followed by a glucose load to prep the heart for FDG uptake and decrease circulating fatty acid levels through endogenous insulin production. Insulin is then injected, based on glucose levels, to decrease the plasma glucose level to help ensure FDG is utilized.

## ■ Diagnosis

Suboptimal patient preparation resulting in incomplete transition to fatty acid metabolism.

## ✓ Pearls

• Myocardium will use the most efficient metabolic fuel, generally fatty acids in the aerobic fasting state.
• With appropriate patient prep, F-18 FDG can be used for cardiac viability and inflammation evaluation.

• Regional decreased cardiac F-18 FDG uptake on a general oncologic exam is likely physiologic.

## Suggested Readings

Dilsizian V, Bacharach SL, Beanlands RS, et al. ASNC imaging guidelines/SNMMI procedure standard for positron emission tomography (PET) nuclear cardiology procedures. J Nucl Cardiol. 2016; 23(5):1187–1226

Inglese E, Leva L, Matheoud R, et al. Spatial and temporal heterogeneity of regional myocardial uptake in patients without heart disease under fasting conditions on repeated whole-body 18F-FDG PET/CT. J Nucl Med. 2007; 48(10):1662–1669

Kumar P, Patel CD, Singla S, Malhotra A. Effect of duration of fasting and diet on the myocardial uptake of F-18–2-fluoro-2-deoxyglucose (F-18 FDG) at rest. Indian J Nucl Med. 2014; 29(3):140–145

# Part 4

Lung

# Case 36

*Ely A. Wolin*

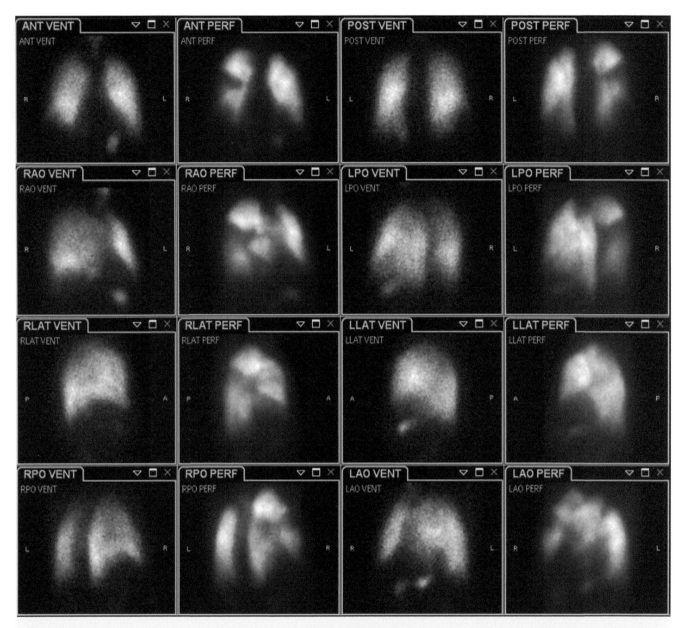

**Fig. 36.1** Planar images from a pulmonary ventilation and perfusion (VQ) scan using aerosolized Technetium-99m (Tc-99m) diethylenetriamine pentaacetic acid (DTPA) and Tc-99m macroaggregated albumin (MAA) show large segmental perfusion defects in the posterior segment of the right upper lobe, the lateral segment of the right middle lobe, and the apicoposterior segment of the left upper lobe, all without an associated ventilation abnormality. Greater than two large mismatched perfusion defects is high probability for pulmonary embolism (PE). Additional right basilar perfusion defects have a matching ventilation abnormality and also correlate with an opacity suggestive of scarring on chest radiographs (not shown).

■ **Clinical History**

91-year-old male with shortness of breath referred for evaluation for pulmonary embolism (▶Fig. 36.1).

# ■ Key Finding

Segmental defect on pulmonary perfusion scan

# ■ Top 3 Differential Diagnoses

- **PE.** The clinical diagnosis of PE is difficult as the classic presentation is rare. Untreated PE has high mortality, but anticoagulation therapy has inherent risks. The nuclear medicine evaluation for PE is a pulmonary ventilation (V) and perfusion (Q) scan. This involves inhalation of a radioactive gas (i.e., Xenon-133) or radioaerosol (i.e., Tc-99m DTPA) for ventilation evaluation, and intravenous administration of radioactive particles which are trapped by the capillary bed (i.e., Tc-99m macroaggregated albumin) for perfusion. A PE should lead to a segmental perfusion defect which extends to the pleural surface with normal ventilation, labeled a mismatched defect. Using classic probabilistic reporting criteria, such as Prospective Investigation of Pulmonary Embolism Diagnosis (PIOPED) and PIOPED II, a scan is high probability for PE if there are at least two large mismatched perfusion defects, or the equivalent of allowing for summation of two moderate defects to equal one large defect. Overall probability depends on pretest probability as well; slightly more than half of high-probability VQ scans are due to PE in the setting of low clinical probability. Other criteria such as PISAPED and perfusion-only modified PIOPED II use a radiograph for ventilation evaluation, and do not use probabilistic reporting, replacing "high probability for PE" with "PE present." The addition of single-photon emission computed tomography (SPECT) imaging may improve diagnostic accuracy.
- **Ventilation abnormality.** Pulmonary ventilation and perfusion are coupled with gravity resulting in more perfusion and ventilation in the bases. Decreased aeration leads to reflex vasoconstriction allowing for blood to be shunted to aerated portions of the lungs. Therefore, processes primarily causing ventilation abnormalities, such as pneumonia, atelectasis, pulmonary edema, and chronic obstructive pulmonary disease (COPD), often result in matched defects. Probability of PE in this case is based on the number and size of matched defects ranging from very low to intermediate probability, using modified PIOPED criteria. Decreased perfusion can result in reflex bronchoconstriction, but it is transient. Comparison to a chest radiograph is important as a triple match, a VQ defect with a similar in size or smaller matched radiographic abnormality, is intermediate probability for PE if in the lower lungs. Emphysema can present with perfused lung between the defect and the pleura, known as the "stripe sign."
- **Mass effect.** Mass effect from effusion, tumor, or adenopathy can result in a VQ defect which is usually not, but may be, segmental. Effusion can cause compressive atelectasis resulting in reflex vasoconstriction and a matched defect. When an effusion layers within a fissure, it can result in a linear perfusion defect running along the fissure, known as the "fissure sign." The concept of a triple match remains important with effusion as around one-third of patients with PE have anipsilateral effusion.

# ■ Diagnosis

High probability for PE.

# ✓ Pearls

- At least two large segmental mismatched defects on a VQ scan is a sign of high probability for PE.
- Triple matched defect is intermediate probability for PE in the lower lungs, and low probability in the upper region.
- Perfused lung between a defect and the pleura (stripe sign) is seen with emphysema and not PE.

# Suggested Readings

Parker JA, Coleman RE, Grady E, et al; Society of Nuclear Medicine. SNM practice guideline for lung scintigraphy 4.0. J Nucl Med Technol. 2012; 40(1):57–65

Roach PJ, Bailey DL, Harris BE. Enhancing lung scintigraphy with single-photon emission computed tomography. Semin Nucl Med. 2008; 38(6):441–449

Tunariu N, Gibbs SJ, Win Z, et al. Ventilation-perfusion scintigraphy is more sensitive than multidetector CTPA in detecting chronic thromboembolic pulmonary disease as a treatable cause of pulmonary hypertension. J Nucl Med. 2007; 48(5):680–684

# Case 37

*Cameron C. Foster*

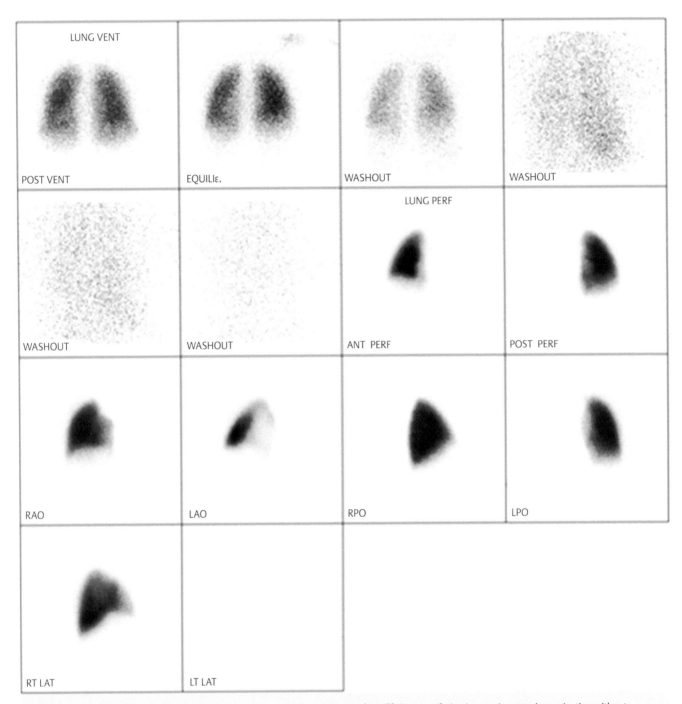

**Fig. 37.1** Ventilation-perfusion scintigraphy demonstrates normal inspiratory and equilibrium ventilation images in posterior projection without evidence of tracer (Xenon-133 [Xe-133] gas) retention on washout images. Perfusion imaging in multiple obliquities demonstrates unilateral absence of tracer (Tc-99m macroaggregated albumin [MAA]) in the left lung with normal distribution of tracer within the right lung.

■ Clinical History

54-year-old male with shortness of breath (▶ Fig. 37.1).

## ■ Key Finding

Unilateral absent lung perfusion

## ■ Top 3 Differential Diagnoses for Perfusion Worse Than Ventilation

- **External compression (tumor, fibrosing mediastinitis).** Unilateral absence of lung perfusion is a rare finding. A ventilation (V)/perfusion (Q) scan cannot determine the cause on its own. However, extrinsic compression of the pulmonary artery is the most common cause of a perfusion defect which is worse than ventilation. Typically, it is from a central lung tumor. Fibrosing mediastinitis is another entity that could lead to pulmonary artery occlusion and absence of perfusion. Cross-sectional imaging is essential to determine the presence of external compression.
- **Pulmonary artery anomalies or corrected congenital heart disease.** Pulmonary artery atresia, severe pulmonary artery stenosis, or pulmonary webs may cause unilateral absence of perfusion with perfusion defect worse than ventilation. Additionally, corrected congenital heart disease may produce similar findings on V/Q scan. Dedicated contrast-enhanced cross-sectional imaging via CT or MRI/MRA can greatly improve detection, as well as correlation for prior surgical history.
- **Massive unilateral pulmonary embolism and aortic dissection.** While massive unilateral pulmonary embolism (PE) can produce unilateral absent perfusion, it is less likely in comparison to other causes. Massive PE of this magnitude will often have more than one V/Q mismatch affecting both lungs. Absent perfusion of an entire lung is low probability of PE as per PIOPED II criteria. Hemorrhage from aortic dissection can result in pulmonary artery compression.

## ■ Top 3 Differential Diagnoses for Ventilation Worse Than Perfusion

- **Mucus plug.** It may obstruct ventilation with compensatory vasoconstriction of the pulmonary arteries. The degree of accompanying perfusion abnormality will increase with time with continued obstruction due to arteriolar constriction induced by local hypoxia. As this is primarily an airway abnormality, the ventilation defect will be larger than the perfusion defect.
- **Unilateral diffuse parenchymal disease.** Diffuse air space disease, atelectasis, or large pneumothorax involving an entire lung will result in decreased or absent ventilation with compensatory vasoconstriction of the pulmonary arteries. The degree of lung involvement will determine the degree of perfusion and ventilation defects.
- **Endobronchial lesion (mass or foreign body).** They can cause a ventilation defect which is larger than perfusion. Central lesions can cause diminished activity within an entire lung. The relative decrease in ventilation to perfusion is an indicator of the extent of luminal involvement.

## ■ Diagnosis

Extrinsic compression (left hilar malignancy).

## ✓ Pearls

- Ventilation scan may be performed with Xe-133 gas or Tc-99m diethylenetriamine pentaacetic acid (DTPA) aerosol.
- Wedge-shaped (peripheral), segmental mismatched perfusion defects are concerning for PE.
- Unilateral absent or decreased lung perfusion or ventilation is usually seen with nonembolic etiologies.

## Suggested Readings

Pickhardt PJ, Fischer KC. Unilateral hypoperfusion or absent perfusion on pulmonary scintigraphy: differential diagnosis. AJR Am J Roentgenol. 1998; 171(1):145–150

Slonim SM, Molgaard CP, Khawaja IT, Seldin DW. Unilateral absence of right-lung perfusion with normal ventilation on radionuclide lung scan as a sign of aortic dissection. J Nucl Med. 1994; 35(6):1044–1047

White RI, Jr, James AE, Jr, Wagner HN, Jr. The significance of unilateral absence of pulmonary artery perfusion by lung scanning. Am J Roentgenol Radium Ther Nucl Med. 1971; 111(3):501–509

# Case 38

*Ely A. Wolin*

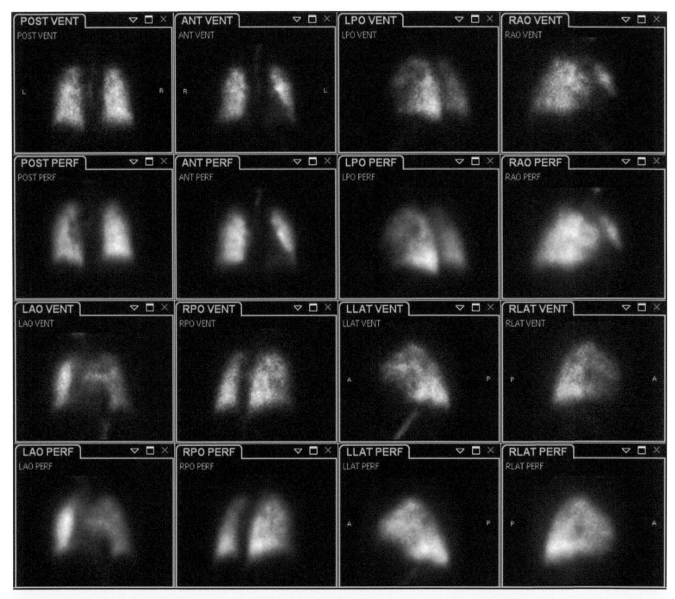

**Fig. 38.1** Multiple planar projection from a pulmonary ventilation and perfusion scan utilizing aerosolized Tc-99m diethylenetriamine pentaacetic acid (DTPA) and Tc-99m macroaggregated albumin (MAA) show diffuse heterogeneous pulmonary perfusion and ventilation in a patient with known chronic obstructive pulmonary disease and pulmonary hypertension. No segmental ventilation perfusion mismatches to suggest pulmonary embolism.

■ **Clinical History**

80-year-old female with pulmonary hypertension referred for pulmonary ventilation and perfusion scan to evaluate for evidence of chronic thromboembolic disease (▶Fig. 38.1).

## ■ Key Finding

Heterogeneous pulmonary perfusion

## ■ Top 3 Differential Diagnoses

• **Primary pulmonary hypertension (PPH).** Elevation of the pulmonary arterial pressure due to elevated pressures in the pulmonary arterial system itself is known as primary (or precapillary) pulmonary hypertension. This condition has multiple etiologies, but can be idiopathic. The common feature for all causes is a progressive vasculopathy involving the pulmonary arterioles, responsible for the heterogeneous pattern of perfusion. There may also be a reversal of the normal gradient with the apices receiving more blood flow. It is progressive and can be fatal. A right heart catheterization with a mean pulmonary arterial pressure of 25mm Hg or greater is diagnostic. Ventilation and perfusion (VQ) scans are usually done to exclude chronic thromboembolic disease as a cause of pulmonary hypertension utilizing the same diagnostic criteria as for acute pulmonary embolism (PE). A normal VQ scan essentially excludes chronic thromboembolic disease as the etiology.

• **Congestive heart failure.** Postcapillary pulmonary hypertension can be caused by anything that leads to elevated pulmonary venous pressures. In congestive heart failure, the increased pressure in the left ventricle leads to increased pressure in the left atrium and subsequently increased pulmonary venous pressure. This physiology is responsible for the characteristic radiographic findings including vascular enlargement and indistinctness. If left untreated, the process can lead to arteriolar damage from prolonged increased pressure, a combined pre- and postcapillary picture.

• **Vasculitis/fat emboli.** Pulmonary vasculitis can be seen in the setting of many systemic and primary pulmonary conditions such as systemic lupus erythematosus, rheumatoid arthritis, and polyarteritis nodosa. Any of the vasculitides affecting the small- and medium-sized vessels will result in a heterogeneous pattern. Fat emboli are usually seen in the setting of long bone fracture.

## ■ Additional Considerations

• **COPD:** As COPD progresses, the normal perfusion scan can become heterogeneous due to reflex vasoconstriction as well as parenchymal destruction.

• **Quantum mottle:** Ensure correct radioisotope window, collimator, patient to camera distance, and imaging time. Can also occur if there is not enough radiopharmaceutical at the target site.

## ■ Diagnosis

COPD with pulmonary arterial hypertension.

## ✓ Pearls

• A normal perfusion scan excludes chronic thromboembolism as the cause of pulmonary hypertension.
• COPD will have normal perfusion early but heterogeneous perfusion as disease progresses.

• Poor imaging statistics (quantum mottle) can simulate heterogeneous pulmonary perfusion.

## Suggested Readings

Fukuchi K, Hayashida K, Nakanishi N, et al. Quantitative analysis of lung perfusion in patients with primary pulmonary hypertension. J Nucl Med. 2002; 43(6):757–761

Peña E, Dennie C, Veinot J, Muñiz SH. Pulmonary hypertension: how the radiologist can help. Radiographics. 2012; 32(1):9–32

Tunariu N, Gibbs SJR, Win Z, et al. Ventilation-perfusion scintigraphy is more sensitive than multidetector CTPA in detecting chronic thromboembolic pulmonary disease as a treatable cause of pulmonary hypertension. J Nucl Med. 2007; 48(5):680–684

# Case 39

*Ely A. Wolin*

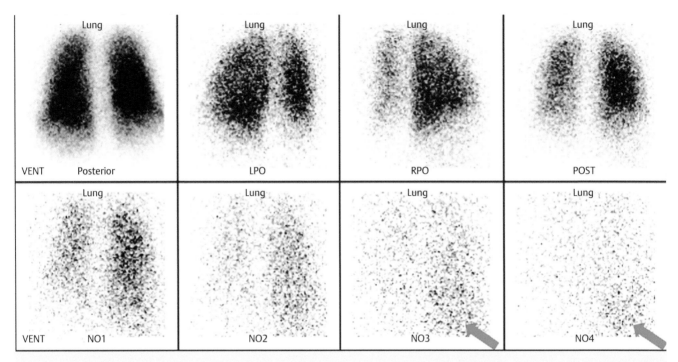

**Fig. 39.1** Images from a pulmonary ventilation scan performed with Xenon-133 as part of a pulmonary perfusion and ventilation scan show faint uptake in the region of the liver, best seen on the late washout images (*red arrows*).

## ■ Clinical History

44-year-old female who presented with chest tightness, shortness of breath, and left lower extremity edema after recent long-distance travel. Left lower extremity ultrasound demonstrated a deep venous thrombosis in the distal superficial femoral vein (▶ Fig. 39.1).

## ■ Key Finding

Liver uptake on Xenon-133 pulmonary ventilation scan

## ■ Diagnosis

• **Hepatic steatosis.** Xenon-133 (Xe-133) is a radioactive noble gas which is produced by the fission of Uranium-235. It is one of the agents commonly used for pulmonary ventilation imaging. Administration of Xe-133 involves delivery of the gas through a closed system. The patient is first instructed to take a breath in and hold it for an initial breath-hold image, then free breaths Xe-133 for 3–5 minutes while additional images are obtained. The Xe-133 is then shut off and the patient continues to breathe for an additional 3–5 minutes allowing for washout imaging. Some of the radioactive gas will enter the alveolar walls and pulmonary capillaries leading to the pulmonary venous system. Once in the blood stream, organ-specific uptake of Xe-133 is determined by blood flow and tissue solubility. Xe-133 is highly soluble in fat. With diffuse fatty liver, slow progressive hepatic uptake will be seen toward the end of the ventilation study. Xe-133 has been used to both diagnose and assess fatty liver disease. It has proven utility for both alcoholic and nonalcoholic fatty

liver disease (NAFLD) and has been shown to be more sensitive and specific than ultrasound. While liver biopsy remains the gold standard for diagnosis of NAFLD, an Xe-133 scan offers a reliable and noninvasive way to evaluate for this disease. This is increasingly relevant as NAFLD has become the most common cause of chronic liver dysfunction in Western countries. Qualitative assessment of liver uptake involves visually comparing the uptake in the liver seen on washout images to the peak activity seen in the lungs. Mechanisms for quantitative assessment have also been used, some of which require a technetium-99m sulfur colloid (Tc-99m SC) scan to be performed after the washout phase of the Xe-133 study to verify positioning of the liver for proper region of interest placement. Quantitative measures have been shown to accurately predict the level of fatty replacement. Despite the utility of Xe-133 in the evaluation of fatty liver disease, it is not performed frequently as the noninvasive evaluation has mostly been replaced by ultrasound, CT, and MRI.

## ■ Diagnosis

Hepatic steatosis.

## ✓ Pearls

• Xe-133 enters the blood stream through alveolar walls and the pulmonary capillary bed, and is fat soluble.
• Liver uptake with Xe-133 can provide an accurate means to quantify fatty replacement.

• Xe-133 scan has mostly been replaced by anatomic imaging for the evaluation of fatty liver disease.
• Xe-133 uptake in the liver can be confused for pulmonary retention in the right lung base.

## Suggested Readings

Al-Busafi SA, Ghali P, Wong P, Novales-Diaz JA, Deschênes M. The utility of Xenon-133 liver scan in the diagnosis and management of nonalcoholic fatty liver disease. Can J Gastroenterol. 2012; 26(3):155–159

Ma X, Holalkere NS, Kambadakone R A, Mino-Kenudson M, Hahn PF, Sahani DV. Imaging-based quantification of hepatic fat: methods and clinical applications. Radiographics. 2009; 29(5):1253–1277

Yeh SH, Wu LC, Wang SJ, et al. Xenon-133 hepatic retention ratio: a useful index for fatty liver quantification. J Nucl Med. 1989; 30(10):1708–1712

# Case 40

*Ely A. Wolin*

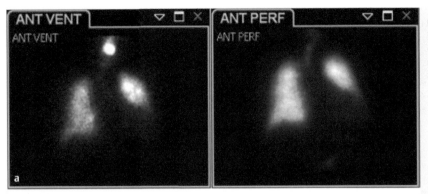

Fig. 40.1 Anterior ventilation and perfusion (VQ) images (a) show a matched defect in the expected region of the anteromedial left lower lobe basal segment which is due to prominent epicardial fat, as seen on correlative coronal CT image (b).

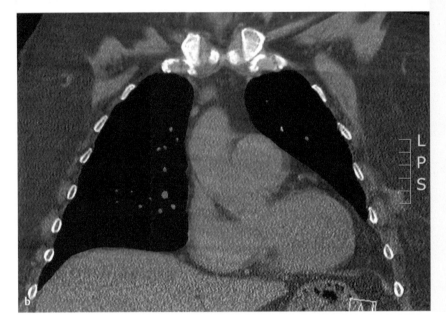

## ■ Clinical History

82-year-old female referred for pulmonary embolism evaluation
(▶Fig. 40.1).

## ■ Key Finding

Nonsegmental pulmonary perfusion defect

## ■ Top 3 Differential Diagnoses

- **Anatomy.** It is important to have a good understanding of anatomy when interpreting pulmonary VQ scans. Several anatomic structures result in apparent nonsegmental defects on the scan, particularly when they are enlarged or tortuous. Standard pulmonary perfusion imaging performed with Tc-99m macroaggregated albumin (MAA) involves planar images obtained in the anterior, posterior, right lateral, left lateral, right anterior oblique, left anterior oblique, right posterior oblique, and left posterior oblique projections. Knowledge of the normal location for anatomic defects in each projection is imperative. The heart and hilar vessels are most commonly responsible for apparent nonsegmental defects. When the heart is enlarged, it can cause a larger-than-expected area of photopenia. Apparent defects from enlarged hilar vessels can be particularly confusing on the oblique projections. Correlation with chest radiographs, which should be obtained within 24 hours of the VQ scan when evaluating for pulmonary embolism (PE), may be helpful. Single-photon emission computed tomography (SPECT) imaging also provides additional problem-solving capabilities.

- **Hilar mass.** A hilar mass can result in a nonsegmental perfusion defect, similar in appearance to that of enlarged hilar vessels. As the hilar mass enlarges, the associated compression and/or occlusion of the adjacent vasculature may lead to a whole lobe or whole lung perfusion defect, as discussed in the unilateral decreased pulmonary perfusion case (case 37).
- **Airspace disease.** This is frequently the cause of a nonsegmental perfusion defect and illustrates the importance of having a comparison chest radiograph. Physiologic mechanisms lead to reflect vasoconstriction in areas of hypoxia, attempting to shunt blood to more aerated lung. This reflex vasoconstriction is long lasting contrary to reflex bronchoconstriction which is temporary in the setting of a perfusion abnormality. Thus, airspace disease will usually result in a matched ventilation and perfusion defect, making PE less likely whether the defect is segmental or not, particularly if the perfusion abnormality is smaller than the correlative radiographic abnormality.

## ■ Additional Considerations

- **Attenuation:** Overlying structures can prevent gamma rays emitting from the patient from reaching the gamma camera, usually resulting in a well-defined, nonsegmental perfusion and ventilation defect. Implanted cardiac pacemakers/defibrillators and central venous access ports are the most common attenuation defects, clinically.

## ■ Diagnosis

Nonsegmental pulmonary perfusion defect due to prominent epicardial fat.

## ✓ Pearls

- Knowing the appearance of normal anatomy from all projections is important for VQ interpretation.
- The addition of SPECT imaging helps with evaluating perfusion defects from enlarged anatomy.

- Airspace disease will usually result in a matched VQ defect due to reflex vasoconstriction.
- Nonsegmental perfusion defects are of very low probability for PE based on the PIOPED II criteria.

## Suggested Readings

Gottschalk A, Stein PD, Sostman HD, Matta F, Beemath A. Very low probability interpretation of V/Q lung scans in combination with low probability objective clinical assessment reliably excludes pulmonary embolism: data from PIOPED II. J Nucl Med. 2007; 48(9):1411–1415

Roach PJ, Schembri GP, Bailey DL. V/Q scanning using SPECT and SPECT/CT. J Nucl Med. 2013; 54(9):1588–1596

Sostman HD, Miniati M, Gottschalk A, Matta F, Stein PD, Pistolesi M. Sensitivity and specificity of perfusion scintigraphy combined with chest radiography for acute pulmonary embolism in PIOPED II. J Nucl Med. 2008; 49(11):1741–1748

# Case 41

*Ely A. Wolin*

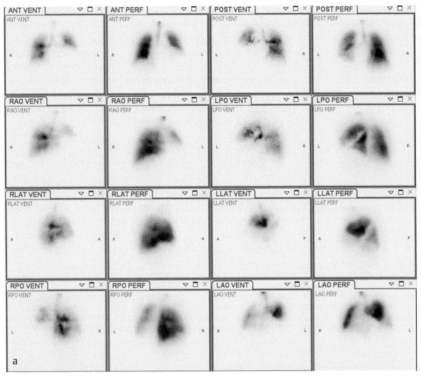

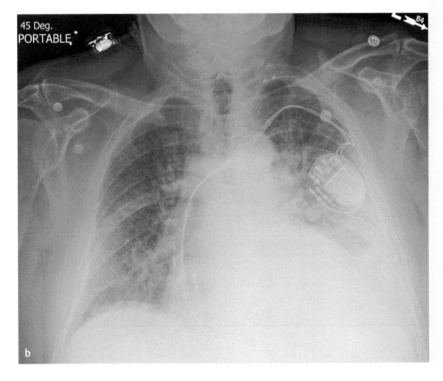

**Fig. 41.1** Images from a pulmonary ventilation and perfusion scan utilizing aerosolize Tc-99m diethylenetriamine pentaacetic acid (DTPA) and intravenous Tc-99m macroaggregated albumin (MAA) **(a)** show a matched large perfusion and ventilation defect in the left lung base with a correlative pleural effusion and retrocardiac opacity on same day portable chest radiograph **(b)**. Heterogeneity seen on the ventilation greater than perfusion images is likely secondary to the known cardiogenic pulmonary edema.

## ■ Clinical History

81-year-old male with new onset shortness of breath, borderline tachycardia on beta blocker, and worsening cardiogenic pulmonary edema (▶Fig. 41.1).

## ■ Key Finding

Triple match on ventilation and perfusion (VQ) scan

## ■ Top 2 Differential Diagnoses

- **Intermediate (or indeterminate) probability for pulmonary embolism (PE).** A triple matched defect is defined as a perfusion defect, that is at least moderate in size, and has a matched ventilation abnormality along with a radiographic abnormality that is of the same size or smaller than the perfusion abnormality. Evaluation of the PIOPED criteria showed that roughly one-fourth of triple match defects overall, and one-third of triple match defects in the lower lung zones, were due to PE. This makes a triple match in the lower lung zone intermediate probability, which usually delineates either a 20–80% or 10–80% chance of PE, depending on criteria used and without taking pretest probability into account. The ventilation and radiographic abnormality in the setting of a PE is due to associated infarct and/or hemorrhage, which is why the radiographic abnormality cannot be greater in size than the perfusion abnormality to fit within this diagnostic criterion. A triple match in the lower lung zone is more concerning because PE is more likely to occur in the lower lung zones, which is more frequently dependent.

- **Low (or very low) probability for PE.** A triple matched defect in the middle or upper lung zones has low (or very low) probability for PE, with PE occurring in around 10% in the PIOPED data. As noted above, PE is more likely to occur in the lower lung zone. Triple match in the mid or upper lung zone is more likely to be due to a parenchymal abnormality than PE with associated infarct. Pneumonia, lung carcinoma, fibrosis, and atelectasis are all examples of nonembolic causes of a triple match seen in the PIOPED data.

## ■ Diagnosis

Intermediate probability VQ scan for PE.

## ✓ Pearls

- Triple match is intermediate (or indeterminate) probability for PE in the lower lung zones.
- Triple match has low (or very low) probability for PE in the middle and upper lung zones.
- Radiographic opacity in triple match is due to infarct and/or hemorrhage when due to PE.
- Radiographic opacity must be the same size or smaller than perfusion defect to be a triple match.

## Suggested Readings

Miniati M, Sostman HD, Gottschalk A, Monti S, Pistolesi M. Perfusion lung scintigraphy for the diagnosis of pulmonary embolism: a reappraisal and review of the Prospective Investigative Study of Acute Pulmonary Embolism Diagnosis methods. Semin Nucl Med. 2008; 38(6):450–461

Stein PD, Gottschalk A. Review of criteria appropriate for a very low probability of pulmonary embolism on ventilation-perfusion lung scans: a position paper. Radiographics. 2000; 20(1):99–105

Worsley DF, Kim CK, Alavi A, Palevsky HI. Detailed analysis of patients with matched ventilation-perfusion defects and chest radiographic opacities. J Nucl Med. 1993; 34(11):1851–1853

# Case 42

*Ely A. Wolin*

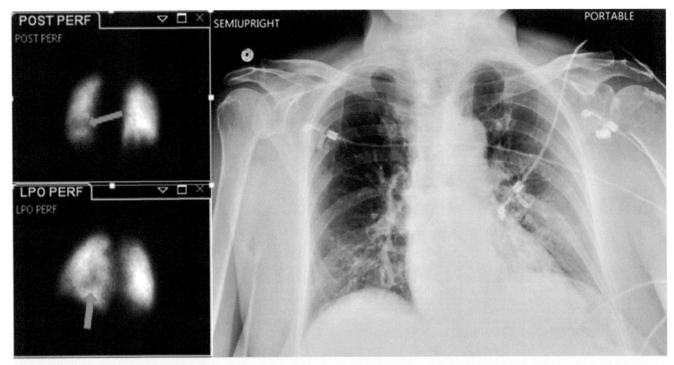

**Fig. 42.1** Posterior and LPO planar images from a pulmonary perfusion scan obtained after the intravenous administration of Tc-99m macroaggregated albumin (MAA) show a perfusion defect in the anteromedial basal segment of the left lower lobe with a stripe of peripherally perfused lung (*red arrows*). There was a similar defect on ventilation images, not shown, and a correlative patchy retrocardiac opacity on same day chest radiograph. The patient was treated with Levaquin with resolution of symptoms and normalization of the chest radiograph.

■ **Clinical History**

84-year-old female with shortness of breath, possible pulmonary embolism (PE) (▶ Fig. 42.1).

## Key Finding

Stripe of normally perfused lung between a perfusion defect and the pleural surface; "stripe sign"

## Top 3 Differential Diagnoses

- **Emphysema.** This is the most common entity associated with the stripe sign on pulmonary perfusion imaging. Peripheral perfusion is believed to be preserved primarily because the peripheral lung is less susceptible to destruction from smoking-related centrilobular emphysema. Peripheral branches of the pulmonary arterioles may also not be affected by centrilobular emphysema.
- **Pneumonia.** It should cause both ventilation and perfusion defects, with the ventilation defect often the larger of the two. The defect will also frequently not be segmental, making PE less likely. Depending on the location of pneumonia, there may be normally perfused lung between the infection and the pleural surface resulting in a stripe sign.
- **PE.** While very unlikely in the setting of a peripheral strip of perfused lung, occurring less than 10% of the time, PE is possible. The peripheral perfusion may be from reperfusion of a portion of a segment affected by PE. Pulmonary hypertension is also theorized to result in enough pressure to push the MAA particles beyond an embolus.

## Additional Consideration

- **Shine through:** Traditional pulmonary perfusion imaging is performed by obtaining planar images in the anterior, posterior, bilateral lateral, and bilateral anterior and posterior oblique projections. It is possible for activity from normally perfused lung to shine through a perfusion defect simulating a stripe sign. This is most likely to occur on the lateral projections, which should not be used on their own to identify a strip sign. Single-photon emission computed tomography (SPECT) imaging prevents this possibility.

## Diagnosis

Pneumonia.

## ✓ Pearls

- Stipe sign refers to normally perfused lung between a segmental perfusion defect and the pleural surface.
- Stripe sign is most commonly seen with smoking-related emphysema.
- SPECT imaging can help identify a stripe sign and prevent confusion from shine through.
- Stripe sign has very low probability for PE in the absence of other concerning perfusion abnormalities.

## Suggested Readings

Bajc M, Neilly JB, Miniati M, Schuemichen C, Meignan M, Jonson B; EANM Committee. EANM guidelines for ventilation/perfusion scintigraphy: Part 1. Pulmonary imaging with ventilation/perfusion single photon emission tomography. Eur J Nucl Med Mol Imaging. 2009; 36(8):1356–1370

Bajc M, Neilly B, Miniati M, Mortensen J, Jonson B. Methodology for ventilation/perfusion SPECT. Semin Nucl Med. 2010; 40(6):415–425

Ergün EL, Volkan B, Caner B. Stripe sign in pulmonary embolism: a review of the causes. Ann Nucl Med. 2003; 17(2):145–148

# Case 43

*Ely A. Wolin*

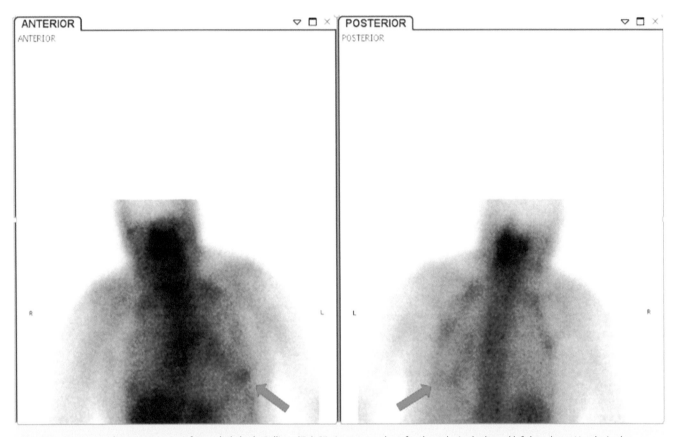

**Fig. 43.1** Anterior and posterior images from whole body Gallium (Ga)-67 citrate scan show focal uptake in the lateral left lung base. Uptake in the cervical spine was similar in intensity and distribution to uptake on Tc-99m medronic acid (MDP) bone scan and likely due to arthropathy.

## ■ Clinical History

83-year-old female with bacteremia and known occiput-C3 fusion with inflammatory changes concerning for infection referred for whole-body gallium scan to evaluate for osteomyelitis (▶ Fig. 43.1).

## ■ Key Finding

Gallium uptake in lungs

## ■ Top 3 Differential Diagnoses

- **Neoplasm.** Ga-67 is a cyclotron produced radionuclide that decays via electron capture with a physical half-life of approximately 78 hours. It emits four primary photon energies of 93, 184, 296, and 388 keV (easier to remember as about 90, 190, 290, and 390). For imaging it is primarily administered in the form of Ga-67 citrate. Gallium itself behaves similar to iron. Ga-67 is cleared very slowly with a biologic half-life of around 25 days. Physiologic distribution of Ga-67 citrate includes liver, bone and bone marrow, spleen, and variable nasopharynx, lacrimal gland, and salivary gland uptake. Clearance is through the kidneys for the first 24 hours and then through the gastrointestinal (GI) tract. First clinical uses for Ga-67 were for tumor imaging, even though it was developed as a bone agent. Ga-67 was used for imaging of lymphoma but has mostly been replaced by fluorine-18 fluorodeoxyglucose (F-18 FDG) positron emission tomography/computed tomography (PET/CT). However, Ga-67 citrate is a nonspecific tumor imaging agent and uptake can be seen in multiple neoplasms including primary lung cancer.

- **Bacterial pneumonia.** Ga-67 citrate circulates bound to transferrin. However, it has a higher binding affinity for lactoferrin, which is released from dead leukocytes, and also binds to bacterial siderophores. Focal pulmonary parenchymal uptake is suggestive of bacterial pneumonia in the appropriate clinical setting.
- **Opportunistic infection.** Ga-67 citrate can be useful for the detection of infections which are unique to the immunocompromised patient. A negative gallium scan has a high negative predictive value, particularly in an untreated patient. Diffuse pulmonary uptake in a patient with human immunodeficiency virus (HIV) is suggestive of *Pneumocystis jiroveci* pneumonia. Less intense diffuse pulmonary uptake, graded relative to hepatic uptake, can be seen with cytomegalovirus and fungal pneumonias. Ga-67 citrate can be useful, particularly when used in conjunction with thallium-201, to help differentiate between *P. jiroveci* infection and Kaposi's sarcoma which will not show Ga-67 avidity.

## ■ Additional Consideration

- **Inflammation:** As inflammatory processes increase lactoferrin production, they will be associated with increased Ga-67 citrate avidity. Pulmonary uptake of Ga-67 citrate can be seen with sarcoidosis, hypersensitivity pneumonitis, idiopathic pulmonary fibrosis, and other inflammatory processes. Postprocedural inflammation, such as after surgery or radiation therapy, will also show uptake.

## ■ Diagnosis

Pneumonia.

## ✓ Pearls

- Ga-67 citrate is a nonspecific inflammation, infection, and malignancy marker.
- A normal Ga-67 citrate scan in an HIV-positive patient with an abnormal chest X-ray suggests Kaposi's sarcoma.

- Focal pulmonary Ga-67 uptake in a patient with fever of unknown origin may be pneumonia or neoplasm.
- Renal activity on a Ga-67 scan is abnormal after 24 hours at which point clearance is primarily GI.

## Suggested Readings

Al-Suqri B, Al-Bulushi N. Gallium-67 scintigraphy in the era of positron emission tomography and computed tomography: tertiary center experience. Sultan Qaboos Univ Med J. 2015; 15(3):e338–e343

Love C, Palestro CJ. Radionuclide imaging of inflammation and infection in the acute care setting. Semin Nucl Med. 2013; 43(2):102–113

Palestro CJ, Broen ML, Forstrom LA, et al. Society of nuclear medicine procedure guideline for gallium scintigraphy in inflammation version 3.0. http://snmmi.files.cms-plus.com/docs/Gallium_Scintigraphy_in_Inflammation_v3.pdf. Accessed 10/4/2016

# Case 44

*Kamal D. Singh*

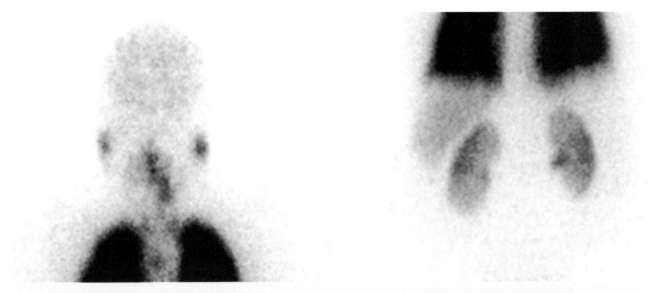

**Fig. 44.1** Static images from a lung perfusion scan with Tc-99m macroaggregated albumin (MAA) demonstrate intracranial, thyroid, liver, and kidney activity. There is also activity seen in the salivary glands, swallowed activity in the esophagus, and expected lung activity.

■ **Clinical History**

56-year-old male with cirrhosis, alcohol abuse, and hypoxemia
(▶Fig. 44.1).

## ■ Key Finding

Extrapulmonary activity on lung perfusion scan

## ■ Top 3 Differential Diagnoses

- **Free Tc-99m pertechnetate.** It is the result of poor labeling of the radiopharmaceutical. The free Tc-99m pertechnetate passes through the pulmonary capillary bed and into systemic circulation. Its normal biodistribution includes the choroid plexus, salivary glands, thyroid, stomach/intestines, kidneys, urinary collecting system, and bladder. Determination of unbound or free Tc-99m within a radiopharmaceutical preparation can be done by thin-layer chromatography (TLC) with acetone as solvent. Regulatory standards require at least 95% radiolabeling efficiency.
- **Right-to-left shunt.** Intrapulmonary or intracardiac shunting can be detected on perfusion imaging when Tc-99m MAA particles bypass the lungs and localize in systemic capillary beds. Cerebral cortical activity distinguishes shunting from other causes of extrapulmonary uptake, such as free Tc-99m. Hence imaging over the brain improves specificity when shunting is suspected. Unlike free Tc-99m, the renal uptake in shunting is primarily within the renal cortex, and collecting system excretion and bladder activity are absent. Quantification of shunt can be performed by whole-body imaging to determine ratio of systemic counts to whole body counts, which is proportional to the shunt size. Shunting greater than 5–10% is generally considered significant. A lung perfusion scan is normally accomplished with 2–5 mCi of Tc-99m MAA containing 200,000–500,000 particles. In cases of known or suspected shunt, the number of particles should be reduced to 100,000. Reduced number of particles also applies for children, pregnant patients, and those with known pulmonary hypertension or history of pneumonectomy. Superior vena cava obstruction is a much less likely possible cause for shunting to the systemic circulation.
- **Retained activity from a different radiotracer study.** Knowledge of any recent nuclear medicine scans is helpful to avoid interfering activity, which may especially be an issue for radiotracers with long half-lives.

## ■ Diagnosis

Right-to-left shunt (23% shunt fraction by quantitative analysis), possible hepatopulmonary syndrome.

## ✓ Pearls

- Image the brain and bladder if extrapulmonary activity is seen on perfusion scan to assess for shunt.
- Right-to-left shunts can be detected and quantified on lung perfusion scan with Tc-99m MAA.
- Left-to-right shunts are identified on first pass radionuclide ventriculography.
- Use reduced particles if known shunt, pregnant/pediatric, pulmonary hypertension, or pneumonectomy.

## Suggested Readings

Esser JP, Oei HY, de Bruin HG, Krenning EP. Liver and vertebral uptake of Tc-99m macroaggregated albumin (MAA). Clin Nucl Med. 2004; 29(12):793–794

Kume N, Suga K, Uchisako H, Matsui M, Shimizu K, Matsunaga N. Abnormal extrapulmonary accumulation of 99mTc-MAA during lung perfusion scanning. Ann Nucl Med. 1995; 9(4):179–184

Parker JA, Coleman RE, Grady E, et al; Society of Nuclear Medicine. SNM practice guideline for lung scintigraphy 4.0. J Nucl Med Technol. 2012; 40(1):57–65

# Case 45

*Ely A. Wolin*

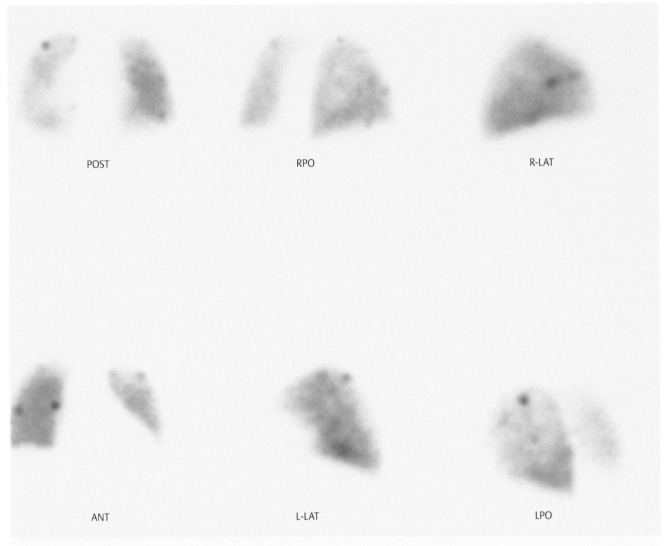

**Fig. 45.1** Images from Technetium-99m (Tc-99m) macroaggregated albumin (MAA) pulmonary perfusion scan show several foci of increased activity in both lungs.

■ **Clinical History**

No clinical history available (▶ Fig. 45.1). (Case courtesy of COL (ret) Ralph Blumhardt, MD.)

## ■ Key Finding

Hot spots on pulmonary perfusion scan

## ■ Diagnosis

- **Radioactive emboli.** This is a well-known artifact seen during MAA perfusion imaging. It is most likely caused by incorrect injection technique. If the individual performing the injection withdraws some blood into the syringe, the Tc-99m MAA particles may combine with it leading to in situ clot formation resulting in "hot clots." When these clots are injected, they travel through the pulmonary circulation until they are trapped by the pulmonary capillary bed and result in a focal area of markedly increased uptake due to the trapped radiolabeled MAA particles. Injecting Tc-99m MAA through an indwelling catheter also results in labeled clots if the catheter is not flushed well prior to injection. This is believed to be secondary to mixing of the radiopharmaceutical with formed thrombus at the tip of the catheter. Central catheter injection can also be problematic. It is possible for a large percentage of the injected radiopharmaceutical to be trapped within thrombus or a fibrin sheath at the end of the catheter. Injection through a central line may also lead to inadequate mixing in the right ventricular outflow tract, and should therefore be avoided.

## ■ Diagnosis

Radioactive emboli.

## ✓ Pearls

- Multiple focal hotspots on Tc-99m MAA lung perfusion scan is pathognomic for radioactive emboli.
- Radioactive emboli can almost entirely be avoided by utilizing proper injection technique.
- Ensure indwelling catheters are appropriately flushed prior to using for radiopharmaceutical injection.
- Avoid utilizing a central catheter for injection.

## Suggested Readings

Parker JA, Coleman RE, Grady E, et al; Society of Nuclear Medicine. SNM practice guideline for lung scintigraphy 4.0. J Nucl Med Technol. 2012; 40(1):57–65

Technetium Tc-99m Albumin Aggregated Injection [package insert]. Kirkland, Quebec, Canada: DRAXIMAGE, Inc; 2002.

# Case 46

*Ely A. Wolin*

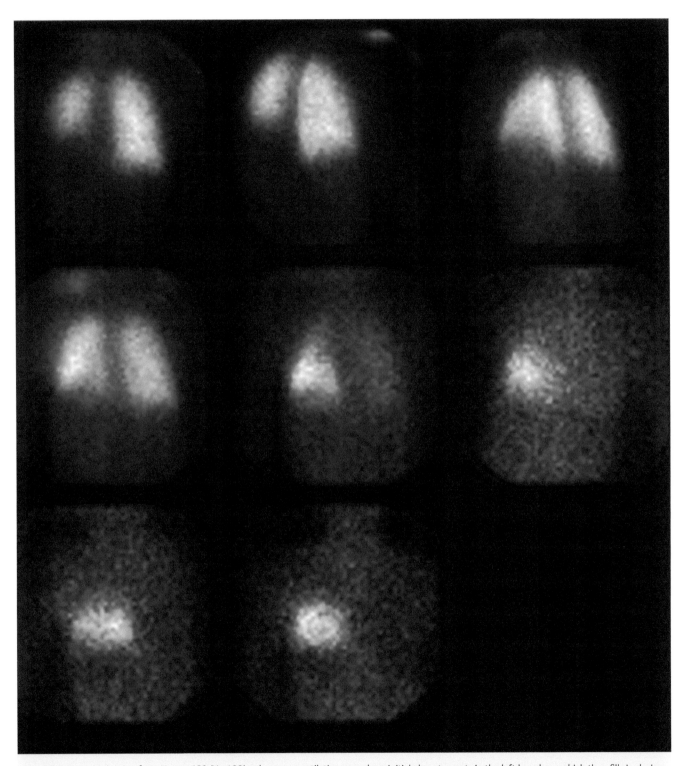

**Fig. 46.1** Posterior images from Xenon-133 (Xe-133) pulmonary ventilation scan show initial absent counts in the left lung base which then fills in during equilibrium and demonstrates trapping on washout images.

## ■ Clinical History

15-year-old male with Swyer–James syndrome referred for pulmonary ventilation and perfusion scan (▶Fig. 46.1).

## Key Finding

Pulmonary retention of Xe-133

## Top 3 Differential Diagnoses

- **COPD.** Xe-133 is a radioactive noble gas, a fission product from uranium-235. It decays via beta-minus decay with a physical half-life of approximately 5.3 days and emits 81 keV gamma. Biologic half-life is only approximately 30 seconds. It is used via inhalation for pulmonary ventilation (V) evaluation during a ventilation and perfusion (Q) scan. A small percentage of the gas is absorbed with the majority remaining within the lungs prior to exhalation. Pulmonary ventilation imaging with Xe-133 involves delivery through a closed system with single breath-hold images obtained followed by equilibrium during free breathing of Xe-133 for 3–6 minutes. The Xe-133 delivery is then discontinued and washout images are obtained. Abnormal distribution at any point in the examination is considered a ventilation defect, with the washout phase the most sensitive. The ability to image physiology through the equilibrium and washout phases is an advantage over the single time point imaging obtained with aerosolized Technetium-99m (Tc-99m) diethylenetriamine pentaacetic acid (DTPA). COPD is associated with progressive airway obstruction as a result of parenchymal destruction and airway inflammation. This prevents expiration of Xe-133 leading to retained activity on the washout images. Retention of Xe-133 can be seen before any abnormal CT findings are evident.
- **Bronchiectasis.** It is abnormal dilation of the bronchial tree. It has many causes including chronic infection, cystic fibrosis, and traction from lung fibrosis. It can be cylindrical, varicose, or cystic in morphology. The dilation, along with damage to the epithelial cilia, make airway clearance ineffective resulting in chronic/recurrent infections. While traction bronchiectasis from pulmonary fibrosis results in a restrictive pattern, most often bronchiectasis shows obstructive physiology on spirometry.
- **Airway obstruction.** Any form of airway obstruction, such as a mass or foreign body, can result in air trapping and retention of Xe-133 on washout images. Initial breath-hold images will also likely be abnormal, as the obstruction prevents inhalation through the affected airway. However, ventilation may normalize during equilibrium imaging as air traverse through the pores of Kohn and canals of Lambert into the postobstructive portion of lung. The obstructed airway will then limit expiration, as it did inspiration, resulting in retention.

## Diagnosis

Swyer–James syndrome.

## Pearls

- An abnormality seen on any stage of Xe-133 ventilation imaging is considered a ventilation defect.
- Xe-133 retention is due to air trapping, most commonly associated with COPD.
- Must be careful not to confuse liver uptake on Xe-133 from steatosis for retention in the lung base.
- While Xe-133 is great for showing physiology, its short biologic half-life limits imaging options.

## Suggested Readings

Milliron B, Henry TS, Veeraraghavan S, Little BP. Brinchiectasis: mechanisms and imaging clues of associated common and uncommon disease. Radiographics. 2015; 35(4):1011–1030

Park EA, Goo JM, Park SJ, et al. Chronic obstructive pulmonary disease: quantitative and visual ventilation pattern analysis at xenon ventilation CT performed by using a dual-energy technique. Radiology. 2010; 256(3):985–997

Yokoe K, Satoh K, Yamamoto Y, et al. Usefulness of 99mTc-Technegas and 133Xe dynamic SPECT in ventilatory impairment. Nucl Med Commun. 2006; 27(11):887–892

# Case 47

*Ely A. Wolin*

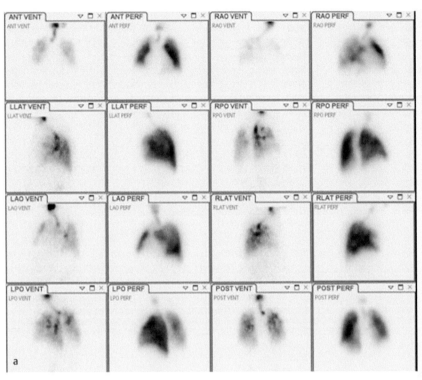

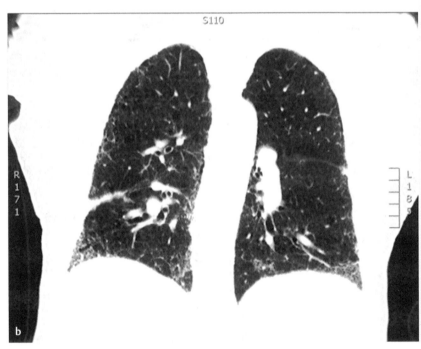

**Fig. 47.1** **(a)** Images from a pulmonary ventilation and perfusion scan utilizing aerosolized Tc-99m diethylenetriamine pentaacetic acid (DTPA) and intravenous Tc-99m macroaggregated albumin (MAA) show diffuse heterogeneous pulmonary ventilation with central clumping. **(b)** Coronal image from a chest CT scan obtained 6 days prior shows apical predominant centrilobular and paraseptal emphysema with basilar predominant subpleural fibrosis.

■ **Clinical History**

78-year-old female referred for evaluation for pulmonary embolus due to shortness of breath (▶Fig. 47.1).

## ■ Key Finding

Heterogeneous pulmonary ventilation

## ■ Top 3 Differential Diagnoses

- **COPD.** Chronic airway obstruction and parenchymal destruction associated with COPD (particularly emphysema) results in alterations in pulmonary ventilation. Normal pulmonary ventilation scintigraphy should show a relatively homogeneous pattern with smooth peripheral activity and an apical to basal gradient. The physiologic alterations associated with COPD lead to abnormal ventilation scintigraphy, usually demonstrating a mix of diffuse inhomogeneity with patchy peripheral activity and central deposition or clumping. The central deposition is due to tapping of the radioactive particles in the large airways secondary to the obstructive physiology. Central deposition may be limited with Technegas (not available in the United States) due to the small particle size.

- **Congestive heart failure.** It can lead to a heterogeneous pattern on both pulmonary perfusion and pulmonary ventilation images. Early congestive heart failure should not show much alteration in either. However, more advanced heart failure will lead to heterogeneity as the vascular and interstitial beds are overwhelmed and fluid begins to fill the alveolar spaces.
- **Multifocal infection.** Multiple airspace opacities will result in a somewhat heterogeneous appearance of pulmonary ventilation. There should be correlative abnormalities on chest radiographs, as well as matched abnormal pulmonary perfusion due to reflex vasoconstriction.

## ■ Additional Considerations

- **Noncardiogenic pulmonary edema:** Noncardiogenic pulmonary edema is generally a result of increased pulmonary capillary permeability. This results in multiple patchy areas of fluid filled alveoli in a distribution atypical for, and without other associated signs of, congestive heart failure. The resultant loss of ventilation capability can lead to heterogeneous pulmonary

scintigraphy. The increased capillary permeability also may result in increased DTPA clearance.
- **Quantum mottle:** As with heterogeneous pulmonary perfusion, incorrect imaging technique can result in a heterogeneous appearance. Ensure correct radioisotope window, collimator, patient to camera distance, and imaging time.

## ■ Diagnosis

COPD.

## ✓ Pearls

- COPD most often results in heterogeneous pulmonary ventilation with central airway deposition/clumping.
- Noncardiogenic pulmonary edema may show heterogeneous ventilation with increased DTPA clearance.

- Radiographic correlation is key for pulmonary scintigraphy, should be completed within 24 hours.
- Incorrect imaging technique can result in quantum mottle mimicking true heterogeneous ventilation.

## Suggested Readings

Cukic V, Begic A. Potential role of lung ventilation scintigraphy in the assessment of COPD. Acta Inform Med. 2014; 22(3):170–173

Milne S, King GG. Advanced imaging in COPD: insights into pulmonary pathophysiology. J Thorac Dis. 2014; 6(11):1570–1585

Roach PJ, Schembri GP, Bailey DL. V/Q scanning using SPECT and SPECT/CT. J Nucl Med. 2013; 54(9):1588–1596

# Part 5

## Hepatobiliary

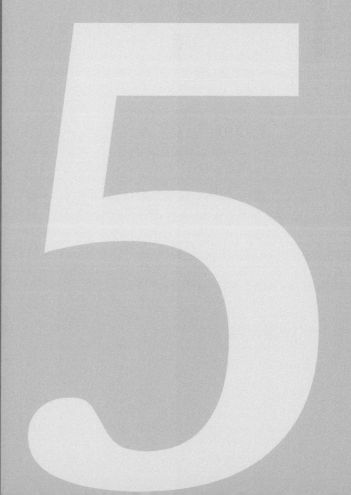

# Case 48

*Ely A. Wolin*

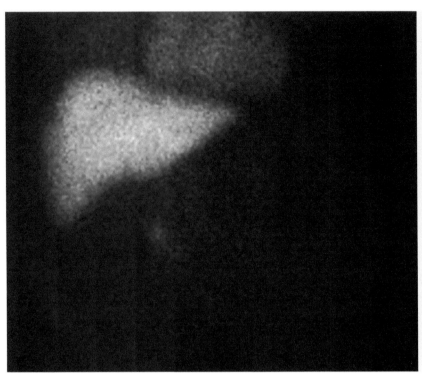

**Fig. 48.1** 60-minute anterior image from dynamic acquisition after the administration of 5.88 mCi Tc-99m mebrofenin shows persistent blood pool activity in the heart. No gallbladder activity is visualized, as well, which persisted on the 4-hour images.

## ■ Clinical History

80-year-old male with methicillin-resistant *Staphylococcus aureus* bacteremia of unknown source, in septic shock, status post endoscopic retrograde cholangiopancreatography (ERCP) with biliary stent placement two days prior with increasing abdominal distention, transaminitis, and hyperbilirubinemia. Referred for hepatobiliary scintigraphy (HBS) to assess for obstruction (▶ Fig. 48.1).

## ■ Key Finding

Delayed clearance of blood pool on HBS

## ■ Diagnosis

- **Hepatic dysfunction.** HBS is performed utilizing iminodiacetic acid (IDA) derivatives tagged with Tc-99m. Currently bromotriethyl-IDA (mebrofenin) and diisopropyl-IDA (disofenin) are used in the United States. These agents remain tightly bound to protein in the blood which limits renal clearance. They dissociate from albumin in the liver and are extracted by hepatocytes, like bilirubin, then secreted unchanged into the biliary canaliculi. The modern IDA derivatives, created through alterations of the benzene ring, have better hepatic uptake allowing for clinical use in patients with higher bilirubin levels. Tc-99m mebrofenin has the highest liver extraction percentage and more rapid biliary clearance and it resists displacement by high bilirubin concentrations.

  HBS, frequently called "HIDA" scan as homage to the first clinically useful IDA derivative, involves anterior dynamic imaging of the abdomen after radiopharmaceutical administration. The dynamic information allows for qualitative assessment of the imaged blood pool, hepatic parenchymal uptake, hepatic transit, biliary ductal system, gallbladder, and biliary-to-bowel transit.

  Hepatic uptake should be diffuse and homogeneous with an abrupt increase in activity as the tracer makes it to the portovenous system, and it should result in rapid clearance of the blood pool. Normally, the blood pool should clear within 5 to 10 minutes. Delayed blood clearance is indicative of hepatocellular dysfunction which may be secondary to multiple causes including cirrhosis, fibrosis, and chronic biliary obstruction. With hepatic dysfunction, there may be vicarious radiopharmaceutical excretion through the kidneys. This is important to differentiate from biliary or bowel activity, particularly when evaluating neonatal jaundice.

  Some quantitative methods have been derived for evaluation of hepatic function, but are not generally part of standard cholescintigraphy. These methods generally involve analysis of time–activity curves from regions of interest drawn around the liver and heart.

  The presence of hepatocellular dysfunction affects the ability to evaluate for cholecystitis with cholescintigraphy. The predictive value of gallbladder visualization and biliary-to-bowel transit within 1 hour requires normal hepatic function. If dysfunction is present, delayed images may be necessary to truly evaluate for cystic duct obstruction or delayed biliary transit.

## ■ Diagnosis

Hepatocellular dysfunction.

## ✓ Pearls

- Hepatic dysfunction results in delayed uptake of IDA derivatives, seen as prolonged blood pool activity.
- Predictive measures of gallbladder visualization within 60 minutes requires normal hepatic function.
- Vicarious renal excretion can simulate biliary or bowel activity when evaluating neonatal jaundice.
- Modern IDA derivatives have better hepatic uptake allowing for usage with higher bilirubin levels.

## Suggested readings

de Graaf W, Bennink RJ, Veteläinen R, van Gulik TM. Nuclear imaging techniques for the assessment of hepatic function in liver surgery and transplantation. J Nucl Med. 2010; 51(5):742–752

Tulchinsky M, Ciak BW, Delbeke D, et al. Society of Nuclear Medicine. SNM practice guideline for hepatobiliary scintigraphy 4.0. J Nucl Med Technol. 2010; 38(4):210–218

Ziessman HA. Hepatobiliary scintigraphy in 2014. J Nucl Med. 2014; 55(6):967–975

# Case 49

*Ely A. Wolin*

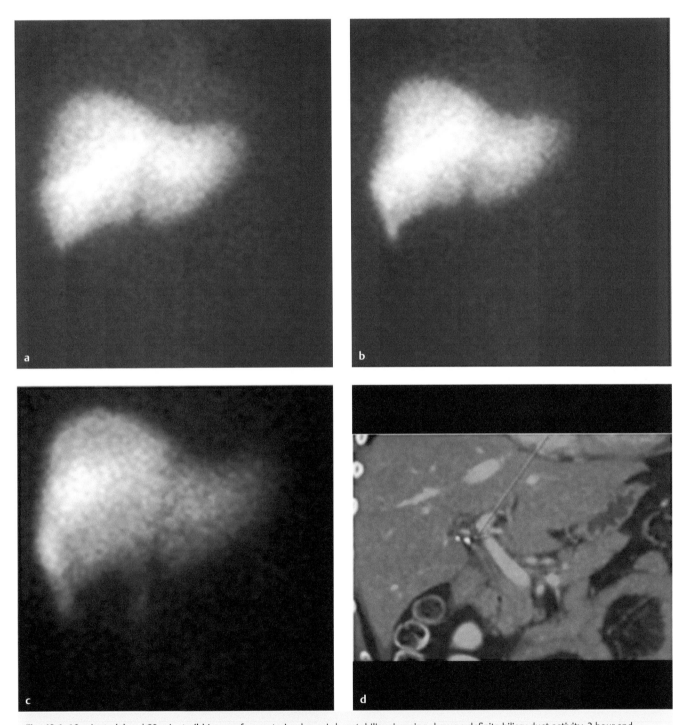

**Fig. 49.1** 10-minute **(a)** and 60-minute **(b)** images from anterior dynamic hepatobiliary imaging show no definite biliary duct activity. 3 hour and 45 minute delayed anterior image **(c)** shows minimal activity within the common bile duct with no definite biliary-to-bowel transit. Correlative coronal CT image **(d)** shows abrupt termination of the common bile duct at a surgical clip.

## ■ Clinical History

26-year-old female postoperative day 2 from laparoscopic cholecystectomy, febrile and tachycardic with increasing total bili- rubin. Referred for evaluation for biliary leak versus obstruction (►Fig. 49.1).

## ■ Key Finding

Delayed biliary clearance on Tc-99m mebrofenin hepatobiliary scintigraphy (HBS)

## ■ Top 3 Differential Diagnoses

- **Biliary obstruction (high grade or partial).** Complete common bile duct obstruction can be missed with anatomic imaging in the acute stage as the gallbladder can collect the undrained bile preventing biliary duct dilation. HBS at this time may appear normal with the exception of absent bowel activity, even on delayed imaging. After about 24 hours, the gallbladder's reservoir capacity will be overwhelmed which then results in increased pressure in, and eventually dilation of, the biliary tree. The increase in pressure impedes bile excretion into the bile canaliculi. At this stage, HBS will likely still show good hepatic extraction and clearance of the blood pool, but no activity will be seen entering the common bile duct, gallbladder, or bowel. If obstruction is not resolved, it will eventually lead to hepatocellular damage. Partial biliary obstruction can be more of a diagnostic challenge with HBS. Findings of partial duct obstruction, depending on chronicity, are in general very nonspecific and can include delayed blood pool clearance, delayed hepatic transit and biliary clearance, and delayed biliary-to-bowel transit. As absent biliary-to-bowel transit may be the only abnormality on HBS with acute complete common bile duct obstruction, some providers will not administer sincalide (cholecystokinin [CCK]-8) in this setting. It is not an absolute contraindication as there are many other causes of delayed biliary-to-bowel transit. CCK-8 should be used with caution if the clinical scenario matches acute biliary obstruction.
- **Hepatic dysfunction.** Hepatocellular function is essential for HBS as the iminodiacetic acid (IDA) derivatives are handled like bile. Decreased hepatic function can affect all stages of HBS, leading to delays in blood pool clearance, biliary duct visualization, and biliary-to-bowel transit, and therefore, can mimic biliary obstruction.
- **Cholestatic jaundice.** Nonobstructive cholestasis can result in a similar pattern of delayed biliary clearance. Patients who are receiving total parenteral nutrition are at risk for this condition, which can lead to acalculous cholecystitis. Cholestasis can also be associated with several medications, the postoperative state, congenital abnormalities, and pregnancy, among other things.

## ■ Diagnosis

Iatrogenic common bile duct obstruction.

## ✓ Pearls

- HBS cannot always distinguish between obstruction, hepatocellular dysfunction, and cholestasis.
- Absent biliary-to-bowel transit may be the only abnormality on HBS with acute biliary obstruction.
- CCK-8 should be administered with caution if biliary-to-bowel transit is not seen within 60 minutes.
- Hepatic function is essential for HBS, decreased function can affect all stages of the exam.

## Suggested Readings

Low CS, Ahmed H, Notghi A. Pitfall and limitations of radionuclide hepatobiliary and gastrointestinal system imaging. Semin Nucl Med. 2015; 45(6):513–529

Roy-Chowdhury N, Roy-Chowdhury J. Diagnostic approach to the adult with jaundice or asymptomatic hyperbilirubinemia. In:UpToDate, Chopra S (Ed), UpToDate, Waltham, MA. (Accessed on November 17, 2016)

Ziessman HA. Nuclear medicine hepatobiliary imaging. Clin Gastroenterol Hepatol. 2010; 8(2):111–116

# Case 50

*Brady S. Davis*

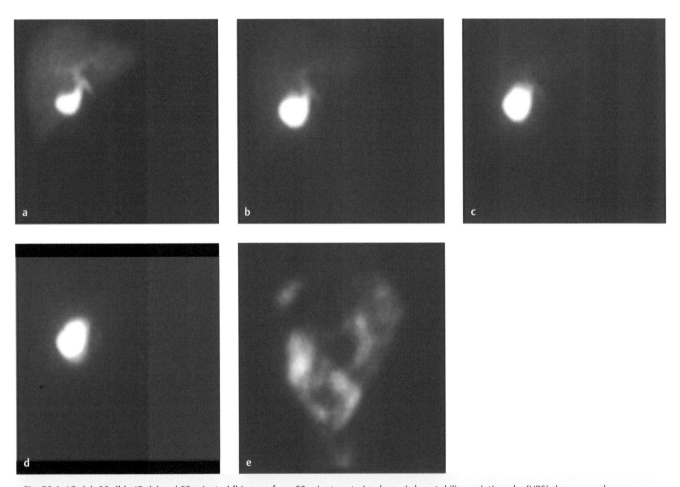

**Fig. 50.1** 15- **(a)**, 30- **(b)**, 45- **(c)** and 60-minute **(d)** images from 60-minute anterior dynamic hepatobiliary scintigraphy (HBS) show normal homogeneous liver activity with prompt biliary duct and gallbladder visualization, but no biliary-to-bowel transit. Representative image from 45 minutes into dynamic imaging during cholecystokinin (CCK) administration **(e)** shows diffuse bowel activity; gallbladder ejection fraction was calculated to be 92%.

■ **Clinical History**

29-year-old male with epigastric pain referred for HBS (▶ Fig. 50.1).

## ▪ Key Finding

Delayed biliary-to-bowel transit on HBS

## ▪ Top 3 Differential Diagnoses

- **Normal variant.** Normally, the hepatobiliary radiotracer is excreted through the bile ducts into the duodenum within 1 hour. However, around one-fifth of healthy patients with normal hepatobiliary function will demonstrate delayed biliary-to-bowel transit. This is likely secondary to physiologic factors relating to fasting state, including the amount of circulating endogenous CCK hormone and the native hypertonicity of the sphincter of Oddi (SO).
- **Biliary obstruction.** There are numerous causes of both low-grade and high-grade biliary obstruction, including stones, benign or malignant strictures, inflammation from pancreatitis or cholangitis, and SO dysfunction (fixed or reversible). Low-grade or partial obstruction is suggested when bowel activity is identified greater than 1 hour, but less than 24 hours. High-grade biliary obstruction can result in a persistent hepatogram with absence of bowel activity at 24 hours. Longstanding obstruction can slowly cause hepatocellular dysfunction that decreases blood pool clearance of radiotracer.
- **Chronic cholecystitis.** Intermittent cystic duct obstruction over a period of time can result in inflammation and fibrosis of the gallbladder wall, termed as chronic cholecystitis. Chronic cholecystitis primarily presents scintigraphically as filling of the gallbladder only on delayed images (2–4 hours) or after morphine augmentation; a less reliable and secondary sign of chronic cholecystitis is delayed biliary-to-bowel transit, possibly due to associated inflammation of the ampulla.

## ▪ Additional Diagnostic Considerations

- **Sphincter of Oddi dysfunction:** Abnormal contraction of the SO, which should normally relax with gallbladder contraction, can lead to delayed biliary-to-bowel transit.
- **Medication effect:** Several medications can result in delayed visualization of small bowel activity on HBS. These include various medications that result in drug-induced cholestasis, as well as opiates due to SO contraction. Pretreatment with CCK can also cause a delay in biliary-to-bowel transit.
- **Hepatocellular dysfunction:** This can result in delayed biliary-to-bowel transit due to associated cholestasis.

## ▪ Diagnosis

Unknown.

## ✓ Pearls

- Delayed biliary-to-bowel transit is a nonspecific finding that can be a normal variant.
- Biliary obstruction and nonobstructive cholestasis can result in delayed biliary-to-bowel transit.
- Delayed biliary-to-bowel transit can be an indicator of chronic cholecystitis.

## Suggested Readings

Lambie H, Cook AM, Scarsbrook AF, Lodge JP, Robinson PJ, Chowdhury FU. Tc99 m-hepatobiliary iminodiacetic acid (HIDA) scintigraphy in clinical practice. Clin Radiol. 2011; 66(11):1094–1105

Tulchinsky M, Colletti PM, Allen TW. Hepatobiliary scintigraphy in acute cholecystitis. Semin Nucl Med. 2012; 42(2):84–100

Ziessman HA. Hepatobiliary scintigraphy in 2014. J Nucl Med. 2014; 55(6): 967–975

# Case 51

*Kamal D. Singh*

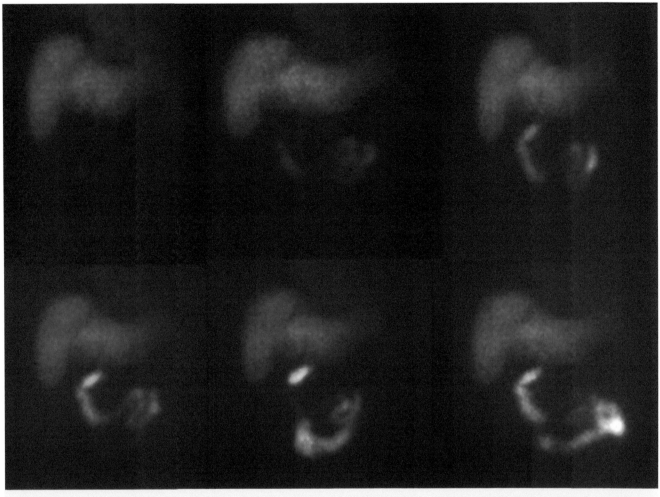

**Fig. 51.1** Representative images from anterior 60-minute dynamic imaging after the administration of technetium-99m (TC-99m) mebrofenin show prompt clearance of the blood pool, normal hepatic transit and biliary-to-bowel transit, with no activity seen in the gallbladder. No evidence of bile leak.

■ **Clinical History**

77-year-old male with known acute cholecystitis post ERCP with concern for bile leak (▶Fig. 51.1).

## ■ Key Finding

Nonvisualization of gallbladder on hepatobiliary imaging

## ■ Top 3 Differential Diagnoses

- **Acute cholecystitis.** Acute cystic duct obstruction is the hallmark of acute cholecystitis. Hepatobiliary imaging has a high specificity (98%) and negative predictive value (99%) and is very useful in cases where ultrasound findings are equivocal. Under normal circumstances, the gallbladder is visualized within 1 hour of radiotracer administration. Nonvisualization of gallbladder activity within 4 hours of radiotracer injection in the setting of normal visualization of biliary and bowel activity is diagnostic of acute cholecystitis. Alternatively, morphine (0.04 mg/kg IV) may be administered after 1 hour of dynamic imaging. Nonvisualization of the gallbladder within 30 minutes of morphine administration is also diagnostic of acute cholecystitis. The "cystic duct" or "nubbin" sign may be seen as focal activity within the cystic duct up to the site of obstruction. Increased pericholecystic hepatic parenchymal activity ("rim sign") can be an ominous sign of complicated/advanced (gangrenous, necrotic, or perforated) cholecystitis necessitating immediate surgical intervention.

- **Chronic cholecystitis.** Delayed visualization of the gallbladder between 1 to 4 hours postinjection, or within 30 minutes after morphine augmentation, is suggestive of chronic cholecystitis. A second injection of radiopharmaceutical, or "booster dose," may be necessary after the initial 60-minute image acquisition, if there is insufficient remaining hepatic or biliary tree activity to permit gallbladder filling.

- **Inadequate patient preparation.** False-positives can occur with insufficient (< 4 hours) or prolonged (>24 hours) fasting, or prolonged hyperalimentation. Pretreatment with cholecystokinin (CCK), 30 minutes prior to injection, is usually recommended for prolonged fasting and hyperalimentation to allow the distended gallbladder to drain. Patients with a recent meal are imaged after fasting for a minimum of 4 hours.

## ■ Additional Diagnostic Considerations

- **Severe hepatocellular disease:** Poor hepatocellular function can result in poor extraction and excretion of the radiotracer, resulting in delayed blood pool clearance (>10 min). False-positive studies occur due to delayed or nonvisualization of gallbladder. The key is to note the delayed blood pool clearance.

- **High-grade biliary obstruction:** Prompt hepatic uptake without biliary excretion of radiotracer ("liver scan" sign) suggests biliary duct obstruction. Delayed 4- and 24-hour imaging is generally obtained to evaluate for bowel activity. The gallbladder may or may not fill depending upon the location and duration of obstruction. CT scan or magnetic resonance cholangiopancreatography (MRCP) may be helpful not only in establishing the diagnosis but also in determining a possible cause of obstruction.

## ■ Diagnosis

Acute cholecystitis.

## ✓ Pearls

- Hepatobiliary scan is highly sensitive and specific for acute calculous cholecystitis.
- False-positives may be seen with recent meal, extended fasting (> 24 hour), and hepatocellular dysfunction.

- The "rim sign" can indicate complicated/advanced (gangrenous, necrotic, or perforated) cholecystitis.

## Suggested Readings

Montini KM, Tulchinsky M. Applied hepatobiliary scintigraphy in acute cholecystitis. Appl Radiol. 2015; 44(5):21–30

Tulchinsky M, Ciak BW, Delbeke D, et al. Society of Nuclear Medicine. SNM practice guideline for hepatobiliary scintigraphy 4.0. J Nucl Med Technol. 2010; 38(4):210–218

Uliel L, Mellnick VM, Menias CO, Holz AL, McConathy J. Nuclear medicine in the acute clinical setting: indications, imaging findings, and potential pitfalls. Radiographics. 2013; 33(2):375–396

# Case 52

*Jonathan Muldermans*

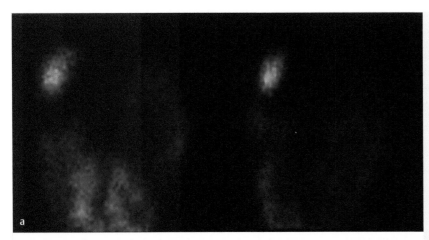

**Fig. 52.1** 1- and 30-minute images from left anterior oblique dynamic imaging during 30-minute cholecystokinin (CCK) injection **(a)**, and associated time-activity curve (TAC) **(c)** for a gallbladder region of interest (ROI) **(b)** show minimal reduction in gallbladder counts over 30 minutes with a calculated gallbladder ejection fraction of 5.59%.

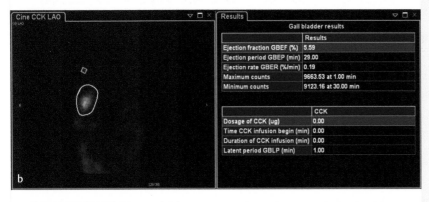

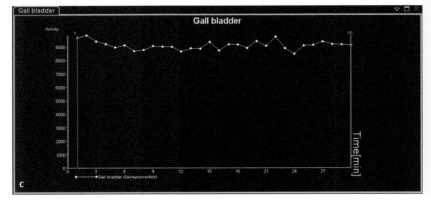

## ■ Clinical History

53-year-old female with prandial/postprandial right upper quadrant abdominal pain, particularly with fatty foods, being evaluated for bariatric surgery with consideration for possible gallbladder removal. Ultrasound was negative for stones. Referred for hepatobiliary scintigraphy (HBS) due to clinical concern for biliary dyskinesia (▶ Fig. 52.1).

## ■ Key Finding

Reduced gallbladder ejection fraction (GBEF)

## ■ Top 3 Differential Diagnoses

- **Chronic acalculous gallbladder disease.** Cholescintigraphy has demonstrated improved diagnostic accuracy over sonography for evaluation of gallbladder disease. In patients with biliary colic, but without cholelithiasis, the clinician may suspect chronic acalculous gallbladder disease (CAGBD), and request evaluation of the GBEF. Various names for this entity are used including cystic duct syndrome, gallbladder spasm, gallbladder dyskinesia, and functional gallbladder disease. It is thought that recurrent biliary colic leads to disorganized smooth muscle contractions in the gallbladder wall, or to increased pressure in the biliary tree due to fibrosis from recurrent infection, either of which will reduce the gallbladder's ability to drain. After the gallbladder is visualized during the initial 1-hour imaging, repeat dynamic images are obtained, usually in the left anterior oblique projection to prevent bowel overlap, during the injection of 0.02 μg/kg of CCK-8 over one hour. An ROI is then drawn around the gallbladder to create a TAC. For a 60-minute injection, a GBEF below 38% is definitely abnormal and above 50% is definitely normal, with the area between possibly normal or abnormal. The lower the GBEF, the more confident the diagnosis of CAGBD. If the diagnosis of CAGBD is made, cholecystectomy is likely to provide symptomatic relief.

- **Medications.** Morphine (or other opioids), atropine, octreotide, ethanol, nicotine, indomethacin, calcium channel blockers, pirenzepine, antihistamines, benzodiazepines, theophylline, and progesterone are some drugs that can reduce the GBEF. Many patients are on one or more of these medications, making reconciliation important. Confounding drugs should be held prior to the procedure, if clinically appropriate.

- **Sphincter of Oddi dysfunction.** This is a rare, poorly understood entity present more commonly in the post-cholecystectomy setting. The term dysfunction includes both stenosis and dyskinesia of the sphincter. Theoretically, increased sphincter tone results in stasis of both biliary and pancreatic secretions leading to recurrent biliary colic, transaminitis, and synchronous or metachronous pancreatitis. Comparison with anatomic imaging studies is helpful and may show dilation of the biliary tree and the main pancreatic duct along with the calcifications and parenchymal atrophy typical of chronic pancreatitis. Endoscopic sphincterotomy is the treatment of choice, as cholecystectomy will not relieve all of the patient's symptoms.

## ■ Diagnosis

Surgical pathology revealed chronic cholecystitis.

## ✓ Pearls

- The preferred dose of CCK-8 is 0.02 μg/kg infused over 60 minutes.
- A GBEF below 38% is abnormal, and diagnostic confidence for CAGBD increases as the GBEF decreases.

- Many medications can reduce gallbladder contractility; these should be held if possible to improve accuracy.
- Sphincter of Oddi (SO) dysfunction should be suspected in patients with biliary colic, transaminitis, and pancreatitis.

## Suggested Readings

Corazziari E. Sphincter of Oddi dysfunction. Dig Liver Dis. 2003; 35(Suppl 3): S26–S29

Ziessman HA, Tulchinsky M, Lavely WC, et al. Sincalide-stimulated cholescintigraphy: a multicenter investigation to determine optimal infusion methodology and gallbladder ejection fraction normal values. J Nucl Med. 2010; 51(2):277–281

Ziessman HA. Hepatobiliary scintigraphy in 2014. J Nucl Med. 2014; 55(6): 967–975

# Case 53

*Kamal D. Singh*

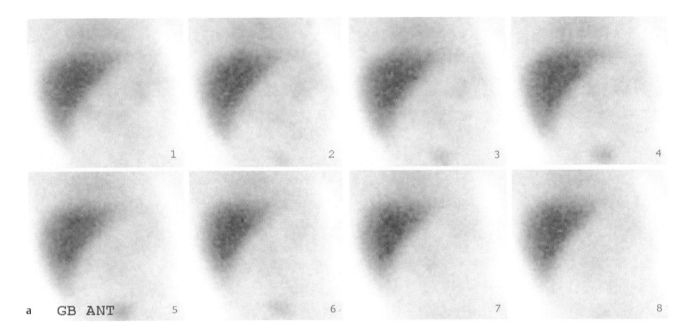

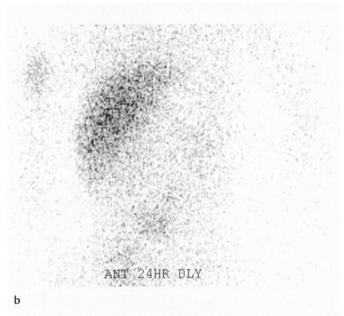

**Fig. 53.1** Hepatobiliary scan with technetium-99m mebrofenin. **(a)** Sequential imaging during the first hour demonstrates no biliary excretion of radiotracer or bowel activity. There is mild persistence of cardiac blood pool activity. No significant change was noted on 4-hour delayed imaging (not included). **(b)** 24-hour delayed anterior static image reveals persistent hepatic parenchymal activity with vicarious genitourinary excretion of radiotracer. There is no evidence of bowel activity.

## ▪ Clinical History

2-week-old neonate with jaundice (▶ Fig. 53.1).

## ■ Key Finding

Persistent hepatogram on neonatal hepatobiliary imaging

## ■ Top 3 Differential Diagnoses

• **Biliary atresia.** Persistent neonatal conjugated hyperbilirubinemia may be due to biliary atresia or neonatal hepatitis. Biliary atresia involves malformation of extrahepatic ducts leading to obstructive cholestasis and jaundice. Despite extrahepatic biliary ductal obstruction, intrahepatic biliary ducts are nondilated due to fibrosis. Prompt diagnosis of biliary atresia is essential, since success rate of the Kasai surgical procedure is highest if performed within the first 2 months of life. Hepatobiliary imaging can exclude biliary atresia by demonstrating patency of the extrahepatic biliary system. Patients are pretreated with phenobarbital (5 mg/kg PO daily for 5 days) in order to optimize biliary excretion. Good hepatic uptake with poor hepatic clearance (persistent hepatogram) and nonvisualization of intestinal activity within 24 hours of radiotracer injection is essentially diagnostic of biliary atresia. Intraoperative cholangiogram, however, remains the gold standard for definitive diagnosis.

• **Neonatal hepatitis.** This condition may be due to a variety of metabolic, congenital, or infectious causes, or it may be idiopathic. Scintigraphic findings include poor hepatic uptake of radiotracer with delayed or decreased biliary excretion secondary to impaired hepatocyte function. On 24-hour delayed imaging, bowel activity is nearly always present confirming patency of the biliary system. Lack of bowel activity may rarely be seen in severe hepatic dysfunction or due to inadequate patient preparation. Hepatic biopsy may further aid in definitive diagnosis prior to medical treatment.

• **Intrahepatic cholestasis from severe parenchymal disease.** Rarely, severe hepatocellular dysfunction or intrahepatic biliary malformation may result in cholestasis with no scintigraphically detectable excretion of radiotracer, resulting in a false-positive study for biliary atresia. A repeat study could theoretically help exclude biliary atresia if the patient's hepatic function improves. However, liver biopsy and/or intraoperative cholangiogram may be necessary for definitive diagnosis.

## ■ Diagnosis

Biliary atresia.

## ✓ Pearls

• Pretreatment with phenobarbital increases biliary secretion of tracer, improving the accuracy of the scan.
• Prompt hepatic uptake without biliary excretion into the bowel over 24 hours suggests biliary atresia.

• Visualization of bowel activity essentially excludes biliary atresia.
• Neonatal hepatitis demonstrates poor hepatic uptake with delayed bowel activity.

## Suggested Readings

Hartley JL, Davenport M, Kelly DA. Biliary atresia. Lancet. 2009; 374(9702): 1704–1713

Kwatra N, Shalaby-Rana E, Narayanan S, Mohan P, Ghelani S, Majd M. Phenobarbital-enhanced hepatobiliary scintigraphy in the diagnosis of biliary atresia: two decades of experience at a tertiary center. Pediatr Radiol. 2013; 43(10): 1365–1375

Shah I, Bhatnagar S, Rangarajan V, Patankar N. Utility of Tc99 m-Mebrofenin hepato-biliary scintigraphy (HIDA scan) for the diagnosis of biliary atresia. Trop Gastroenterol. 2012; 33(1):62–64

# Case 54

*Cathy Zhou*

ANTERIOR

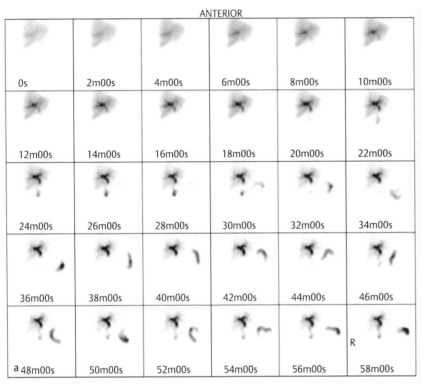

| | | | | | |
|---|---|---|---|---|---|
| 0s | 2m00s | 4m00s | 6m00s | 8m00s | 10m00s |
| 12m00s | 14m00s | 16m00s | 18m00s | 20m00s | 22m00s |
| 24m00s | 26m00s | 28m00s | 30m00s | 32m00s | 34m00s |
| 36m00s | 38m00s | 40m00s | 42m00s | 44m00s | 46m00s |
| a 48m00s | 50m00s | 52m00s | 54m00s | 56m00s | 58m00s |

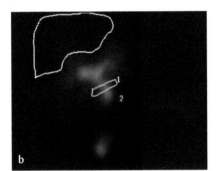

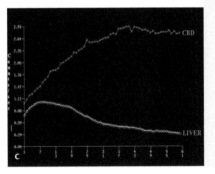

**Fig. 54.1** After Tc-99m-labeled mebrofenin administration, dynamic anterior imaging of the abdomen over 60 minutes demonstrates prompt, homogenous uptake by the liver. There is prominence of the intrahepatic bile ducts. Excretion is seen within the common bile duct (CBD) by 10 minutes and small bowel by 12 minutes **(a)**. Subsequently, cholecystokinin (CCK) was given and imaging continued for 30 minutes. Regions of interest were drawn over the hepatic parenchyma and CBD **(b)**; and then time–activity curves were generated **(c)**. Fractional emptying of the CBD for the duration of the exam is 5% which is less when compared to a normal value of 50% or above.

■ **Clinical History**

58-year-old female with a history of cholecystectomy and chronic right upper quadrant pain (▶ Fig. 54.1).

## ■ Key Finding

Delayed biliary ductal clearance after cholecystectomy

## ■ Top 3 Differential Diagnoses

- **Biliary dyskinesia/sphincter of Oddi dysfunction.** It refers to disordered peristalsis of the biliary tract and/or reduction in speed of biliary tree emptying into the gastrointestinal tract, and includes stenosis (fixed) or dyskinesia (reversible) of the sphincter of Oddi (SO). Patients may experience biliary pain and recurrent pancreatitis. Hepatobiliary scan can provide diagnostic confirmation. A scintigraphic score takes into account the time of peak liver activity, time of biliary and bowel visualization, prominence of the biliary tree, the percentage of CBD emptying, and the ratio of activity between the CBD and liver. A score over 4 indicates SO dysfunction.
- **Cholelithiasis.** Calculi can be found in the gallbladder remnant, cystic duct stump or CBD. Calculi are classified as recurrent if found more than 2 years after surgery, and can form due to biliary stasis. Otherwise they are classified as retained and are presumed to have been present at the time of cholecystectomy. Partial biliary obstruction will have delayed biliary ductal clearance, while high-grade obstruction will demonstrate little to no biliary excretion.
- **Bile duct injury.** One of the most serious complications following cholecystectomy is a bile duct injury, manifesting acutely as a leak or transection with symptoms of abdominal pain, fever, and jaundice. More chronically, bile duct stricture may form with resulting biliary obstruction. These can be discovered on ultrasound or magnetic resonance cholangiopancreatogram (MRCP), and hepatobiliary scan can be used to confirm a biloma or obstruction. These injuries typically require stenting or surgical repair.

## ■ Additional Diagnostic Consideration

- **Malignancy:** Obstruction of the bile ducts from intrinsic narrowing or extrinsic compression can occur in the setting of pancreaticobiliary malignancy and patients will exhibit symptoms related to biliary obstruction, such as jaundice, clay-colored stools, and dark urine. Hepatobiliary scan is not routinely indicated in workup for presumed cancer; CT and cholangiography are preferred. However, if obtained, findings will usually reflect biliary obstruction.

## ■ Diagnosis

SO dysfunction.

## ✓ Pearls

- SO dysfunction can be categorized by Rome criteria.
- Stump or gallbladder remnant cholecystitis are uncommon complications of cholecystectomy.
- Bile duct injuries are more likely in laparoscopic (versus open) cholecystectomy.

## Suggested Readings

Girometti R, Brondani G, Cereser L, et al. Post-cholecystectomy syndrome: spectrum of biliary findings at magnetic resonance cholangiopancreatography. Br J Radiol. 2010; 83(988):351–361

Sostre S, Kalloo AN, Spiegler EJ, Camargo EE, Wagner HN, Jr. A noninvasive test of sphincter of Oddi dysfunction in postcholecystectomy patients: the scintigraphic score. J Nucl Med. 1992; 33(6):1216–1222

Ziessman HA. Hepatobiliary scintigraphy in 2014. J Nucl Med. 2014; 55(6):967–975

# Case 55

*Britain A. Gailliot*

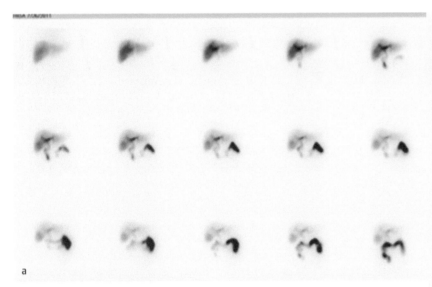

**Fig. 55.1** Initial dynamic hepatobiliary imaging over 60 minutes in the anterior projection demonstrates persistent radiotracer localization with a rounded lesion in the inferior right hepatic lobe. T1 arterial phase contrast-enhanced (Eovist) axial image **(b)** shows a large enhancing lesion in the right lobe of the liver with persistent retention of contrast on 20-minute delayed T1 imaging **(c)**.

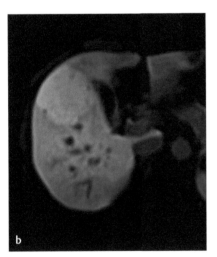

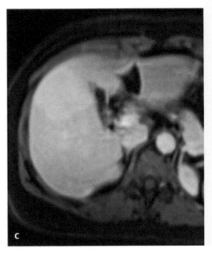

■ **Clinical History**

45-year-old female presenting with right upper quadrant pain (▶Fig. 55.1).

(Case courtesy of Joseph S. Fotos, MD, Penn State Hershey Medical Center.)

## ■ Key Finding

Uptake within a liver mass on hepatobiliary imaging

## ■ Top 3 Differential Diagnoses

- **Focal nodular hyperplasia.** It is a benign hyperplastic process composed of normal hepatocytes with disorganized biliary canaliculi. Hepatobiliary imaging involves the administration of Tc-99m-labeled iminodiacetic acid (IDA) analogs which are taken up by functioning hepatocytes and secreted through the biliary system. Given the presence of normal hepatocytes in focal nodular hyperplasia (FNH), the radiotracer is taken up in a manner similar to the surrounding liver parenchyma. However, approximately 15 minutes after the administration of the radiotracer the remainder of the liver begins to washout while the radiotracer within the FNH cannot be excreted due to the malformed biliary system. This results in persistent activity within the FNH on subsequent imaging.
- **Hepatocellular carcinoma (HCC).** HCC is derived from hepatocytes which contain varying degrees of functionality, depending on the level of differentiation. If there is sufficient functionality, the hepatocytes are capable of taking up enough hepatobiliary radiotracer to appear similar to the adjacent parenchyma. This is analogous to the early imaging obtained when an FNH is present. However, with HCC the radiotracer is actively excreted, making it indistinguishable from the remainder of the liver during washout. Without differentiated functioning hepatocytes, HCC will appear photopenic throughout the exam, which is more common.
- **Hepatic adenoma.** These are benign lesions derived from hepatocytes which demonstrate varying degrees of functionality and, therefore, can appear similar to a well-differentiated HCC with uptake and excretion on hepatobiliary scintigraphy (HBS).

## ■ Diagnosis

Focal nodular hyperplasia.

## ✓ Pearls

- Liver lesions that are of hepatocellular origin may take up hepatobiliary radiotracers.
- FNH shows persistent activity on hepatobiliary scan due to disorganized drainage.
- Around 50% of HCC have sufficient hepatocyte function to take up hepatobiliary radiotracers.
- Technetium-99m sulfur colloid (Tc-99m SC) scan may provide additional differentiating information and prevent biopsy.

## Suggested Readings

Bahirwani R, Reddy KR. Review article: the evaluation of solitary liver masses. Aliment Pharmacol Ther. 2008; 28(8):953–965

Grazioli L, Federle MP, Brancatelli G, Ichikawa T, Olivetti L, Blachar A. Hepatic adenomas: imaging and pathologic findings. Radiographics. 2001; 21(4):877–892, discussion 892–894

Ziessman HA. Hepatobiliary scintigraphy in 2014. J Nucl Med. 2014; 55(6): 967–975

# Case 56

*Ely A. Wolin*

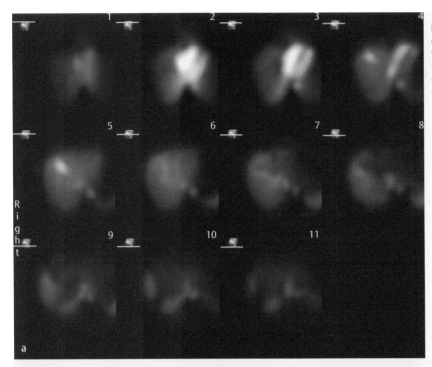

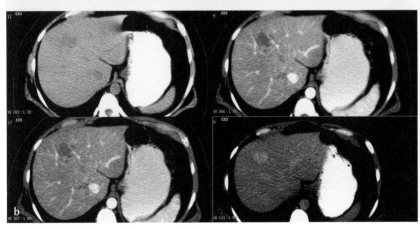

**Fig. 56.1** Axial images from single-photon emission computed tomography (SPECT) acquisition after the administration of 25.2 mCi Tc-99m-labeled red blood cells show focal uptake in the anterior aspect of the liver (a), corresponding to the lesion seen on correlative multiphasic CT scan (b).

## ▪ Clinical History

58-year-old female with a mass in segment 4 of the liver noted incidentally initially on ultrasound, with nonspecific characteristics on follow-up CT scan (▶Fig. 56.1).

## ■ Key Finding

Tagged red blood cells (RBC) uptake in a liver mass

## ■ Diagnosis

- **Hemangioma.** Hepatic hemangioma is thought to be a congenital vascular malformation or hamartoma composed of multiple cavernous vascular spaces. It is the most common benign tumor of the liver. Growth of these lesions is thought to be secondary to ectasia and not true hyperplasia or hypertrophy. They can have a wide range in size, with the lesions greater than 5 cm termed as giant hemangioma. Larger lesions may be symptomatic causing pain or fullness.

  There are imaging characteristics that allow for confident diagnosis of a hemangioma, notably the classic discontinuous nodular peripheral enhancement with centripetal fill-in seen on multiphase contrast-enhanced CT and MRI. However, these imaging features occur in typical hemangiomas and are not always present. Tc-99m-tagged RBC imaging can be helpful to differentiate hemangioma from other solid hepatic tumors.

Typically, on Tc-99m RBC scintigraphy, hemangioma will initially be photopenic, due to the same slow flow responsible for the classic multiphase CT appearance, with a gradual increase in uptake and retention on delayed images. This pattern is known as a perfusion/blood pool mismatch, and is nearly 100% specific for hemangioma, as no other solid liver tumor should retain RBC activity. Hepatocellular Carcinoma (HCC), in contrast, may show an initial mild increased uptake due to the hypervascular nature but will then become photopenic. Absence of uptake does not exclude hemangioma, as some will not show the classic uptake patterns depending on amount of flow and thrombosis in the cavernous vascular spaces. Overall sensitivity is high for lesions greater than 2 cm on planar imaging, 1 cm with single-photon emission computed tomography (SPECT).

## ■ Diagnosis

Hemangioma.

## ✓ Pearls

- Tagged RBC imaging can be useful to confirm hepatic hemangioma in morphologically atypical cases.
- Initial photopenia with subsequent fill-in and retention is nearly 100% specific for hemangioma.

- Planar scintigraphy has good sensitivity for hemangiomas larger than 2 cm, SPECT larger than 1 cm.

## Suggested Readings

Middleton ML. Scintigraphic evaluation of hepatic mass lesions: emphasis on hemangioma detection. Semin Nucl Med. 1996; 26(1):4–15

Prasanna PM, Fredericks SE, Winn SS, Christman RA. Best cases from the AFIP: giant cavernous hemangioma. Radiographics. 2010; 30(4):1139–1144

Tzen KY, Yen TC, Lin WY, Tsai CC, Lin KJ. Diagnostic value of 99 mTc-labeled red blood cell SPET for a solitary solid liver mass in HBV carrier patients with different echogenicities. Hepatogastroenterology. 2000; 47(35):1375–1378

# Case 57

*Vicki Nagano*

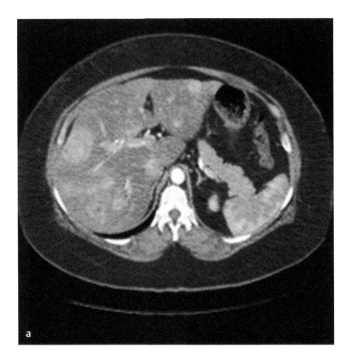

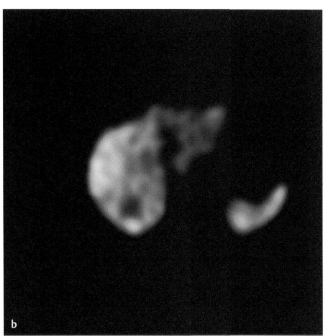

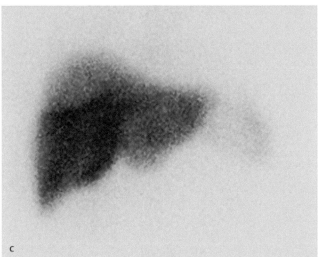

**Fig. 57.1** **(a)** Contrast-enhanced axial CT image through the liver shows multiple hyperdense enhancing lesions in both lobes of the liver. The heterogeneous appearance of the spleen is due to the phase of contrast. **(b)** Technetium-99m sulfur colloid (Tc-99m SC) single-photon emission computed tomography (SPECT) image shows mildly increased uptake in the lateral right lobe and lateral left lobe which is compatible with focal nodular hyperplasia. The large cold defect in the posterior right lobe was diagnosed as a hemangioma on subsequent Tc-99m red blood cells (RBC) scintigraphy (not shown). **(c)** A planar image demonstrating the normal radiopharmaceutical distribution of Tc-99m SC predominantly within the liver with faint activity within the spleen. Breast attenuation creates geographic decreased counts overlying hepatic dome.

■ **Clinical History**

35-year-old female not on birth control pills (▶Fig. 57.1).

## ■ Key Finding

Uptake in a hepatic lesion on SC scan

## ■ Top 3 Differential Diagnoses

- **Focal nodular hyperplasia (FNH).** FNH is a benign hepatic tumor which is most commonly found in women (80%). It typically appears as a solitary solid mass consisting of hepatocytes, bile ducts, and Kupffer cells. Most lesions are 2 to 5 cm in diameter, 20% are multiple, and they are more common in the right lobe of the liver (70%). CT often demonstrates a contrast-enhancing lesion with a central area of scarring. Due to the presence of Kupffer cells, two-thirds of FNH nodules have normal or increased SC uptake. One-third have decreased uptake which may be related to the existence of a large number of fibrotic cells. If the nodule does not accumulate SC, FNH is not ruled out, and the remaining broad differential includes hepatic adenoma, hepatocellular carcinoma (HCC) (including the fibrolamellar variant), and metastases. For radionuclide studies, the practical limits of resolution are 1 to 2 cm for single-photon emission computed tomography (SPECT) imaging and 2 to 3 cm for planar imaging.
- **Superior vena cava syndrome.** In obstruction of the superior vena cava (SVC), collateral vessels return blood via the left internal mammary and left umbilical veins into the quadrate lobe, resulting in a focal hot spot when SC is injected into the upper extremity. Injection in the lower extremity results in a normal scan.
- **Budd–Chiari syndrome.** In this syndrome, obstruction of the hepatic veins results in congestion, hemorrhage, and necrosis of the liver parenchyma. However, the caudate lobe retains its function due to direct venous drainage into the inferior vena cava. On SC imaging, it appears as a hot spot in the caudate lobe of the liver, surrounded by an area of diminished uptake.

## ■ Additional Diagnostic Consideration

- **Regenerating nodular cirrhosis:** Decreased hepatic uptake of SC occurs in cirrhosis due to alteration of the liver's microcirculation. Regenerating nodules are composed primarily of hepatocytes that are surrounded by coarse fibrous septations. They have normal SC uptake and thus appear as relative hot spots surrounded by a region of diminished uptake.

## ■ Diagnosis

Focal nodular hyperplasia.

## ✓ Pearls

- Two-thirds of FNH demonstrate uptake on Tc-99m SC scan.
- Hepatic adenomas, hemangiomas, HCC, metastases, and abscesses are photopenic on Tc-99m SC scan.
- Hemangiomas are cold on Tc-99m SC and hepatobiliary scan, with uptake on delayed Tc-99m RBC scan.
- Regenerating nodules, Budd–Chiari, and SVC syndrome produce focal hepatic uptake on Tc-99m SC scans.

## Suggested Readings

Boulahdour H, Cherqui D, Charlotte F, et al. The hot spot hepatobiliary scan in focal nodular hyperplasia. J Nucl Med. 1993; 34(12):2105–2110

Huynh LT, Kim SY, Murphy TF. The typical appearance of focal nodular hyperplasia in triple-phase CT scan, hepatobiliary scan, and Tc-99 m sulfur colloid scan with SPECT. Clin Nucl Med. 2005; 30(11):736–739

Ziessman HA, O'Malley JP, Thrall JH. Nuclear medicine: the requisites, 4th ed. Philadelphia, PA: Elsevier, 2014

# Case 58

*Ely A. Wolin*

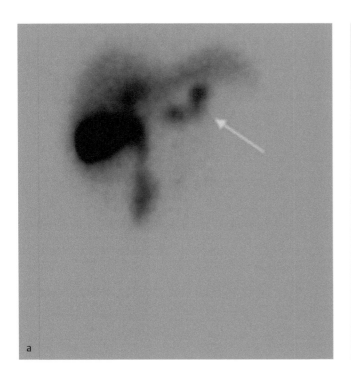

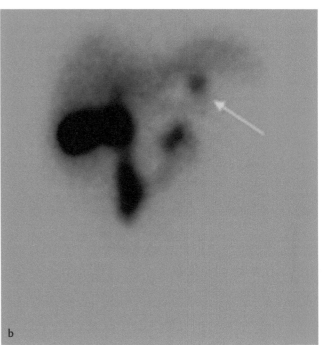

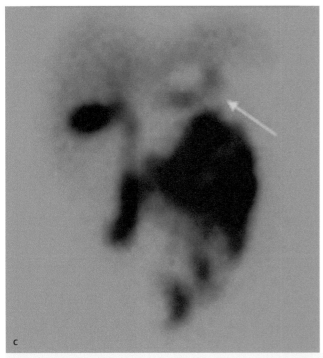

**Fig. 58.1** Gastric activity is seen on representative 1-, 17-, and 43-minute left anterior oblique images (**a** to **c**) from dynamic acquisition during 60-minute cholecystokinin (CCK) administration (*yellow arrows*).

## ■ Clinical History

48 year-old female referred for hepatobiliary scan (▶Fig. 58.1).

## ■ Key Finding

Gastric activity on hepatobiliary scintigraphy (HBS)

## ■ Top 2 Differential Diagnoses

- **Enterogastric reflux.** HBS is most commonly performed for evaluation for cholecystitis. When the clinical concern is for chronic cholecystitis, usually secondary to chronic recurrent biliary colic type symptoms, it is important to recognize enterogastric reflux. Activity from a Tc-99m-tagged iminodiacetic acid (IDA) analog seen in the stomach suggests enterogastric reflux. This can be transient or persistent and may occur before or after CCK-8 augmentation. The finding is important because enterogastric reflux can cause an alkaline gastritis that may mimic chronic cholecystitis clinically. Reflux of bile into the stomach also facilitates *Helicobacter pylori* colonization, and can be associated with chronic inflammation and metaplasia. The reflux may reach the esophagus and may be responsible for cases of refractory gastroesophageal reflux disease. Some have postulated that visualization of enterogastric reflux, or at least worsening of reflux, after CCK-8 injection is more likely to represent a clinically significant finding as this suggests postprandial symptoms similar to cholecystitis. Minimal, transient reflux of activity from the duodenum into the stomach may be a normal finding. Larger quantities and persistent reflux are more likely to be symptomatic. Enterogastric reflux is more common in the postcholecystectomy state, possibly due to the loss of the gallbladder's reservoir capacity leading to increased flow of bile into the duodenum. It can be seen with a variety of etiologies including prior partial gastrectomy, scleroderma, duodenitis, pancreatitis, and after narcotics administration.
- **Free pertechnetate.** If unbound Tc-99m is injected or radiopharmaceutical dissociation occurs, there may be free pertechnetate uptake in the gastric mucosa. While this may mimic enterogastric reflux, it should look different scintigraphically as activity will not be seen flowing in to the stomach on the dynamic images and the uptake will not have transient properties. The physiologic uptake of Tc-99m pertechnetate by gastric mucosa is the reason it is the radiopharmaceutical used for Meckel's diverticulum evaluation.

## ■ Diagnosis

Enterogastric reflux.

## ✓ Pearls

- Enterogastric reflux can result in alkaline gastritis that may mimic chronic cholecystitis clinically.
- Presence of enterogastric reflux facilitates gastric colonization of *H. pylori*.
- Enterogastric reflux visualized after CCK-8 administration may be more clinically significant.
- Efforts to quantify enterogastric reflux with stomach and hepatobiliary regions of interest have been suggested.

## Suggested Readings

Arroyo AJ, Burns JB, Huyghe WA, Dollman AE, Patel YP. Enterogastric reflux mimicking gallbladder disease: detection, quantitation and potential significance. J Nucl Med Technol. 1999; 27(3):207–214

Covington MF, Krupinski E, Avery R, Kuo PH. Classification schema of symptomatic enterogastric reflux utilizing sincalide augmentation on HBS. J Nucl Med Technol. 2014; 42:198–202

# Case 59

*Trevor A. Thompson*

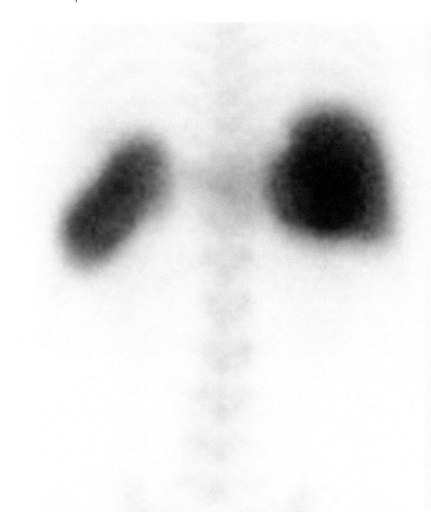

**Fig. 59.1** Posterior planar image from a liver spleen scan utilizing 7.7 mCi of technetium-99m sulfur colloid (Tc-99m SC) shows mildly increased splenic activity which is approaching the intensity of the liver along with more than expected bone marrow uptake.

■ **Clinical History**

68-year-old female with hepatopathy (▶ Fig. 59.1).

## ■ Key Finding

Increased splenic uptake on SC liver–spleen scintigraphy ("colloid shift")

## ■ Top 3 Differential Diagnoses

- **Hepatic metastatic disease.** The normal biodistribution of Tc-99m SC results in greater activity within the liver than spleen. Reversal of this pattern, so called colloid shift, with spleen to liver uptake ratio of greater than 2:1, results from decreased liver uptake or increased splenic uptake. Metastatic disease of the liver, most commonly due to gastrointestinal adenocarcinoma, is the most common cause of colloid shift on SC imaging. Replacement of the liver parenchyma by photopenic malignant tissue results in overall decreased liver uptake. Displacement and distortion of the normal liver architecture may also contribute to decreased colloid uptake. As decreased hepatic uptake has occasionally been reported in those with metastatic disease not involving the liver, secondary effects of systemic malignancy on the reticuloendothelial system (RES) may also play a role.
- **Hepatocyte dysfunction.** This is the second most common cause of colloid shift. Common causes of diffuse hepatocyte dysfunction include cirrhosis (alcoholic and nonalcoholic), hepatic steatosis, and hepatitis. While hepatitis can result in colloid shift, acuity of disease likely plays a role in imaging findings as some patients with acute hepatitis demonstrate a normal liver–spleen uptake ratio. Diabetes mellitus, while commonly associated with fatty liver disease, has been shown to result in colloid shift even in the absence of additional imaging evidence of fatty change within the liver.
- **Reticuloendothelial system overstimulation.** Overstimulation of the extrahepatic RES, most commonly in the setting of anemia, results in increased splenic uptake as well as commonly an associated increase in bone marrow uptake. As the majority of patients with anemia undergoing SC scintigraphy have underlying malignancy or liver disease, it is unclear whether primary anemia in the absence of these comorbidities is truly associated with a measurable colloid shift.

## ■ Additional Diagnostic Considerations

- **Trauma:** Relatively increased splenic uptake has been demonstrated on SC imaging following blunt abdominal trauma, even in the absence of additional evidence of direct splenic injury. Altered uptake has been demonstrated as early as 1 week following trauma and, in some cases, found to persist for greater than 6 months. Generalized posttraumatic stimulation of the extrahepatic RES is postulated to account for acute changes. Tuftsin, a phagocytic stimulator, may be responsible for prolonged findings. The presence of colloid shift in these cases does not correlate with patient prognosis.

## ■ Diagnosis

Hepatocyte dysfunction.

## ✓ Pearls

- Systemic metastatic disease can result in a colloid shift even if there is no direct involvement of the liver.
- Acute hepatitis may demonstrate either a colloid shift or a normal liver–spleen uptake relationship.
- Diabetes mellitus may demonstrate a colloid shift even in the absence of associated hepatic steatosis.
- Colloid shift in the setting of RES overstimulation typically demonstrates increased bone marrow uptake.
- Posttraumatic colloid shift may persist for more than 6 months and does not correlate with prognosis.

## Suggested Readings

Bekerman C, Gottschalk A. Diagnostic significance of the relative uptake of liver compared with spleen in Tc-99m sulfur colloid scintiphotography. J Nucl Med. 1971; 12(5):237–240

Briggs RC, Amberson SM. Colloid shift following blunt trauma. J Nucl Med. 1987; 28(2):188–190

Chakraborty D, Sunil HV, Mittal BR, Bhattacharya A, Singh B, Chawla Y. Role of Tc99 m sulfur colloid scintigraphy in differentiating non-cirrhotic portal fibrosis from cirrhosis liver. Indian J Nucl Med. 2010; 25(4):139–142

Wilson GA, Keyes JW, Jr. The significance of the liver-spleen uptake ratio in liver scanning. J Nucl Med. 2074(15):593–597

# Part 6

**Gastrointestinal**

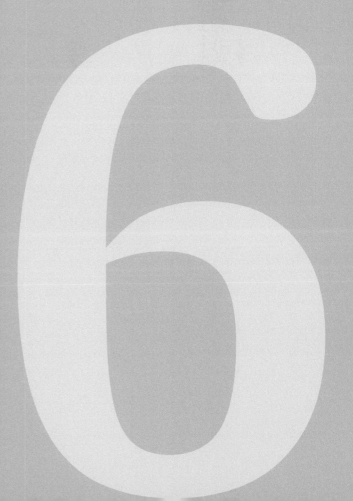

# Case 60

*Ely A. Wolin*

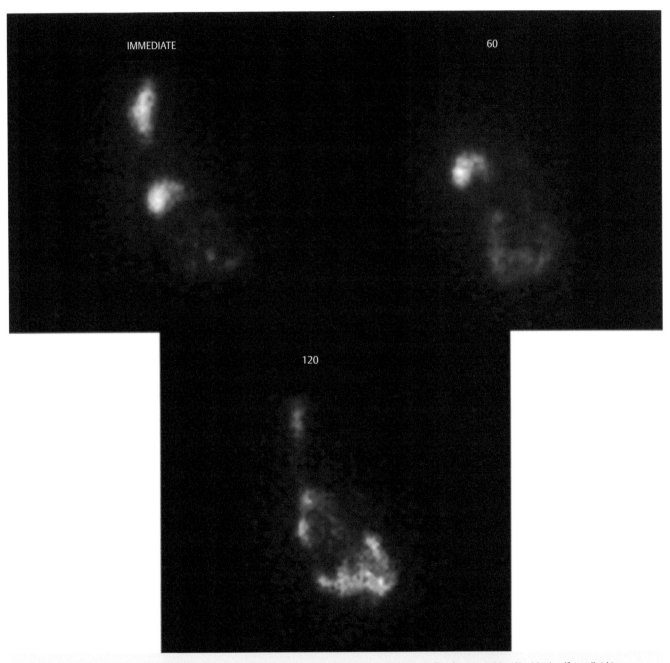

**Fig. 60.1** Immediate, 60-, and 120-minute images from a gastric emptying study using 0.953 mCi of technetium-99m (Tc-99m) sulfur colloid in a standard solid meal show uptake within the mid esophagus on the immediate images, with progression into the stomach and small bowel at 60 minutes, and recurrent high-level esophageal activity seen at 120 minutes.

## ■ Clinical History

88-year-old female with nausea after meals referred for gastric emptying study (▶ Fig. 60.1).

## ▪ Key Finding

Esophageal activity seen on gastric emptying study

## ▪ Top 2 Differential Diagnoses

• **Gastroesophageal reflux disease.** Scintigraphic gastric emptying studies are frequently performed for the evaluation of gastroparesis, and remain the gold standard. While much of the overall impression of a gastric emptying study is derived from the quantitative data, with well-defined normal limits of emptying at predetermined time points, it is very important to analyze the source images when interpreting the exam to ensure that the quantitative data is reliable, and also to evaluate for any other possibly clinically relevant findings. One such finding somewhat commonly seen is esophageal activity. Seeing activity in the esophagus, particularly if only seen on the more delayed images, is pathognomonic for gastroesophageal reflux disease (GERD). This is important to note as GERD may actually be responsible for the symptoms leading to the clinical concern for gastroparesis. Furthermore, there appears to be somewhat of a relationship between gastroparesis and GERD. It is thought that a delay in gastric emptying can either cause or exacerbate GERD. Delayed emptying can lead to distension and increased pressure in the gastric cardia which may shorten the lower esophageal sphincter, making it less effective. Prolonged gastric retention also gives gastric contents more time to reflux, increases gastric acid production, and can lead to higher volume reflux. Delayed gastric emptying has been found in up to one-third of adult patients with GERD. Although scintigraphy is not primarily performed for evaluation of GERD in the adult population, it is useful in the evaluation of suspected GERD in an infant. This does not include a standard gastric emptying evaluation, but instead is performed with a dedicated protocol usually involving 60-minute dynamic imaging of a supine infant after administration of Tc-99m radiolabeled milk or formula. It is a highly sensitive study that uses a normal, physiologic meal and does not require abdominal compression. If GERD is seen, either in an adult or pediatric patient, 24-hour images can be obtained to evaluate for pulmonary activity due to aspiration.

• **Esophageal retention.** Esophageal activity seen on a gastric emptying study may represent radiotracer that never made it into the stomach. If this is the case, activity should be seen in the esophagus on the initial image obtained immediately after oral intake of the radiolabeled meal and should decrease, not increase, on subsequent images.

## ▪ Diagnosis

Early esophageal retention with subsequent gastroesophageal reflux.

## ✓ Pearls

• Images from gastric emptying studies should be evaluated for evidence of gastroesophageal reflux.
• Up to one-third of adults with GERD have been found to have delayed gastric emptying.

• Delayed gastric emptying can both cause and exacerbate GERD.
• Scintigraphy is useful for the evaluation of an infant with suspected GERD.

## Suggested Readings

Abell TL, Camilleri M, Donohoe K, et al. American Neurogastroenterology and Motility Society and the Society of Nuclear Medicine. Consensus recommendations for gastric emptying scintigraphy: a joint report of the American Neurogastroenterology and Motility Society and the Society of Nuclear Medicine. J Nucl Med Technol. 2008; 36(1):44–54

Elbl B, Birkenfeld B, Walecka A, et al. Upper gastrointestinal tract scintigraphy and ultrasonography in diagnosis of gastroesophageal reflux in children. Pol J Radiol. 2011; 76(1):63–67

Fass R, McCallum RW, Parkman HP. Treatment challenges in the management of gastroparesis-related GERD. Gastroenterol Hepatol (N Y). 2009; 5(10, Suppl 18): 4–16

Mariani G, Boni G, Barreca M, et al. Radionuclide gastroesophageal motor studies. J Nucl Med. 2004; 45(6):1004–1028

# Case 61

*Trevor A. Thompson*

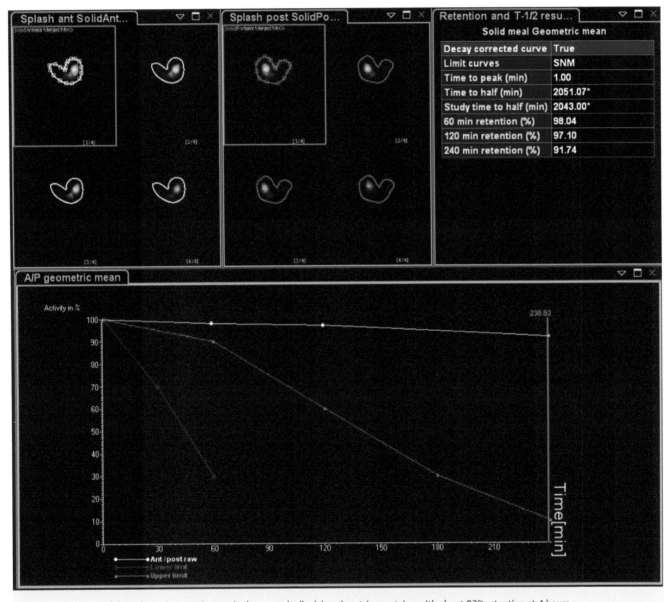

**Fig. 61.1** Standard solid meal gastric emptying study shows markedly delayed gastric emptying with about 92% retention at 4 hours.

■ **Clinical History**

64-year-old female with gastroparesis after Nissen fundoplication (▶Fig. 61.1).

## ■ Key Finding

Delayed solid meal gastric emptying

## ■ Top 3 Differential Diagnoses

- **Diabetic gastroenteropathy.** Gastroparesis, or delayed gastric emptying in the absence of mechanical obstruction, is most commonly caused by diabetes mellitus (DM). It affects approximately 5% of those with type 1 DM and 1% of those with type 2 DM. Diabetic gastroenteropathy is presumed secondary to autonomic neuropathy involving the stomach and is typically seen in the setting of other diabetic complications including retinopathy, nephropathy, and peripheral neuropathy. The hyperglycemia seen in DM also suppresses gastric motility and delays gastric emptying. In fact, rapid gastric emptying (RGE) leading to spikes in serum glucose may precede the onset of DM and gastroparesis. Clinical predictors of diabetic gastroenteropathy include abdominal bloating, female gender, high glucose levels, and high body mass index (BMI).
- **Postsurgical gastroparesis.** Surgical vagotomy, performed for the treatment of refractory peptic ulcer disease, intentionally compromises the vagal innervation to the stomach in an effort to decrease gastric acid secretion. However, decreased vagal (parasympathetic) innervation also significantly prolongs gastric emptying, unless pyloroplasty is performed concurrently. Inadvertent vagal nerve injury may occur as a complication of procedures such as fundoplication and gastric bypass.
- **Viral/postviral gastroparesis.** Gastroparesis can present as an acute symptom related to viral gastroenteritis, most commonly due to norovirus or enterovirus. It may also present in a delayed manner following a prodromal gastrointestinal (GI) or respiratory infection, known as postviral gastroparesis (PVGP), a subtype of idiopathic gastroparesis. While both conditions are typically self-limited, symptoms related to PVGP may be prolonged and persist for months to years. PVGP secondary to cytomegalovirus, Epstein–Barr virus, and varicella zoster virus infection typically result in the longest duration of symptoms.

## ■ Additional Diagnostic Consideration

- **Medications:** Several classes of medication can alter gastric motor function and result in either accelerated or delayed gastric emptying. Prokinetic agents that accelerate gastric emptying, include metoclopramide, tegaserod, erythromycin, and domperidone. Medications that can delay gastric emptying include opiates, benzodiazepines, anticholinergics (i.e., atropine, dicyclomine, tricyclic antidepressants), calcium channel blockers, and aluminum-containing antacids, as well as phenobarbital, progesterone, and octreotide. Discontinuation of these medications for 48 to 72 hours prior to imaging is important to avoid false-positive or false-negative gastric emptying results due to medication effects.

## ■ Diagnosis

Severely delayed gastric emptying; possible vagal nerve injury.

## ✓ Pearls

- Diabetic gastroenteropathy is the most common cause of gastroparesis.
- Gastroparesis can be due to acute viral gastroenteritis or present following a viral prodrome (PVGP).
- Surgical vagal nerve injury results in delayed gastric emptying unless pyloroplasty is also performed.
- Numerous medications can result in false-positive or false-negative findings on gastric emptying studies.

## Suggested Readings

Camilleri M, Parkman HP, Shafi MA, Abell TL, Gerson L. American College of Gastroenterology. Clinical guideline: management of gastroparesis. Am J Gastroenterol. 2013; 108(1):18–37, quiz 38

Mariani G, Boni G, Barreca M, et al. Radionuclide gastroesophageal motor studies. J Nucl Med. 2004; 45(6):1004–1028

Maurer AH. Gastrointestinal motility, part 1: esophageal transit and gastric emptying. J Nucl Med. 2015; 56(8):1229–1238

# Case 62

*Brady S. Davis*

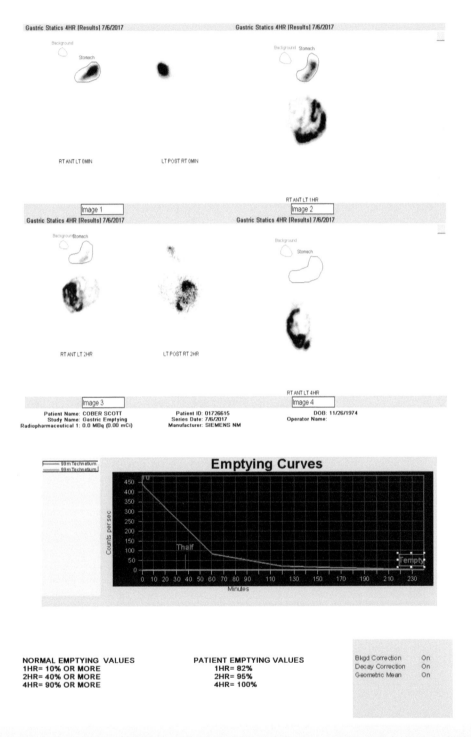

**Fig. 62.1** Anterior and posterior images obtained immediately following technetium-99m sulfur colloid (Tc-99m SC)-labeled international standardized solid meal ingestion, and again at 1, 2, and 4 hours. Qualitatively the emptying appears to be rapid with little retained meal noted at 2 hours. This is confirmed on the elimination curves based on region of interest location on static images, demonstrating 82% gastric emptying at 1 hour (normal is 10–70%). This is consistent with rapid gastric emptying.

## ■ Clinical History

34-year-old female presenting with abdominal discomfort with meals (▶ Fig. 62.1).

(Case courtesy of Joseph S. Fotos, MD, Penn State Hershey Medical Center.)

■ **Key Finding**

Rapid gastric emptying

■ **Top 3 Differential Diagnoses**

- **Gastric surgery.** RGE, or dumping syndrome, can be difficult to distinguish clinically from delayed gastric emptying as they can present with similar symptoms including nausea, vomiting, abdominal bloating, and cramping. Additional symptoms include diarrhea and cold sweats. RGE is defined as less than 70% of radiotracer left in the stomach at 30 minutes, or less than 30% left at 60 minutes, on a gastric emptying study utilizing the standard solid meal. The result is too much undigested, hyperosmolar food reaching the small bowel. While it is decreasing in prevalence, RGE remains a relatively common complication of gastric surgeries such as pyloroplasty, antrectomy, Roux-en-Y gastric bypass, gastrojejunostomy, and Nissen fundoplication (children). These surgeries can all result in RGE due to alteration of the gastric outlet, or altering the reservoir capabilities of the stomach.

- **Diabetes mellitus.** Although DM is classically associated with delayed gastric emptying, early DM, particularly type 2, can present with RGE. This is likely in part due to early vagal nerve damage. RGE may, in fact, precede DM with the rapid emptying and absorption of carbohydrates which may be a possible causative factor for elevated glucose levels.

- **Gastrinoma.** Gastrin hormone is normally produced by G cells in the antrum of the stomach and physiologically increases gastric acid secretion, growth of gastric mucosa, and gastric motility. Gastrinoma is a tumor found in the pancreas (75%) or duodenum (15%) that independently secretes gastrin leading to Zollinger–Ellison syndrome which is characterized by peptic ulcers, diarrhea, and RGE.

■ **Additional Diagnostic Considerations**

- **Medication effect:** Multiple medications can cause RGE such as metoclopramide, domperidone, cisapride, erythromycin, and motilin.
- **Hyperthyroidism:** Thyroid hormone is believed to cause hypermobility of not only the stomach, but also the large and

small bowel. Nearly 15% of poorly controlled hyperthyroid patients experience diarrhea, constipation, or RGE.
- **Additional nonsurgical causes:** RGE can also be seen in association with hypertension, viral illness, and cyclic vomiting syndrome. RGE may also be idiopathic.

■ **Diagnosis**

Rapid gastric emptying, unknown etiology.

✓ **Pearls**

- RGE, while less prevalent, remains a common complication of gastric surgery.
- Rapid, instead of delayed, gastric emptying can be seen with DM and it may possibly precede diabetes.

- Several medications, often used for treatment of gastroparesis, and can result in RGE.

**Suggested Readings**

Balan K, Sonoda LI, Seshadri N, Solanki C, Middleton S. Clinical significance of scintigraphic rapid gastric emptying. Nucl Med Commun. 2011; 32(12):1185–1189

Berg P, McCallum R. Dumping syndrome: a review of the current concepts of pathophysiology, diagnosis, and treatment. Dig Dis Sci. 2016; 61(1):11–18

Cooper CJ, Said S, Bizet J, Alkahateeb H, Sarosiek I, McCallum RW. Rapid or normal gastric emptying as new supportive criteria for diagnosing cyclic vomiting syndrome in adults. Med Sci Monit. 2014; 20:1491–1495

# Case 63

*Ely A. Wolin*

**University Health System**

4502 Medical Drive
San Antonio, Texas 78229

**¹⁴C-Urea Breath Test**                                    February 6, 2018

| Test Date | First Name | Last Name |
|---|---|---|
| DOB | Patient ID# | Referring Dr. |

Confounding Factors: (Check all that apply or NONE)

- [✓] NONE
- [ ] Antibiotics (Last 30 days)
- [ ] Proton Pump Inhibitors (Last 14 days)
- [ ] Bismuth (Last 30 days)
- [ ] Sucralfate (Last 14 days)

Sample CPM: *1012 10*

BKG CPM: *32.0*

Scintillator Efficiency: *94 4*

$$DPM = \frac{Sample\ CPM - BKG\ CPM}{Scintillator\ Efficiency}$$

DPM Result: *1038.20*

| INTERPRETATION | RESULTS |
|---|---|
| < 50 DPM | NEGATIVE |
| 50-199 DPM | INDETERMINATE |
| ≥ 200 DPM | POSITIVE |

**Fig. 63.1** Results from urea breath test show 1038.20 disintegrations per minute.

## ■ Clinical History

51-year-old male with DM type 2, hypertension, and obesity with complaints of abdominal pain for several weeks (▶Fig. 63.1).

(Case courtesy of Umber Salman, M.D., University of Texas Health San Antonio.)

## ■ Key Finding

Positive urea breath test

## ■ Top 2 Differential Diagnoses

- **_Helicobacter pylori_ infection.** It is a Gram-negative bacteria that leads to chronic inflammation of the gastric mucosa that is known to be associated with duodenal and gastric ulcers, and gastric cancer. The bacteria have high urease activity allowing them to survive in the acidic environment of the stomach by converting urea to alkaline ammonia and carbon dioxide ($CO_2$). Diagnosis is often performed by endoscopy with biopsy, as well as with serum immunoglobulin titers and stool antigen testing. However, the urea breath test (UBT) offers a noninvasive and reliable test for the presence of _H. pylori._ UBT involves the oral administration of a capsule containing urea tagged with carbon-14 (C-14), which is a beta emitter with a physical half-life of around 5,730 years and maximum energy of 160 keV. Depending on the method used, about 10 minutes after ingesting the dose the patient exhales a deep breath through a straw into a mylar balloon. The air from the balloon is then transferred with a pump and tubing into a scintillation vial containing a trapping solution. The blue fluid turns clear after trapping 1 mmol of $CO_2$ and is then mixed with scintillation fluid. The samples, a normal breath sample and a C-14 standard sample, are all counted in a liquid scintillation counter (LSC). This process is frequently performed off site at a laboratory with the appropriate facilities. The background and LSC efficiency corrected disintegrations per minute (DPM) are calculated. Increased DPM indicates the presence of radioactive $CO_2$ due to the incorporation of C-14. This occurs in the presence of urease enzyme which is not present in normal breath. The enzyme hydrolyzes the urea into ammonia and $^{14}CO_2$. This $^{14}CO_2$ is absorbed and brought to the lungs for exhalation. DPM greater than or equal to 200 at 10 minutes is considered positive for _H. pylori._ Several medications are known to cause a false-negative result, including antibiotics, bismuth, sucralfate, and proton pump inhibitors. UBT is especially useful for follow up after eradication therapy as it is sensitive enough to detect patchy colonization which might be missed with biopsy. A Carbon-13 tagged urea can also be used for the test, but requires use of a mass spectrometer or infrared spectrophotometer instead of an LSC.
- **Other urease-producing microorganisms.** Bacteria other that _H. pylori_ with urease activity can be found in both the oral cavity and the stomach that may lead to a false-positive exam. Such bacteria include _Proteus mirabilis, Klebsiella pneumoniae,_ and _Staphylococcus aureus._

## ■ Diagnosis

_Helicobacter pylori_ infection.

## ✓ Pearls

- UBT is a noninvasive test for the presence of _H. pylori_, particularly useful after eradication.
- Patient should fast for 6 hours and discontinue antibiotics and bismuth for 30 days prior to UBT.
- Hold proton pump inhibitors for 14 days and $H_2$ blockers for 24 hours prior to UBT.
- UBT is less sensitive after partial gastric resection, likely due to more rapid gastric transit.

## Suggested Readings

Dede F, Civen H, Dane F, et al. Carbon-14 urea breath test: does it work in patients with partial gastric resection? Ann Nucl Med. 2015; 29(9):786–791

Ferwana M, Abdulmajeed I, Alhajiahmed A, et al. Accuracy of urea breath test in Helicobacter pylori infection: meta-analysis. World J Gastroenterol. 2015; 21(4):1305–1314

Patel SK, Pratap CB, Jain AK, Gulati AK, Nath G. Diagnosis of Helicobacter pylori: what should be the gold standard? World J Gastroenterol. 2014; 20(36):12847–12859

# Case 64

*Kamal D. Singh*

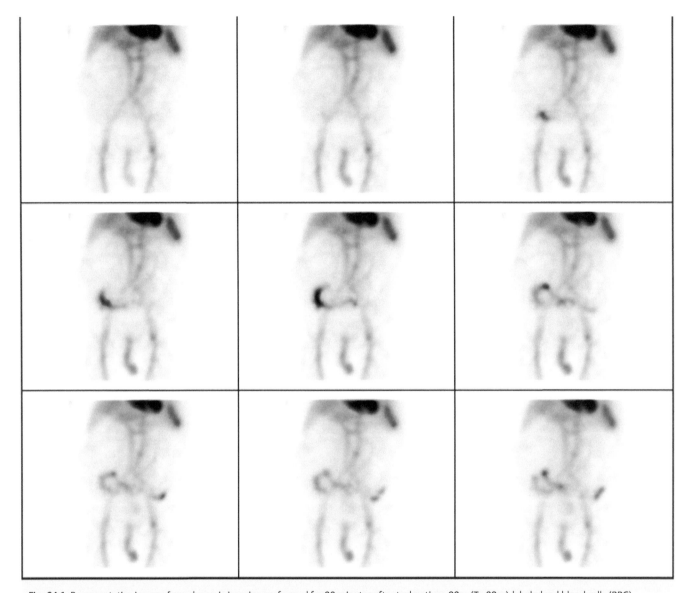

**Fig. 64.1** Representative images from dynamic imaging performed for 90 minutes after technetium-99m (Tc-99m)-labeled red blood cells (RBC) administration show the appearance of extravascular activity in the right lower quadrant which appears to conform to bowel, progresses in intensity, and demonstrates both retrograde and antegrade movement.

■ **Clinical History**

89-year-old male with lower GI bleed with only diverticuli noted on colonoscopy 6 weeks prior (▶ Fig. 64.1).

## ■ Key Finding

Intra-abdominal activity on Tc-99m-labeled RBC scan

## ■ Top 3 Differential Diagnoses

- **Active gastrointestinal (GI) bleed.** Tc-99m RBC scan is obtained for confirmation and localization of an active lower GI bleed (hematochezia or bright red blood per rectum) prior to angiographic intervention. In contrast, patients with hematemesis from an upper GI bleed (proximal to ligament of Treitz) typically undergo endoscopy for diagnosis and management. Common causes of lower GI bleed include diverticulosis, angiodysplasia, inflammatory bowel disease (IBD), and neoplasm. After IV administration of the Tc-labeled RBC, dynamic imaging is performed for 60 to 90 minutes. Classic findings for active lower GI bleed include a focus of activity which appears and conforms to bowel anatomy, increases in activity over time, and demonstrates peristalsis (intraluminal antegrade or retrograde transit). Scintigraphy is highly sensitive and can detect bleeding rates as low as 0.1 mL/min, compared to 1 mL/min for angiography. Given the intermittent nature of most GI bleeds, Tc-labeled RBC scan allows for delayed imaging up to 24 hours from the time of initial injection. However, if bleeding is only detected on the delayed static imaging, precise localization is not possible.
- **Neoplasm or IBD.** Hypervascular intestinal tumors and vascular malformations or IBD may be detected on a Tc-99m-labeled RBC scan as focal or segmental static activity that does not change in position over time. Cross-sectional imaging or colonoscopy may aid in definitive diagnosis.
- **Genitourinary activity.** An area of activity that is fixed in location is not typical of an active GI bleed. Common causes of fixed activity include urinary tract activity, especially within the bladder, due to renal excretion of Tc-RBC. In addition, penile activity in a male and uterine activity in a menstruating female can mimic rectosigmoid bleeding. Static lateral views are useful in distinguishing these entities from an active GI bleed.

## ■ Additional Diagnostic Consideration

- **Free technetium:** The in vitro technique for Tc-RBC allows for higher labeling efficiency (98%) compared to the modified in vivo (90%) or the in vivo (80%) methods. A higher labeling efficiency results in less free or unbound technetium in the bloodstream. Excess free technetium accumulates in the gastric mucosa and may enter the small bowel through peristalsis, simulating an active GI bleed. Imaging over the neck to detect thyroid activity can confirm presence of free technetium.

## ■ Diagnosis

Active lower GI bleed.

## ✓ Pearls

- In vitro labeling of RBC has high labeling efficiency and is the preferred method for GI bleed scan.
- If bleeding is not detected on initial dynamic imaging, delayed images can be obtained up to 24 hours.
- Technetium-99m sulfur colloid (Tc-99m SC) scan has shorter prep time but does not offer the flexibility of delayed imaging.
- Etiologies of false-positive scans usually present as focal activity without peristalsis.

## Suggested Readings

Currie GM, Kiat H, Wheat JM. Scintigraphic evaluation of acute lower gastrointestinal hemorrhage: current status and future directions. J Clin Gastroenterol. 2011; 45(2):92–99

Mariani G, Pauwels EKJ, AlSharif A, et al. Radionuclide evaluation of the lower gastrointestinal tract. J Nucl Med. 2008; 49(5):776–787

Uliel L, Mellnick VM, Menias CO, Holz AL, McConathy J. Nuclear medicine in the acute clinical setting: indications, imaging findings, and potential pitfalls. Radiographics. 2013; 33(2):375–396

# Case 65

*Kamal D. Singh*

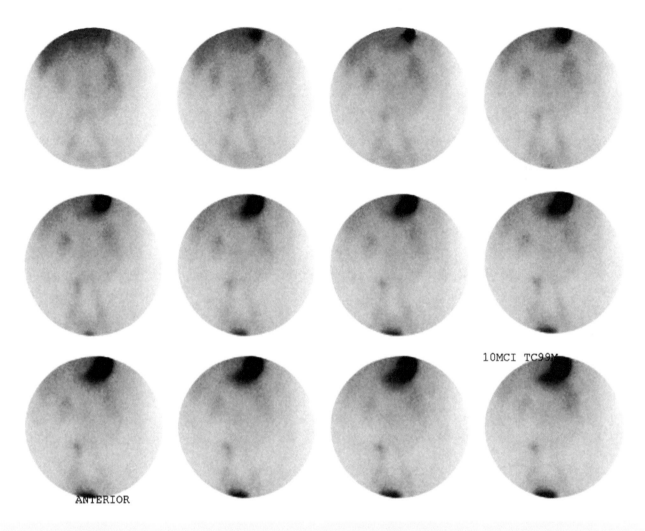

**Fig. 65.1** Sequential images from a Meckel's scan with technetium-99m (Tc-99m) pertechnetate demonstrate focal uptake in the right lower quadrant which appears at the same time as the physiologic gastric mucosal activity and intensifies over time without evidence of peristalsis. The anterior intra-abdominal location of this activity was confirmed on a static lateral projection (not included). Physiologic urinary excretion of radiotracer is also noted.

## ■ Clinical History

8-year-old male with chronic abdominal discomfort and history of intermittent lower GI bleeding (▶ Fig. 65.1).

## ■ Key Finding

Focal intra-abdominal activity on pertechnetate imaging

## ■ Top 3 Differential Diagnoses

- **Meckel's diverticulum.** It is the congenital persistence of the omphalomesenteric (vitelline) duct. It occurs in 2% of the population, has a 2:1 male-to-female ratio, occurs 2 feet from the ileocecal valve, and generally affects children within 2 years of age (rule of 2's). Although not all Meckel's diverticula have gastric mucosa, the vast majority of symptomatic cases do. Patients may present with bleeding, obstruction, intussusception, or volvulus. Tc-99m pertechnetate is taken up by mucin-producing cells and can detect enteric diverticula with ectopic gastric mucosa. Proper patient preparation can improve sensitivity of a Meckel scan, which includes nothing by mouth (nil per os, NPO) for at least 4 hours with possible pretreatment with cimetidine (blocks radiotracer release from ectopic mucosa), pentagastrin (enhances ectopic mucosal uptake), and glucagon (decreases small bowel peristalsis). Focal activity in the right lower quadrant, which appears at the same time as physiologic gastric uptake, intensifies over time and is nonperistaltic, is diagnostic of a Meckel's diverticulum. Uptake usually appears within 30 minutes but may take up to 60 minutes depending upon the amount of gastric mucosa present. False-negative studies may be due to absence of gastric mucosa (no radiotracer uptake mechanism) or secondary to diverticular ischemia/necrosis.

- **Focal intra-abdominal infectious or inflammatory processes.** False-positive studies may occur in the setting of focal infectious or inflammatory intra-abdominal processes, or with heterotopic gastric mucosa, such as GI duplication cyst with heterotopic gastric mucosa, inflammatory bowel disease, appendicitis, and focal enteritis/colitis. Hypervascular masses, such as arteriovenous malformations and other neoplasms, may also be seen as focal regions of increased activity on a Meckel scan. With the exception of duplication cyst with heterotopic gastric mucosa, the remainder of these entities demonstrate increased blood pool activity which fades over time, rather than focal activity that mirrors physiologic gastric activity. Correlation with cross-sectional imaging may be necessary in some cases to differentiate these conditions from a true Meckel's diverticulum.
- **Physiologic renal/urinary activity.** Additional static lateral views can confirm whether focal activity is intra-abdominal or retroperitoneal in location. Upright and postvoid imaging can also help distinguish physiologic activity within a distended renal pelvis, ureter, ectopic kidney, or bladder diverticulum from a Meckel's diverticulum.

## ■ Diagnosis

Meckel's diverticulum.

## ✓ Pearls

- Tc-99m pertechnetate scan detects Meckel's diverticulum with ectopic gastric mucosa.
- Focal intra-abdominal activity that intensifies over time without peristalsis suggests a Meckel's diverticulum.

- False-positives include urinary tracer excretion and intra-abdominal inflammatory/infectious processes.

## Suggested Readings

Emamian SA, Shalaby-Rana E, Majd M. The spectrum of heterotopic gastric mucosa in children detected by Tc-99m pertechnetate scintigraphy. Clin Nucl Med. 2001; 26(6):529–535

Lin S, Suhocki PV, Ludwig KA, Shetzline MA. Gastrointestinal bleeding in adult patients with Meckel's diverticulum: the role of technetium 99 m pertechnetate scan. South Med J. 2002; 95(11):1338–1341

Treves ST, Grand RJ. Gastrointestinal bleeding. In: Treves ST, ed. Pediatric Nuclear Medicine. New York, NY: Springer-Verlag; 1995

# Case 66

*Ely A. Wolin*

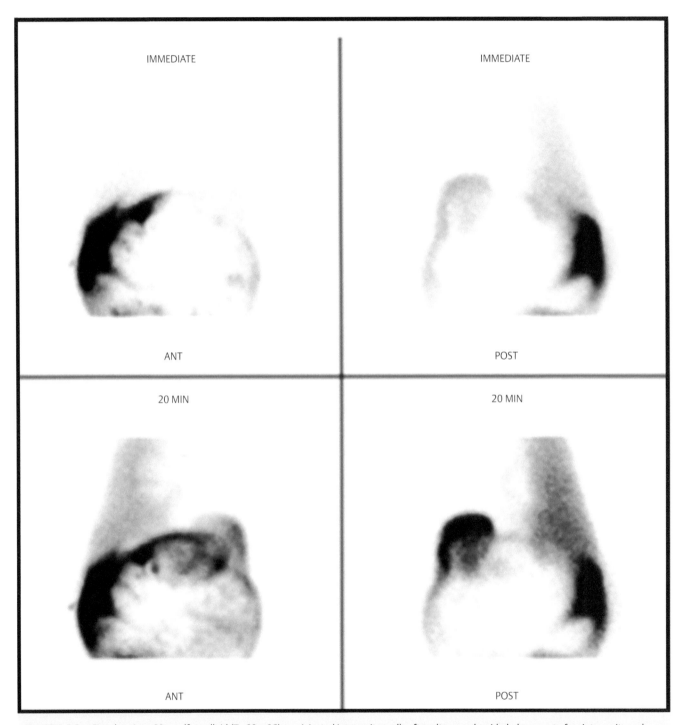

**Fig. 66.1** 3.3 mCi technetium-99m sulfur colloid (Tc-99m SC) was injected intraperitoneally after ultrasound-guided placement of an intraperitoneal catheter. Immediate and 20-minute anterior and posterior planar images show radiotracer dispersed throughout intraperitoneal ascites, the majority in the perihepatic region near the site of injection along with homogenous activity throughout the right hemithorax.

■ **Clinical History**

.................................................................................

80-year-old female cirrhotic with recurrent hydrothorax and ascites (▶ Fig. 66.1).

## ■ Key Finding

Pleural activity on peritoneal scintigraphy

## ■ Top 2 Differential Diagnoses

- **Diaphragmatic defect.** Peritoneal scintigraphy can be performed using either Tc-99m SC or Tc-99m macroaggregated albumin (MAA). The radiopharmaceutical is injected directly into the peritoneal cavity using aseptic technique. This is generally performed for evaluation of patency of a peritoneovenous (PV) shunt. If the shunt is intact, serial images over 1 to 2 hours will show activity in the liver and spleen (for Tc-99m SC) or in the lungs (for Tc-99m MAA). Pleural activity is an abnormal finding and suggests the presence of a diaphragmatic defect, either congenital fenestration or traumatic perforation. This is a known complication of chronic peritoneal dialysis as well.
- **Hepatic hydrothorax.** A pleural effusion in the setting hepatic failure and ascites raises the concern for hepatic hydrothorax.

This occurs in around 10% of cirrhotic patients. The etiology is not definitively known, but likely results from ascitic fluid transiting through small, possibly microscopic, diaphragmatic defects or via lymphatic channels. Hepatic hydrothorax can occur without significant ascites as well, likely due to the negative intrathoracic pressure during inspiration. These patients can present with dyspnea, cough, and pleuritic chest pain. Peritoneal scintigraphy is not usually required for diagnosis, but can be performed in uncertain cases. If needed, it is best to do this study after thoracentesis to prevent a false-negative exam due to pressure from the pleural effusion. Hepatic hydrothorax is suggested in patients with a large transudative pleural effusion, usually on the right side, with no primary cardiopulmonary or malignant process.

## ■ Diagnosis

Hepatic hydrothorax.

## ✓ Pearls

- Peritoneal scintigraphy can be used to document the patency of a PV shunt.
- A patent PV shunt will result in Tc-99m SC activity in liver/spleen or Tc-99m MAA activity in lungs.
- Hepatic hydrothorax can occur without ascites due to negative intrathoracic pressure on inspiration.
- Peritoneal scintigraphy can be used to diagnose hepatic hydrothorax in uncertain cases.

## Suggested Readings

Badillo R, Rockey DC. Hepatic hydrothorax: clinical features, management, and outcomes in 77 patients and review of the literature. Medicine (Baltimore). 2014; 93(3):135–142

Bhattacharya A, Mittal BR, Biswas T, et al. Radioisotope scintigraphy in the diagnosis of hepatic hydrothorax. J Gastroenterol Hepatol. 2001; 16(3):317–321

Shimbo A, Matsuda S, Tejima K, et al. Induced negative pressure proposed as a new method for diagnosing hepatic hydrothorax involving minor leaks. Clin Case Rep. 2014; 2(6):296–302

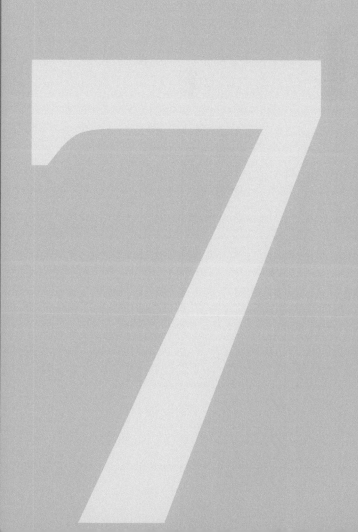

# Part 7

## Genitourinary

# Case 67

*Ely A. Wolin*

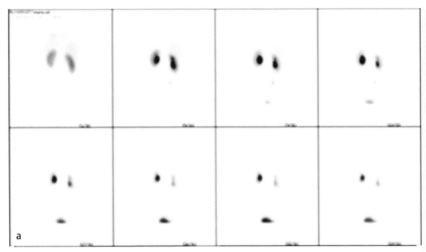

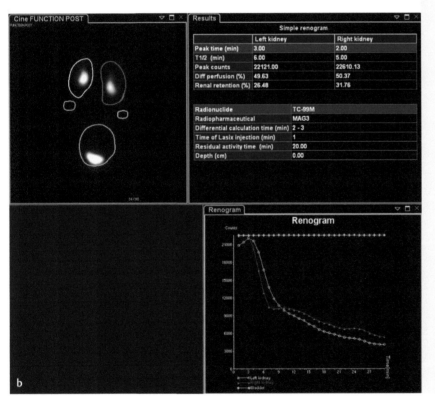

**Fig. 67.1** **(a)** Compressed 4-minute images from Tc-99m mercaptoacetyltriglycine (MAG3) dynamic renography shows hold up of activity in the proximal left renal collecting system. **(b)** Quantitative data from subsequent dynamic imaging after the intravenous administration of Lasix shows prompt washout with a washout half time of 6 minutes on the left.

■ **Clinical History**

16-year-old female found to have bilateral hydronephrosis on renal ultrasound after evaluation for urinary tract infection (UTI) (▶ Fig. 67.1).

## ■ Key Finding

Delayed washout on a Tc-99m MAG3 renography without diuretic augmentation

## ■ Top 3 Differential Diagnoses

• **Mechanical obstruction.** When a patient is noted to have hydronephrosis on anatomic imaging, it is important to be able to delineate if the collecting system dilation is due to a mechanical obstruction, i.e., secondary to stricture, mass, or stone. This is the main reason behind performing diuretic renography in nuclear medicine. A collecting system that shows delayed washout on standard Tc-99m MAG3 renography, usually considered a half emptying time greater than 15 minutes, should be given a diuretic with continued dynamic assessment of the kidneys. If the collecting system washout remains delayed, it is suggestive of mechanical obstruction.

• **Vesicoureteral reflux (VUR).** Not all cases of collecting system dilation are secondary to a mechanical obstruction. Urine is propagated from the renal pelvis, down the ureter, and into the bladder by smooth muscle cells. Any failure in this propagation can result in collecting system dilation even without the presence of a mechanical obstruction. This is known as a functional obstruction or functional retention. In these patients, the collecting system washout time will normalize after the administration of a loop diuretic as the resultant increased hydrostatic pressure (assuming functioning nephrons) overcomes the functional obstruction. A washout half time of less than 10 minutes after diuretic administration is definitely normal and less than 15 minutes is likely normal. VUR can cause a dilated but otherwise normal collecting system. Associated recurrent infection/inflammation can also lead to reduced ureteral peristalsis resulting in a functional obstruction.

• **Prior obstruction or infection.** Previous but resolved mechanical obstruction or infection of the upper urinary tract can result in a dilated, but not obstructed, collecting system secondary to a patulous system with decreased peristalsis.

## ■ Additional Diagnostic Consideration

• **Primary megaureter:** It is a term used to describe multiple entities involving a congenital abnormality of the distal ureter and ureterectasis. Primary megaureter can be refluxing, obstructing, or nonrefluxing and nonobstructing. Obstructed primary megaureter is thought to be secondary to an aperistaltic, possibly aganglionotic segment of the distal ureter similar to Hirschsprung's disease in the colon. The adynamic segment results in proximal dilation from relative obstruction which may be overcome by increased hydrostatic pressure.

## ■ Diagnosis

Patulous extrarenal pelvis post UTI.

## ✓ Pearls

• Diuretic renography is used to evaluate for a mechanical obstruction in a patient with hydronephrosis.

• Increased hydrostatic pressure from the diuretic can normalize washout in a functional obstruction.

• A dilated nonobstructed system can be from VUR, prior obstruction/infection, and primary megaureter.

• Collecting system half washout in under 10 minutes after diuretic administration is not obstructed.

## Suggested Readings

Berrocal T, López-Pereira P, Arjonilla A, Gutiérrez J. Anomalies of the distal ureter, bladder, and urethra in children: embryologic, radiologic, and pathologic features. Radiographics. 2002; 22(5):1139–1164

Taylor AT. Radionuclides in nephrourology, Part 2: pitfalls and diagnostic applications. J Nucl Med. 2014; 55(5):786–798

# Case 68

*Ely A. Wolin*

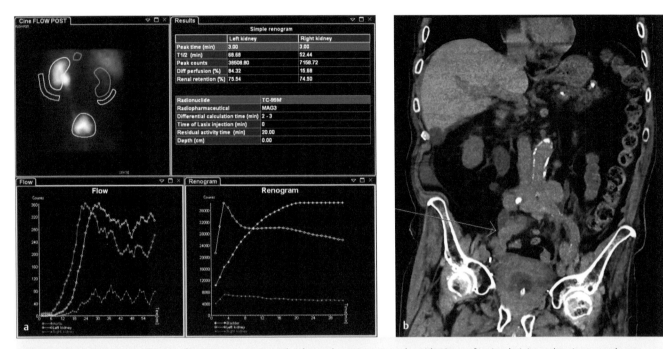

**Fig. 68.1** **(a)** Quantitative evaluation of Tc-99m mercaptoacetyltriglycine dynamic renography with 40 mg of Lasix administered at time zero shows markedly delayed and diminished flow to the right kidney with no right renal excretion. Left kidney shows normal flow with delayed washout concerning for obstruction. **(b)** Coronal image from correlative CT scan shows right hydroureter with abrupt cutoff at the level of enlarged lymph nodes (*arrow*). (Quality control: the left renal region of interested should have included the proximal collecting system.)

■ **Clinical History**

91-year-old male with recurrent metastatic prostate cancer admitted for urosepsis and acute renal failure with concern for ureteral obstruction (▶Fig. 68.1).

## ▪ Key Finding

Decreased renal perfusion on dynamic renography

## ▪ Top 3 Differential Diagnoses

- **Renal artery stenosis.** Renal perfusion is evaluated by the dynamic acquisition of 1 to 5 second images for the initial 60 seconds of renal scintigraphy. Visually, activity should be in the renal arteries within seconds of activity in the aorta, usually around the same time activity reaches the aortic bifurcation. Semiquantitative evaluation is done using whole kidney and aorta regions of interest (ROI). The time–activity curve (TAC) for each kidney should show rapid climb, within seconds of a similar rapid climb in the aorta, and then peak and level off at a level similar to each other and above the level of the aorta. Decreased flow to either kidney may be secondary to renal artery stenosis (RAS), most frequently caused by atherosclerotic disease and fibromuscular dysplasia. External compression on the renal artery, such as from tumor or fibrosis, can appear similar. Angiotensin-converting enzyme inhibitor (ACEI)-augmented renography can be performed in the evaluation of renovascular hypertension (RVH).

- **Ureteral obstruction.** It is important to identify ureteral obstruction and treat it as it can lead to obstructive nephropathy. Obstruction of urinary outflow results in increased intrarenal resistance due to both pressure and reactive vasoconstriction. Eventually, this results in decreased glomerular filtration rate (GFR) and, if left untreated, renal atrophy and fibrosis. Decreased renal flow on renal scintigraphy will not be the first sign of ureteral obstruction, but it is important to note along with other parameters indicating residual renal function.

- **Renal vein thrombosis.** The inability for blood to drain out of the kidney can lead to pressure extending across the renal vascular bed that increases resistance to arterial flow. Renal vein extension from tumor, such as in renal cell carcinoma and Wilms tumor, is important to exclude with anatomic imaging.

## ▪ Additional Diagnostic Considerations

- **Renal artery dissection:** Dissection is not a frequent cause of decreased renal perfusion. Renal perfusion may be completely absent if there is resultant acute complete occlusion of the renal artery. If a perfused kidney is not seen in the renal fossa, ectopia and prior resection should be excluded first.

- **Poor injection technique:** Poor injection bolus can result in a false positive for delayed flow. With a poor bolus, the TACs for the aorta and both kidneys will have a slow initial rise.

- **Subcapsular collection:** A high-pressure subcapsular collection can result in increased renal resistance and manifestations similar to RAS, the so-called Page kidney.

## ▪ Diagnosis

Likely prolonged right ureteral obstruction from pelvic adenopathy.

## ✓ Pearls

- Decreased renal perfusion can result from slow blood in, slow blood out, or slow urine out.
- It is important to ensure an adequate bolus of the radiopharmaceutical when evaluating renal perfusion.

- Exclude renal ectopia or prior resection if a perfused kidney is not seen in the renal fossa.

## Suggested Readings

Taylor AT. Radionuclides in nephrourology, Part 2: pitfalls and diagnostic applications. J Nucl Med. 2014; 55(5):786–798

Wolin EA, Hartman DS, Olson JR. Nephrographic and pyelographic analysis of CT urography: differential diagnosis. AJR Am J Roentgenol. 2013; 200(6): 1197–1203

# Case 69

*Brady S. Davis*

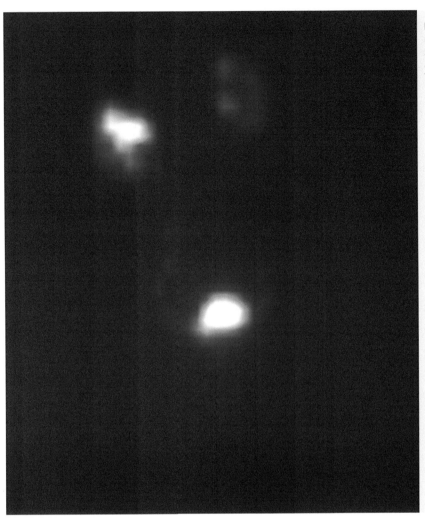

Fig. 69.1 30-minute posterior image from Tc-99m mercaptoacetyltriglycine dynamic renography with Lasix given at time zero shows significant residual activity in the proximal left renal collecting system. Washout T ½ was 56 minutes.

## ■ Clinical History

75-year-old female with chronic left hydronephrosis complaining of left lower back and flank pain (▶ Fig. 69.1).

### ▪ Key Finding

Delayed washout of the genitourinary collecting system on diuretic renography

### ▪ Top 2 Differential Diagnoses

• **Mechanical obstruction.** Evaluating a dilated genitourinary collecting system for mechanical obstruction is best done with diuretic renography. This involves performance of standard nuclear medicine renography with Tc-99m MAG3 with the addition of a diuretic, usually furosemide. The diuretic can be administered either 15 minutes prior to the radiopharmaceutical, at the same time as the radiopharmaceutical (time 0), or 20 minutes later after delayed clearance has already been shown without the diuretic. A TAC is created using either a whole kidney or collecting system ROI for generation of quantitative data. Washout will be delayed if a system is dilated secondary to mechanical obstruction, and the delay will persist despite the increased hydrostatic pressure from diuretic effect. A postdiuretic half emptying time (either from peak to half peak or from time of diuretic administration to half that level, depending on the protocol utilized) greater than 20 minutes is consistent with mechanical obstruction, whereas less than

10 minutes is normal. The 10- to 20-minute area is a nonspecific zone with many interpreting 10 to 15 minutes as "likely not obstructed" and 15 to 20 minutes as "likely obstructed." Mechanical obstruction carries a broad differential, including stones, blood clots, sloughed papilla, crossing of iliac vessels, and benign or malignant strictures.

• **False positive for mechanical obstruction.** A patulous collecting system will result in delayed washout of radiotracer but should normalize after diuretic administration. However, this requires an adequate response to the diuretic. Patients with dehydration or poor baseline renal function may fail to mount a full response. A larger dose of furosemide might also be needed to overcome the so-called reservoir effect in a markedly patulous system. A full or neurogenic urinary bladder increases back pressure into the collecting system and can also mimic obstruction. This can be relieved with catheterization, if the patient is unable to empty their bladder spontaneously.

### ▪ Diagnosis

Obstructed left renal collecting system.

### ✓ Pearls

• Diuretic renography can help delineate if genitourinary collecting system dilation is due to obstruction.
• Washout half time over 20 minutes on diuretic renography is suggestive of mechanical obstruction.

• Renal failure and dehydration can cause a false-positive exam due to poor diuretic response.
• Furosemide dose is typically around 40 mg for adults, based on renal function, and 1 mg/kg for children.

### Suggested Readings

Boubaker A, Prior JO, Meuwly JY, Bischof-Delaloye A. Radionuclide investigations of the urinary tract in the era of multimodality imaging. J Nucl Med. 2006; 47(11):1819–1836

McQuillan BF, Zelasko S, Wolin EA. Nuclear medicine genitourinary imaging in native kidneys. J Am Osteopath Coll Radiol. 2016; 5:14–20

Taylor A, Jr, Nally JV. Clinical applications of renal scintigraphy. AJR Am J Roentgenol. 1995; 164(1):31–41

# Case 70

*James J. Gullo*

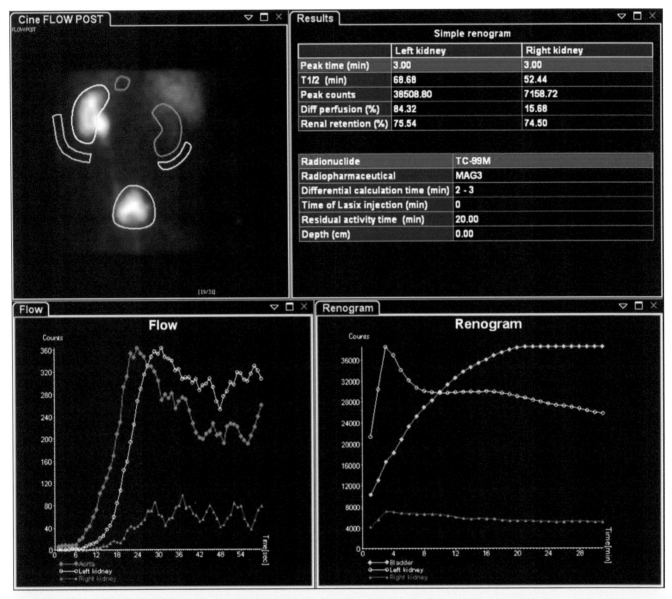

**Fig. 70.1** Quantitative analysis from diuretic enhanced Technetium-99m (Tc-99m) mercaptoacetyltriglycine dynamic renography utilizing cortical regions of interest shows increased bilateral cortical retention at 20 minutes, approximately 38% on the left and 44% on the right.

■ **Clinical History**

46-year-old male with history of pyeloplasty 2 years prior for congenital ureteropelvic junction (UPJ) obstruction with improved but persistent right flank and testicular pain (▶Fig. 70.1).

## ■ Key Finding

Increased cortical retention on MAG3 renal scan

## ■ Top 2 Differential Diagnoses

- **Acute renal failure.** TC-99m MAG3 is excreted almost entirely by tubular secretion. MAG3 is removed from the blood by a transporter located in the basolateral membrane of the proximal tubule. It then accumulates in the cells of the proximal renal tubule before being transported to the lumen of the tubule by organic ion transporters in the apical membrane. In renal failure, the apical membrane transporter is impaired more than the basolateral transporter and MAG3 can be extracted into the tubule cells with a greater efficiency than it is transported to the tubular lumen, resulting in retained cortical activity. Furthermore, any insult to the kidney will usually result in decreased GFR prior to decreased tubular function. This allows for radiotracer to continue to reach the tubules and be secreted into the tubular lumen, but decreased GFR results in decreased filtrate washing out the tubules, visible as cortical retention on scintigraphy. In acute renal failure, MAG3 renal scintigra-phy will demonstrate preserved renal blood flow during the flow phase of the study. There will be cortical retention with retained cortical activity at 20 min possibly approaching 100%. Normally, at 20 min the retained activity should be less than 30% of the peak activity. The TAC will demonstrate a gradually rising slope well past the point where the cortical activity would be expected to decrease.
- **Chronic renal failure.** While chronic renal failure will also demonstrate delayed cortical retention during renal scintigraphy, the TAC will usually demonstrate a plateau as opposed to gradually rising slope as is seen with acute renal failure due to loss of function of both the basolateral and apical membrane transporters in the renal tubule cells. There may also be decreased renal blood flow with reduced extraction of tubular agents such as MAG3. The kidneys may appear smaller than normal.

## ■ Diagnosis

Chronic nephron dysfunction from prior UPJ obstruction.

## ✓ Pearls

- Increased 20-minute cortical retention is a nonspecific indicator of acute or chronic nephron dysfunction.
- Acute renal failure will usually show preserved flow with retention resulting in a rising slope on TAC.
- Chronic renal failure may show reduced flow, plateauing of the TAC, and a small kidney.
- A cortical ROI may be required to evaluate for cortical retention if there is collecting system retention.

## Suggested Readings

Sfakianaki E, Sfakianakis GN, Georgiou M, Hsiao B. Renal scintigraphy in the acute care setting. Semin Nucl Med. 2013; 43(2):114–128

Taylor AT. Radionuclides in nephrourology, part 1: Radiopharmaceuticals, quality control, and quantitative indices. J Nucl Med. 2014; 55(4):608–615

Taylor AT. Radionuclides in nephrourology, part 2: pitfalls and diagnostic applications. J Nucl Med. 2014; 55(5):786–798

# Case 71

*Cameron C. Foster*

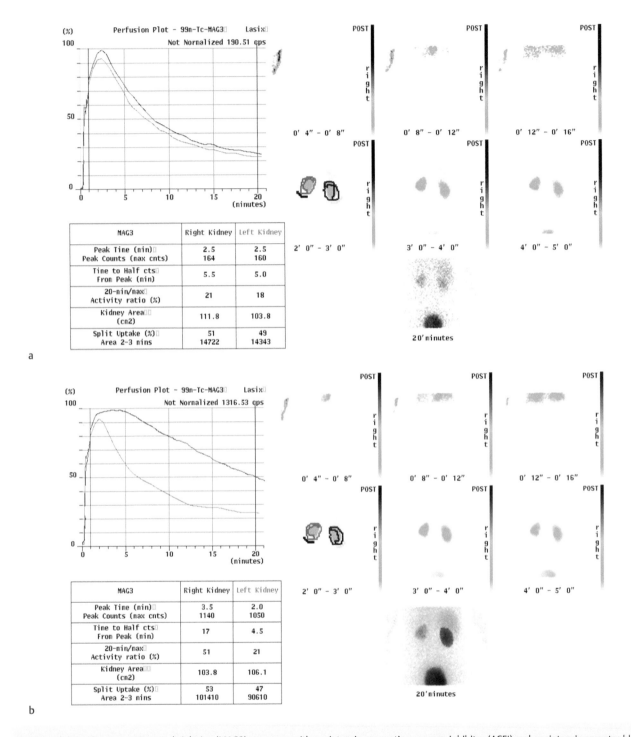

**Fig. 71.1** **(a)** Baseline mercaptoacetyltriglycine (MAG3) renogram with angiotensin-converting enzyme inhibitor (ACEI) and angiotensin receptor blocker medication held demonstrates normal bilateral renal function. Normal faint activity is seen in both kidneys on final image at 20 minutes. **(b)** Captopril MAG3 renogram demonstrates normal left renal function and marked increase in 20/max, T ½, peak time, and generalized rightward shift of the renal curve on the right. Asymmetrically increased right renal activity is seen on final image at 20 minutes.

■ **Clinical History**

61-year-old female with hypertension (▶Fig. 71.1).

## ■ Key Finding

Worsening renal function on MAG3 renal scan following captopril administration

## ■ Top 3 Differential Diagnoses

- **Renal artery stenosis (RAS).** Renovascular hypertension (RVH) accounts for approximately 1 to 4% of all hypertension cases. It is most commonly due to atherosclerosis or fibromuscular dysplasia. Although other modalities such as magnetic resonance angiography (MRA) may be better at detecting an actual stenosis, ACE inhibition renography is very specific for functional RVH. Narrowing of the afferent renal artery greater than 60% typically is the low-end cutoff for causing RVH via the renin–angiotensin cascade. ACEI is administered before radiotracer injection, and the patient is monitored hemodynamically during imaging. MAG3 imaging is considered positive by curvilinear changes due to cortical retention (increase in time to peak cortical activity and 20/max, decreased split function, rightward shift of the curve, etc.) when compared to a baseline scan. When appropriately performed, the test approaches 90% sensitivity and 95% specificity. A positive study generally predicts improvement of hypertension upon revascularization.
- **Unilateral urinary obstruction.** Differentiating between unilateral urinary obstruction and RAS by MAG3 renography is usually done by appearance of an obstructive curve (poor/delayed excretion) on the baseline scan that does not improve with Lasix administration. If the affected kidney is already demonstrating significant renal impairment, the response to Lasix as well as response to the ACEI challenge may be diminished, which results in reduced sensitivity and specificity for both entities. This is because ACEIs cause a decrease in glomerular filtration rate (GFR) which does not affect the uptake or secretion of MAG3, since it is a tubular agent.
- **False-positive scan in patients on calcium channel blocker.** False-positive renal impairment on a MAG3 renogram with ACEI challenge study can be seen in patients who are on chronic calcium channel blockers. This effect should be bilateral and symmetric (except in cases of existing unilateral renal impairment or nephrectomy). In the setting of bilateral renal decline on a renogram in the presence of calcium channel-blocking medication, the study should be repeated after discontinuance of these medications.

## ■ Diagnosis

Renal artery stenosis (right-sided).

## ✓ Pearls

- Adequate fluid hydration prior to and blood pressure monitoring during captopril scan is important.
- A positive scan suggests hemodynamically significant RAS and predicts benefit from revascularization.
- Baseline renal scan with MAG3 is compared to a postcaptopril renal scan with MAG3 for diagnosis.
- False positives can result from dehydration, obstruction, hypotension, and calcium channel blockers.

## Suggested Readings

Ludwig V, Martin WH, Delbeke D. Calcium channel blockers: a potential cause of false-positive captopril renography. Clin Nucl Med. 2003; 28(2):108–112

Soulez G, Oliva VL, Turpin S, Lambert R, Nicolet V, Therasse E. Imaging of renovascular hypertension: respective values of renal scintigraphy, renal Doppler US, and MR angiography. Radiographics. 2000; 20(5):1355–1368, discussion 1368–1372

Taylor AT, Jr, Fletcher JW, Nally JV, Jr, et al; Society of Nuclear Medicine. Procedure guideline for diagnosis of renovascular hypertension. J Nucl Med. 1998; 39(7):1297–1302

# Case 72

*Trevor A. Thompson*

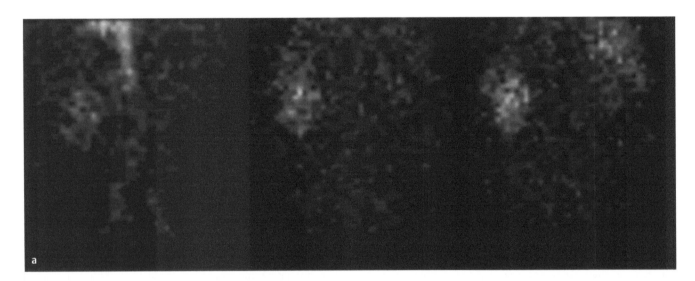

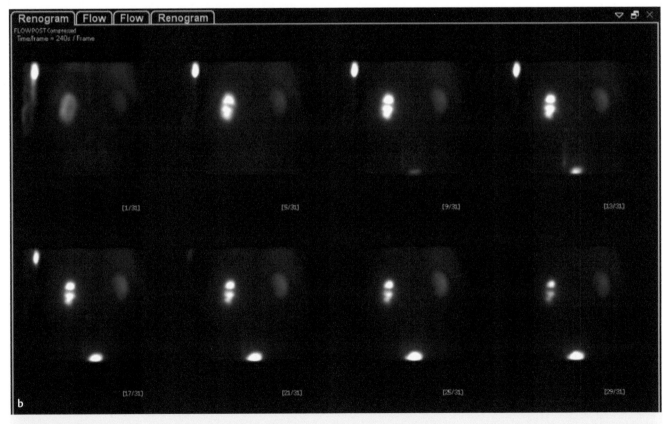

**Fig. 72.1** **(a)** Select 23-, 40-, and 60-second images from initial 60-second posterior dynamic acquisition, 1 second per frame, after the administration of Tc-99m mercaptoacetyltriglycine (MAG3) (*top row*) shows markedly delayed and diminished flow to the right kidney. **(b)** Five-minute compressed images from remainder of the 30 minutes of dynamic renography shows a slowly progressive right renogram.

■ Clinical History

68-year-old male with right renal artery stenosis (RAS) and hypertension (▶Fig. 72.1).

## ■ Key Finding

Delayed/persistent nephrogram on standard MAG3 renography in native kidneys

## ■ Top 3 Differential Diagnoses

- **Acute tubular necrosis (ATN).** In native kidneys, acute tubular necrosis is most commonly encountered as a result of diabetes mellitus, especially in the setting of recent iodinated IV contrast material administration. Additional common causes of ATN in native kidneys include renal ischemia and nephrotoxic medications. Classically, ATN appears as relatively maintained renal perfusion with markedly decreased excretion resulting in prolonged cortical retention (e.g., a persistent nephrogram). While preservation of renal perfusion can help distinguish this from other causes of acute renal injury on MAG3 renography, renal perfusion may be impaired in severe cases of ATN. ATN involving the native kidneys is typically bilateral.
- **Ureteral obstruction.** This condition may occur due to a variety of causes that vary on the basis of patient age. Congenital and developmental causes, such as ureteral duplication and ureteropelvic junction (UPJ) obstruction, are most frequent in children; while ureterolithiasis and malignancy should be considered in adult patients. Findings of ureteral obstruction on MAG3 renography are dependent on chronicity and severity of obstruction. Initially, ureteral obstruction will only affect collecting system washout of MAG3 as glomerular filtration is affected before renal plasma flow. If untreated, the obstruction will eventually result in delayed cortical transit, delayed cortical uptake, and decreased perfusion. Diuretic renography is commonly used to distinguish ureteral obstruction from a nonobstructed dilated collecting system.
- **Renal artery/vein thrombosis.** Thrombosis of native renal vessels, whether arterial (RAT) or venous (RVT), is most commonly secondary to a hypercoagulable state with malignant invasion or underlying vascular abnormality (i.e., atherosclerotic plaque) being less common causes of thrombosis. RAT and RVT typically appear scintigraphically similar, as both frequently demonstrate decreased or absent renal perfusion and cortical uptake with delayed cortical transit. Prolonged cortical retention is typically seen in acute RVT, which can be confirmed with duplex Doppler ultrasound.

## ■ Additional Diagnostic Consideration

- **RAS:** Basic MAG3 renography in the setting of RAS is most typically performed for baseline imaging in the evaluation of renovascular hypertension (RVH). In this setting, RAS is most commonly due to atherosclerosis or fibromuscular dysplasia. RAS can result in decreased renal perfusion with decreased cortical uptake and delayed cortical transit, depending on severity. Comparison with MAG3 renography following angiotensin-converting enzyme inhibitor (ACEI) administration, demonstrating worsening renal function, is required to confirm RAS as this scintigraphic appearance is nonspecific.

## ■ Diagnosis

Renal artery stenosis.

## ✓ Pearls

- Bilateral persistent nephrograms with relatively maintained renal perfusion suggest ATN.
- Ureteral obstruction, depending on chronicity and severity, can present with persistent nephrograms.
- RAT/RVT and RAS can also result in persistent nephrograms.

## Suggested Readings

Blaustein DA, Myint MM, Babu K, Avram MM, Chandramouli BS. The role of technetium-99 m MAG3 renal imaging in the diagnosis of acute tubular necrosis of native kidneys. Clin Nucl Med. 2002; 27(3):165–168

Soulez G, Oliva VL, Turpin S, Lambert R, Nicolet V, Therasse E. Imaging of renovascular hypertension: respective values of renal scintigraphy, renal Doppler US, and MR angiography. Radiographics. 2000; 20(5):1355–1368, discussion 1368–1372

Uliel L, Mellnick VM, Menias CO, Holz AL, McConathy J. Nuclear medicine in the acute clinical setting: indications, imaging findings, and potential pitfalls. Radiographics. 2013; 33(2):375–396

# Case 73

*Britain A. Gailliot*

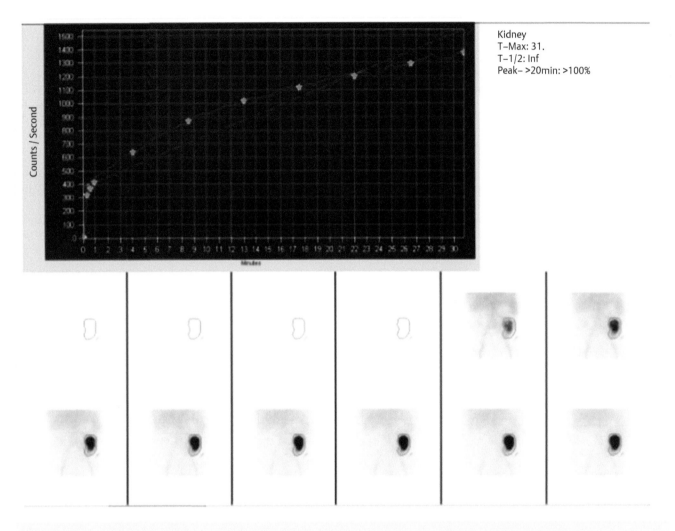

Kidney
T–Max: 31.
T–1/2: Inf
Peak– >20min: >100%

**Fig. 73.1** Tc-99m mercaptoacetyltriglycine (MAG3) renography shows persistent increased activity in a left lower quadrant (anterior imaging) transplant kidney with no visualized collecting system activity. Perfusion was normal.

■ **Clinical History**

Patient referred for renal transplant evaluation (▶Fig. 73.1). (Case courtesy of Joseph Fotos, MD, Penn State Hershey Medical Center.)

## ■ Key Finding

Abnormal transplant renogram with Tc-99m MAG3

## ■ Top 3 Differential Diagnoses

- **Acute Tubular Necrosis (ATN).** Renal scintigraphy is often the first line imaging modality when ATN is suspected following renal transplantation. ATN typically occurs during the first few days postoperatively. Perfusion is preserved, or minimally decreased, with nearly simultaneous appearance of activity within the transplanted kidney and adjacent iliac artery. However, in severe cases of ATN, perfusion may be markedly decreased, similar to findings seen in acute rejection (AR). Radiotracer uptake and excretion is significantly delayed, demonstrated as progressively increasing activity. ATN is usually of little consequence as complete recovery is expected with steady improvement of kidney function on future renal scintigraphy.

- **Rejection.** Rejection is the other primary concern in the setting of decreased transplant renal function. Rejection is characterized on renal scintigraphy by decreased perfusion with delayed uptake and excretion. As previously mentioned, similar findings can be seen with severe ATN, in which case the timing of onset can help determine the correct diagnosis; AR typically presents between the first week to first few months postoperatively. Ultimately, a biopsy may be required.
- **Drug toxicity.** Nephrotoxicity as a result of immunosuppressive therapy typically presents in the second or third month postoperatively as the medication is titrated and may reach supratherapeutic levels. Renal scintigraphy findings are non-specific in this setting and can mimic ATN or rejection. Timing and medication history are important considerations.

## ■ Additional Diagnostic Consideration

- **Surgical complications:** Common surgical complications include ureteral obstruction, urine leak, and vascular compromise. Ureteral obstruction and urine leak have scintigraphic findings similar to these processes occurring in a native kidney. Vascular compromise is also similar in appearance to a native kidney with the exception of venous thrombosis which presents with absent/reduced perfusion and function as well as delayed uptake due to the absence of collateral drainage. Doppler ultrasound should be performed when vascular compromise is suspected.

## ■ Diagnosis

Acute tubular necrosis.

## ✓ Pearls

- ATN is most often characterized by persistent uptake and reduced excretion with preserved perfusion.
- Postop presentation: ATN first few days, AR 1 week to a few months, drug toxicity 2 to 3 months.

- This discussion is for Tc-99m MAG3, and does not apply if the glomerular filtration rate (GFR) agent Tc-99m diethylenetriamine pentaacetic acid (DTPA) is used.

## Suggested Readings

Akbar SA, Jafri SZ, Amendola MA, Madrazo BL, Salem R, Bis KG. Complications of renal transplantation. Radiographics. 2005; 25(5):1335–1356

Uliel L, Mellnick VM, Menias CO, Holz AL, McConathy J. Nuclear medicine in the acute clinical setting: indications, imaging findings, and potential pitfalls. Radiographics. 2013; 33(2):375–396

Yazici B, Yazici A, Oral A, Akgün A, Toz H. Comparison of renal transplant scintigraphy with renal resistance index for prediction of early graft dysfunction and evaluation of acute tubular necrosis and acute rejection. Clin Nucl Med. 2013; 38(12):931–935

# Case 74

*James J. Gullo*

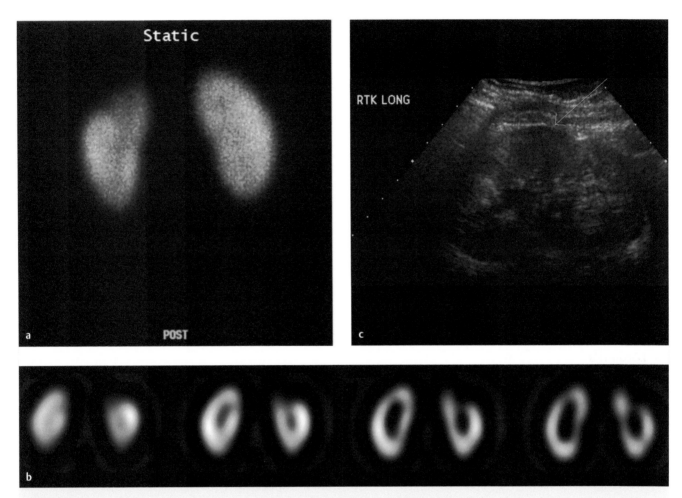

**Fig. 74.1** Posterior planar **(a)** and coronal single photon emission computed tomography (SPECT) images **(b)** from Tc-99m dimercaptosuccinic acid (DMSA) renogram shows normal radiotracer uptake in the region of concern in the mid right kidney, shown on correlative ultrasound image **(c;** arrow). Focal wedge-shaped defect in the upper pole left kidney is consistent with scarring versus focal pyelonephritis.

## ■ Clinical History

9-year-old female with recurrent UTIs with recent renal ultrasound suggesting fetal lobulation versus scarring (▶ Fig. 74.1).

## ■ Key Finding

DMSA uptake in a renal mass

## ■ Top 3 Differential Diagnoses

- **Hypertrophied column of Bertin.** In the typical kidney, there are thin bands of cortical tissue between the renal pyramids. When the polar parenchyma is underabsorbed during embryogenesis, this band appears thickened and extends deeper into the renal sinus than normal. This is referred to as a hypertrophied column of Bertin. This finding can mimic a renal mass on ultrasound. DMSAscintigraphy is an excellent method to assess the renal cortex. DMSA localizes to the renal cortex by binding to sulfhydryl groups in the proximal tubules of functioning, normal renal parenchyma. With a hypertrophied column of Bertin, DMSA scintigraphy will show uptake in the hypertrophied column that is identical to the rest of the renal cortex, while a more aggressive process will have abnormal decreased uptake. The renal contour over this column will be smooth. The typical location is in the middle third of the left kidney although this finding can appear at any location in either kidney. It is an incidental finding and requires no follow-up imaging once diagnosed.
- **Persistent fetal lobulation.** The kidneys develop as multiple lobulations. Each lobule comprises a single renal pyramid supplied by an artery and vein with overlying cortex. This leads to the characteristic multilobular appearance of the kidneys in the fetus and neonate. As a child ages, the lobules fuse resulting in the smooth renal cortex typical of the adult kidney. In 5% of adults, fusion is incomplete leaving one or more persistent lobulations. DMSA renal scintigraphy will show normal appearing, functional renal tissue with one or multiple shallow, smooth indentations of the renal cortex between the renal pyramids that can be present in any location on either kidney. Persistent fetal lobulation is considered a normal variant and is often an incidental finding.
- **Dromedary hump.** A dromedary hump is a prominent bulge at the lateral border of the left kidney due to impression of the adjacent spleen. It can mimic a renal mass but will demonstrate uptake identical to normal renal parenchyma on DMSA scintigraphy. While fetal lobulation and column of Bertin can be seen in either kidney, a dromedary hump will only be located on the left kidney. It is an incidental finding of no clinical significance. This finding is named after the dromedary (*Camelus dromedarius*) which has a single hump as opposed to the two humped Bactrian camel (*Camelus ferus*).

## ■ Diagnosis

Persistent fetal lobulation.

## ✓ Pearls

- Hypertrophied column of Bertin will have identical appearance to renal cortex on DMSA scintigraphy.
- Fetal lobulation will have normal cortical uptake on scintigraphy with smooth, shallow cortical lobulations.
- Dromedary hump is a prominent bulge at the lateral border of the left kidney due to splenic impression.
- DMSA uptake in a renal "mass" indicates normal functioning renal tissue, a sign of benignity.

## Suggested Readings

Bhatt S, MacLennan G, Dogra V. Renal pseudotumors. AJR Am J Roentgenol. 2007; 188(5):1380–1387

Fretzayas A, Moustaki M, Alexopoulou E, Nicolaidou P. Differential diagnosis of renal mass. Columns of Bertin. Pediatr Nephrol. 2010; 25(3):441–444

Grüning T, Drake BE, Freeman SJ. Single-photon emission CT using (99 m)Tc-dimercaptosuccinic acid (DMSA) for characterization of suspected renal masses. Br J Radiol. 2014; 87(1039):20130547

# Case 75

*Trevor A. Thompson*

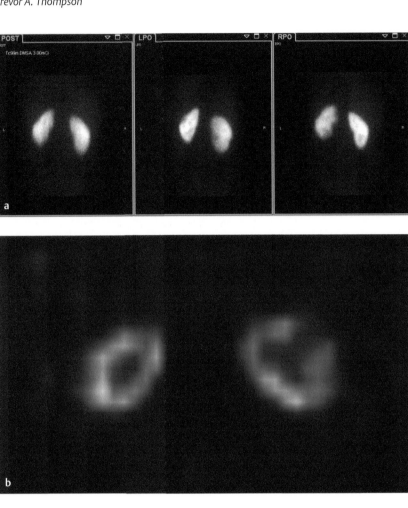

**Fig. 75.1** Planar **(a)** and axial single-photon emission computed tomography (SPECT) **(b)** images from Tc-99m dimercaptosuccinic acid (DMSA) renography show a focal area of photopenia in the upper pole left kidney. **(c)** Correlative axial contrast-enhanced CT image shows a left renal cyst.

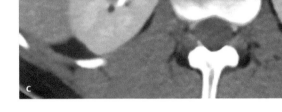

■ Clinical History
.......................................................................

30-year-old female with history of vesicoureteral reflux (VUR) (▶ Fig. 75.1).

## ■ Key Finding

Defect on renal cortical scintigraphy

## ■ Top 3 Differential Diagnoses

- **Scar.** Technetium-99m DMSA is the imaging agent of choice for renal cortical scintigraphy and is most commonly utilized in the pediatric setting. In children, renal cortical scarring is most commonly due to VUR, urinary tract infection (UTI), or a combination of both. In adults, scarring is typically due to infection or infarction, commonly secondary to atherosclerotic disease or thromboembolism. Cortical scarring appears as solitary or multiple peripheral photopenic defects on cortical scintigraphy. In the pediatric setting, cortical imaging is used to detect, quantify, and monitor areas of scarring while voiding cystourethrography (VCUG) or radionuclide cystography (RNC) is employed to differentiate between the causative etiologies of renal scarring.
- **Pyelonephritis.** This condition is present in approximately 60% of children with febrile UTI. While renal cortical imaging is more sensitive than renal ultrasound for the detection of acute pyelonephritis, American College of Radiology Appropriateness Criteria recommend ultrasonography as the initial imaging modality of choice in uncomplicated first cases of suspected pyelonephritis in children given the radiation dose associated with cortical imaging. Renal cortical imaging, however, can be performed in the setting of atypical response to therapy, recurrent infection, or 4 to 6 months following UTI for detection of resultant cortical scarring. In adults, imaging of pyelonephritis is reserved for those with suspected complication (i.e., renal abscess), atypical/severe presentation, or if initial therapy has failed. In these cases, CT or ultrasound is preferred as these modalities provide highly specific information on potential complications as well as extent of extrarenal disease when compared to cortical scintigraphy. On cortical imaging, pyelonephritis may present as solitary or multiple focal defects or as diffusely decreased cortical activity involving one or both kidneys.
- **Space-occupying lesion.** A space-occupying lesion within the renal parenchyma may present as a focal defect on renal cortical scintigraphy. This includes both benign and malignant etiologies such as a cortical cyst, abscess, or neoplasm. The benefit of renal cortical scintigraphy in these cases is to exclude normal variant anatomy, such as a prominent column of Bertin, dromedary hump, or fetal lobulation, which may mimic neoplasia on anatomic imaging but demonstrate normal uptake of Tc-99m DMSA.

## ■ Additional Diagnostic Consideration

- **Attenuation:** Attenuation of cortical uptake by overlying structures can result in artifactual defects on renal cortical scintigraphy. However, review of additional projections typically demonstrates the artifactual nature of these findings. If planar projections are inconclusive, single-photon emission computed tomography (SPECT) imaging can also be performed.

## ■ Diagnosis

Renal cyst.

## ✓ Pearls

- Cortical scintigraphy is often used to evaluate renal scarring in children that commonly occurs due to VUR or UTI.
- Imaging of acute pyelonephritis depends upon patient age as well as suspicion of associated complication.
- Normal cortical uptake helps distinguish benign anatomic variants from true space-occupying lesions.
- Multiplanar image acquisition or SPECT can differentiate artifactual attenuation from a true cortical defect.
- At the time of writing this, DMSA is unfortunately not available for clinical use.

## Suggested Readings

Craig WD, Wagner BJ, Travis MD. Pyelonephritis: radiologic-pathologic review. Radiographics. 2008; 28(1):255–277, quiz 327–328

Jang SJ. Nuclear Medicine in Pediatric Urology. Child Kidney Dis. 2015; 19(1): 14–22

McQuillan BF, Zelasko S, Wolin EA. Nuclear medicine genitourinary imaging in native kidneys. J Am Osteopath Coll Radiol. 2016; 5(3):14–20

# Case 76

*Ely A. Wolin*

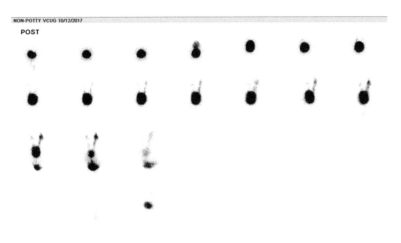

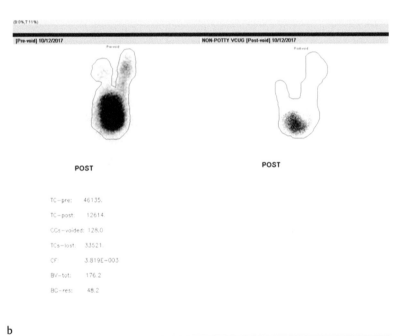

a

b

**Fig. 76.1** Posterior images from the third phase of bladder filling with Tc-99m sulfur colloid-labeled saline demonstrate bilateral vesicoureteral reflux (grade 3 on right and grade 2 on the left). Patient began to void midway in this filling phase. Pre- and postvoid posterior images demonstrate persistent bilateral reflux after voiding, with a small amount of residual urine.

## ■ Clinical History

10-month-old female with history of recurrent fevers (▶Fig. 76.1).

(Case courtesy of Joeph S. Fotos, M.D., Penn State Hershey Medical Center.)

## ■ Key Finding

Upper collecting system activity on RNC

## ■ Top 2 Differential Diagnoses

• **Vesicoureteral reflux.** Radionuclide cystography (RNC) is a great tool for the evaluation of vesicoureteral reflux (VUR). While fluoroscopic VCUG is still the primary study used for evaluation, particularly in males due to the ability to demonstrate posterior urethral valves, RNC has an important role for follow-up imaging and for evaluation of at-risk siblings.

RNC is performed by injection of a small amount of radiopharmaceutical mixed with saline, usually Tc-99m sulfur colloid, into the urinary bladder through a catheter while the patient is supine on an imaging table. Enough volume needs to be instilled to ensure adequate distension of the bladder which can be estimated according to the patient's age. Posterior dynamic images are obtained during bladder filling and voiding. At least one cycle is necessary, but imaging for three cycles of filling and voiding provides the greatest sensitivity.

The dynamic acquisition during RNC provides the main advantage over VCUG. VCUG provides evaluation for upper collecting system only at a limited number of single time points when the imager decides to look. This means any transient reflux may be missed. With RNC, the collecting system is evaluated throughout the entire cycle of filling and voiding allowing for capture of any moments of reflux into the upper collecting system, even if low volume and transient. Multiple episodes of reflux are frequently seen on RNC.

As RNC does not provide detailed anatomic information, the traditional grading system for VUR cannot be used. Instead, reflux is called mild if it involves only the ureter, moderate if it reaches the pelvicalyceal system, and severe if there is apparent dilation of the pelvicalyceal system with ureteral tortuosity.

• **Activity from prior injection.** Visualization of upper collecting system activity on RNC is pretty much pathognomic for VUR. However, it is important to ensure that the patient did not receive a recent injection of a renally cleared radiopharmaceutical resulting in excreted activity in the collecting system.

## ■ Diagnosis

Bilateral vesicoureteral reflux.

## ✓ Pearls

• RNC is more sensitive than VCUG and preferred for follow up and evaluation of at-risk siblings.
• Imaging through three cycles of bladder filling and voiding increased sensitivity for VUR.

• Traditional grading system for VUR is not used for RNC due to lack of anatomic detail.
• Posterior urethral valves cannot be identified with RNC.

## Suggested Readings

Dalirani R, Mahyar A, Sharifian M, Mohkam M, Esfandiar N, Ghehsareh Ardestani A. The value of direct radionuclide cystography in the detection of vesicoureteral reflux in children with normal voiding cystourethrography. Pediatr Nephrol. 2014; 29(12):2341–2345

Joaquim AI, de Godoy MF, Burdmann EA. Cyclic direct radionuclide cystography in the diagnosis and characterization of vesicoureteral reflux in children and adults. Clin Nucl Med. 2015; 40(8):627–631
McQuillan BF, Zelasko S, Wolin EA. Nuclear medicine genitourinary imaging in native kidneys. J Am Osteopath Coll Radiol. 2016; 5(3):14–20

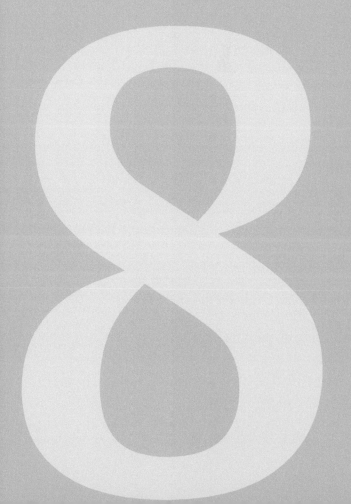

# Part 8

## Bone

# Case 77

*Kamal D. Singh*

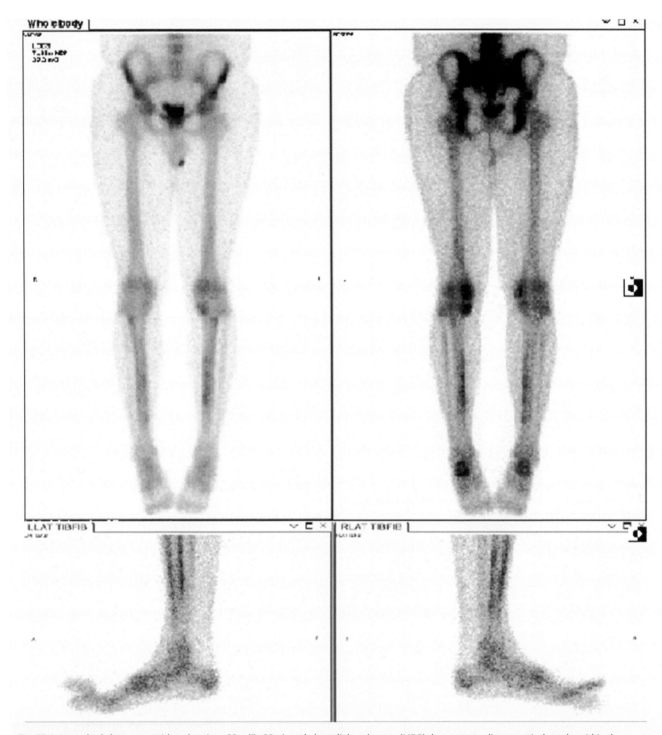

**Fig. 77.1** Lower body bone scan with technetium-99m (Tc-99m) methylene diphosphonate (MDP) demonstrates linear cortical uptake within the bilateral posteromedial mid tibial diaphysis in a "tram-track" pattern.

### ■ Clinical History

23-year-old male with bilateral shin pain for over a year, symptoms worsening to lower tibia (▶Fig. 77.1).

■ **Key Finding**

Symmetric "tram-track" cortical uptake of long bones

■ **Top 3 Differential Diagnoses**

- **Hypertrophic osteoarthropathy (HOA).** Secondary HOA is a clinical syndrome of symptomatic periostitis of long bones due to various neoplastic and non-neoplastic pulmonary and extrapulmonary disorders. Common pulmonary causes include bronchogenic carcinoma, fibrous tumor of the pleura, mesothelioma, and chronic pulmonary infection/inflammation; as a result, a chest radiograph should be obtained in patients with scintigraphic evidence of HOA. Extrapulmonary etiologies include inflammatory bowel disease, cyanotic congenital heart disease, and thyroid acropachy. The exact pathophysiology of HOA remains unclear; however, vasoactive agents and hormones secreted by tumors and other inflammatory/infectious processes have been implicated. Scintigraphic findings of bilateral symmetric upper and lower extremity parallel cortical activity in a "tram-track" configuration often precede plain film evidence of undulating periosteal proliferation. There may be associated increased activity within the scapula, mandible/maxilla, and periarticular regions. Patients usually report painful swelling of the affected limb, stiff joints, and demonstrate digital clubbing on physical exam. The radiographic and scintigraphic findings usually resolve after treatment of the underlying disease.

- **Shin/quadriceps splints.** Severe bilateral shin and quadriceps splints may produce increased parallel cortical activity within the lower extremities of physically active patients with lower leg pain related to exertion of overuse. Shin splints (medial tibial stress syndrome) result in unilateral or bilateral posteromedial tibial cortical periostitis. These patients present with dull aching leg pain. Unlike stress fractures that appear as focal regions of increased uptake on all three phases of a bone scan, splints are generalized linear or longitudinal activity along the diaphysis, usually the middle third, detected on delayed phase imaging. While stress fractures may coexist in a patient with shin or quadriceps splints, there has been no evidence to suggest a progression of splints to stress fracture.

- **Chronic venous stasis.** Chronic venous insufficiency can lead to soft-tissue edema, associated skin changes (including stasis ulcers), and thick undulating or nodular periosteal proliferation of the affected extremity due to local hypoxia. Physical examination can help differentiate this entity from other causes of increased parallel long bone activity within an extremity by noting overlying skin changes. In the setting of cellulitis and chronic venous stasis, it may be difficult to exclude superimposed osteomyelitis.

■ **Diagnosis**

Bilateral shin splints.

✓ **Pearls**

- Benign and malignant etiologies can lead to HOA; obtain a chest X-ray to evaluate for underlying tumor.
- Shin and quadriceps splints are common in athletes and result in cortical periostitis with linear activity.

- Chronic venous stasis may lead to undulating periosteal proliferation due to hypoxia.

**Suggested Readings**

Love C, Din AS, Tomas MB, Kalapparambath TP, Palestro CJ. Radionuclide bone imaging: an illustrative review. Radiographics. 2003; 23(2):341–358

Ali A, Tetalman MR, Fordham EW, et al. Distribution of hypertrophic pulmonary osteoarthropathy. AJR Am J Roentgenol. 1980; 134(4):771–780

Rana RS, Wu JS, Eisenberg RL. Periosteal reaction. AJR Am J Roentgenol. 2009; 193(4):W259–72

# Case 78

*John P. Lichtenberger*

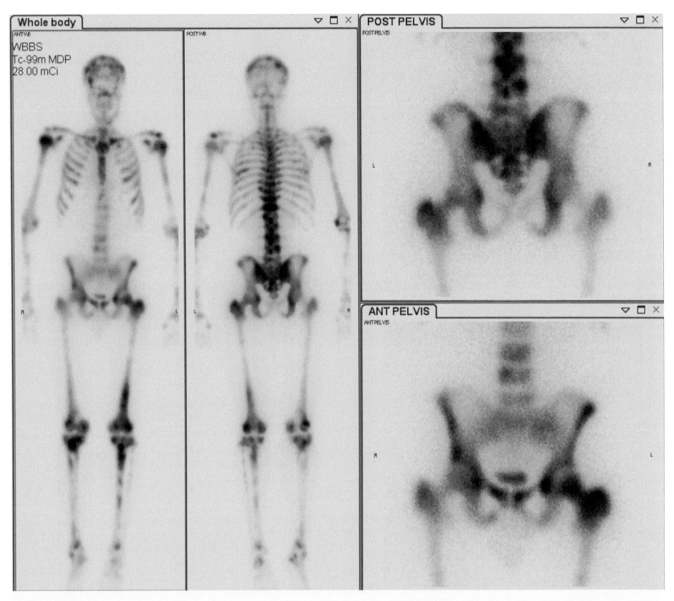

**Fig. 78.1** Whole-body bone scan with technetium-99m (Tc-99m) methylene diphosphonate (MDP) shows diffuse increased skeletal uptake with multiple areas of focally increased activity and no significant soft-tissue or renal activity.

## ■ Clinical History

65-year-old male with metastatic prostate cancer (▶ Fig. 78.1).

■ Key Finding

Superscan

■ Top 3 Differential Diagnoses

• **Metastatic disease.** A superscan refers to increased skeletal uptake on bone scan with decreased or absent renal and soft-tissue activity. Diffuse osseous metastatic disease is the most common cause of a superscan, most commonly metastatic prostate cancer. With metastatic disease, the skeletal activity is typically inhomogeneous and centered primarily within the axial and proximal appendicular skeleton. Distinct metastatic foci may be discernible.

• **Metabolic bone disease.** Although somewhat varied in scintigraphic appearance, metabolic diseases, such as renal osteodystrophy, hyperparathyroidism, and osteomalacia, may result in generalized increased activity in the skeleton relative to the kidneys and soft tissues. Features that suggest metabolic disease include uniform distribution of activity, involvement of the appendicular skeleton, and disproportionate increased calvarial uptake. The osseous manifestations of renal osteodystrophy result from altered vitamin D metabolism and secondary hyperparathyroidism. This diagnosis is suggested on bone scan by prominent activity along the costochondral junctions, involvement of distal long bones, "railroad tracking" and bowing of the femurs, and sternal activity. Pseudofractures may be seen in the setting of osteomalacia.

• **Paget's disease.** Intense activity and expansion of bones are characteristic of Paget's disease, most commonly involving the pelvis, femora, spine, and skull. When multifocal or widespread, concentration of radiopharmaceutical in the skeletal lesions and increase in target-to-soft-tissue ratio may result in an apparent superscan.

■ Additional Diagnostic Consideration

• **Myeloproliferative/marrow infiltrative disorder:** A superscan from myeloproliferative diseases, such as lymphoma, mastocytosis, and myelofibrosis, usually manifests as uniform and homogeneous radiotracer uptake within both the axial and appendicular skeleton, similar to a metabolic superscan. Appropriate history and laboratory values aid in distinguishing between myeloproliferative/marrow infiltrative disorders and metabolic disease.

■ Diagnosis

Diffuse osteoblastic metastatic disease.

✓ Pearls

• Superscan refers to increased skeletal with decreased or absent renal and soft-tissue activity on bone scan.
• Metastatic disease is the most common cause of a superscan and typically involves the axial skeleton.
• Metabolic bone disease involves both the axial and appendicular skeleton and is usually homogeneous.
• Paget's disease may result in a superscan when widespread.

Suggested Readings

Buckley O, O'Keeffe S, Geoghegan T, et al. 99 mTc bone scintigraphy superscans: a review. Nucl Med Commun. 2007; 28(7):521–527

Cheng TH, Holman BL. Increased skeletal:renal uptake ratio: etiology and characteristics. Radiology. 1980; 136(2):455–459

Love C, Din AS, Tomas MB, Kalapparambath TP, Palestro CJ. Radionuclide bone imaging: an illustrative review. Radiographics. 2003; 23(2):341–358

# Case 79

*William T. O'Brien, Sr.*

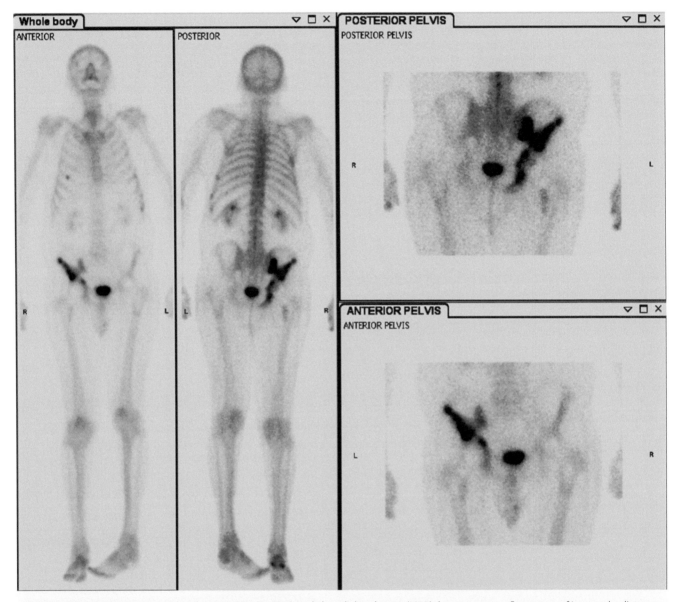

**Fig. 79.1** Whole-body bone scan with technetium-99m (Tc-99m) methylene diphosphonate (MDP) demonstrates confluent areas of increased radiotracer uptake involving the right iliac bone, acetabulum, and ischium. Additional foci of increased uptake are noted in the right 6th rib and left 7th, 9th, and 10th ribs.

■ Clinical History

78-year-old male with metastatic prostate cancer prior to Xofigo therapy (▶ Fig. 79.1).

## ■ Key Finding

Increased activity and osseous expansion in the pelvis

## ■ Top 2 Differential Diagnoses in an Adult

- **Paget's disease.** This condition most commonly occurs in middle-aged to older men. The cause is unknown. On bone scans, Paget's disease exhibits increased activity, often with apparent expansion. Distribution is monostotic in 10 to 35% cases most commonly affecting the pelvis, spine, sacrum, femur, and cranium. Osteoporosis circumscripta, a classic lytic lesion of the skull, will have uptake at the margins. Paget's disease progresses from one end of a long bone to the other with a sharp demarcation from the involved to the uninvolved portion, rendering the classic "blade of grass" appearance. Bone scan uptake is typically increased during all three phases of the disease (lytic, mixed, and sclerotic). Bone scan is more sensitive than radiography, and useful for identifying polyostotic disease. Sarcomatous degeneration may initially result in increasing focal activity, but may later appear photopenic due to lesional necrosis.

- **Metastases.** Bone scan is the most useful imaging modality to search for osteoblastic metastatic disease. Although usually multifocal, metastases may occasionally be monostotic. The axial skeleton is most commonly involved. Sclerotic metastases are most likely due to prostate cancer in men and breast cancer in women. Metastatic disease typically presents as multifocal regions of increased activity on bone scan, with the activity often from the body's reaction to the tumor. The involved bone may be enlarged secondary to tumor burden. Lesions may demonstrate increased activity within the first 6 months after chemotherapy, referred to as the "flare phenomenon," as a result of a healing osteoblastic response. Increasing activity after 6 months should be considered progression of the disease.

## ■ Top 3 Differential Diagnoses in a Child

- **Ewing's sarcoma.** It is the second most common primary bone tumor in children (after osteosarcoma), usually involving the pelvis or femur. Patients typically present with progressive pain. Bone scans demonstrate increased activity and bone expansion may also be seen. Osseous metastases occur in approximately half of patients; therefore, follow-up imaging is warranted to evaluate for disease progression.
- **Lymphoma.** Lymphoma can mimic Ewing's sarcoma clinically and radiographically but has a more favorable prognosis. Increased activity and bony expansion may be seen on bone

scan. The pelvis is commonly involved. Biopsy is warranted to confirm the diagnosis but should be coordinated with the pediatric surgeon as the tract used for biopsy may alter the surgical approach.
- **Fibrous dysplasia (FD).** This condition may be monostotic or polyostotic (McCune–Albright syndrome). The lesions may be lucent having a ground glass matrix or may be sclerotic. Bony expansion is common. Increased uptake is noted in involved bones. Common locations include long bones, pelvis, craniofacial bones, spine, and ribs.

## ■ Diagnosis

Metastatic prostate cancer.

## ✓ Pearls

- Paget's disease most commonly affects the pelvis; bone scan may help identify sarcomatous degeneration.
- Paget's disease and FD can be monostotic or polyostotic.

- Correlation with anatomic imaging can be paramount in distinguishing benign from malignant disease.

## Suggested Readings

Abdelrazek S, Szumowski P, Rogowski F, Kociura-Sawicka A, Mojsak M, Szorc M. Bone scan in metabolic bone diseases. Review. Nucl Med Rev Cent East Eur. 2012; 15(2):124–131

Kumar AA, Kumar P, Prakash M, Tewari V, Sahni H, Dash A. Paget's disease diagnosed on bone scintigraphy: Case report and literature review. Indian J Nucl Med. 2013; 28(2):121–123

Orzel JA, Sawaf NW, Richardson ML. Lymphoma of the skeleton: scintigraphic evaluation. AJR Am J Roentgenol. 1988; 150(5):1095–1099

# Case 80

*Kamal D. Singh*

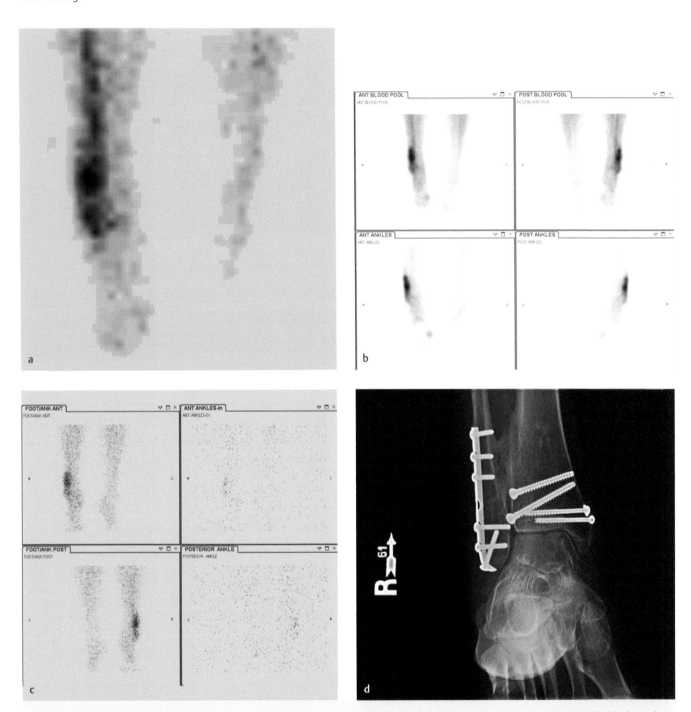

Fig. 80.1 Flow image (a) and blood pool and delayed images (b) from a three-phase bone scan (TPBS) of ankles with technetium-99m (Tc-99m) reveal diffuse hyperemia on the right with matched blood pool and delayed uptake in the region of the distal right fibula. Images from an Indium-111 (In-111) white blood cell (WBC) and technetium-99m sulfur colloid (Tc-99m SC) scan (c) show increased sulfur colloid uptake in the region of the bone scan abnormality, greater than minimal WBC activity. Correlative ankle radiograph (d).

## ■ Clinical History

67-year-old female with history of open reduction and internal fixation (ORIF) of the right ankle presenting with right lateral ankle cellulitis, refractory to outpatient treatment, swelling and tenderness to palpation, with healed scab over later malleolus (▶Fig. 80.1).

## ■ Key Finding

Three-phase positive bone scan

## ■ Top 3 Differential Diagnoses

- **Trauma.** A TPBS involves dynamic flow imaging for the first minute after radiopharmaceutical injection, static blood pool imaging for next few minutes, and subsequent static delayed imaging at 2 to 4 hours. Although a TPBS is classically performed for determination of osseous infection, increased uptake on all three phases is a nonspecific finding and can be seen in setting of acute fracture or recent surgery. Approximately 80% of fractures demonstrate increased activity within 24 hours and over 95% of fractures demonstrate increased activity by 3 days. A healed extremity fracture may have persistent focal increased activity on the delayed phase of the bone scan for over a year.
- **Osteomyelitis.** TPBS not only has a high sensitivity and negative predictive value for acute osteomyelitis, but it may also detect abnormalities 1 to 2 weeks earlier than radiographic manifestations. False-negative bone scans, however, are often

seen in the setting of disrupted blood supply and abscess formation, especially in neonates and infants with hematogenously acquired osteomyelitis. Specificity is decreased in the setting of recent surgery, trauma, or orthopedic hardware. Dual-isotope imaging with indium-111-labeled white blood cells (In-111 WBC; for infection) and technetium-99m sulfur colloid (Tc-99m SC; for normal bone marrow mapping) can aide in assessment of osteomyelitis. Focal uptake on an In-111 WBC scan, which is spatially discordant from Tc-99m SC bone marrow scan, is suggestive of infection.
- **Bone tumor.** Primary or secondary malignant bone tumors may demonstrate increased activity on all three phases. Although most benign osseous neoplasms will not demonstrate increased flow or blood pool activity, osteoid osteomas (OO) contain a three-phase positive nidus with a "target sign" on delayed imaging.

## ■ Additional Diagnostic Consideration

- **Complex regional pain syndrome:** This condition typically occurs after trauma or surgery and is characterized by pain, swelling, and vasomotor instability out of proportion to the degree of injury. Periarticular swelling and osteopenia may be seen on plain radiographs. Early or acute complex regional pain syndrome (CRPS) classically demonstrates unilateral increased flow and blood pool activity with periarticular

increased radiotracer activity on delayed images. This classic pattern is only seen in two-thirds of affected patients. The flow and blood pool activity may normalize in chronic or long-standing CRPS. Interestingly, CRPS in children commonly demonstrates normal or even decreased activity (so-called cold CRPS).

## ■ Diagnosis

Reactive bone marrow post ORIF.

## ✓ Pearls

- Flow, blood pool, and delayed imaging at 2 to 4 hours make up a TPBS.
- Three-phase positive scans may be seen with acute fractures, osteomyelitis, OOs, and CRPS.
- In-111 WBC scan with Tc-99m SC scan is highly specific for hardware osteomyelitis.
- CRPS presents with periarticular osteopenia and corresponding increased activity on TPBS.

## Suggested Readings

Love C, Din AS, Tomas MB, Kalapparambath TP, Palestro CJ. Radionuclide bone imaging: an illustrative review. Radiographics. 2003; 23(2):341–358

Kozin F, Soin JS, Ryan LM, Carrera GF, Wortmann RL. Bone scintigraphy in the reflex sympathetic dystrophy syndrome. Radiology. 1981; 138(2):437–443

# Case 81

*Kamal D. Singh*

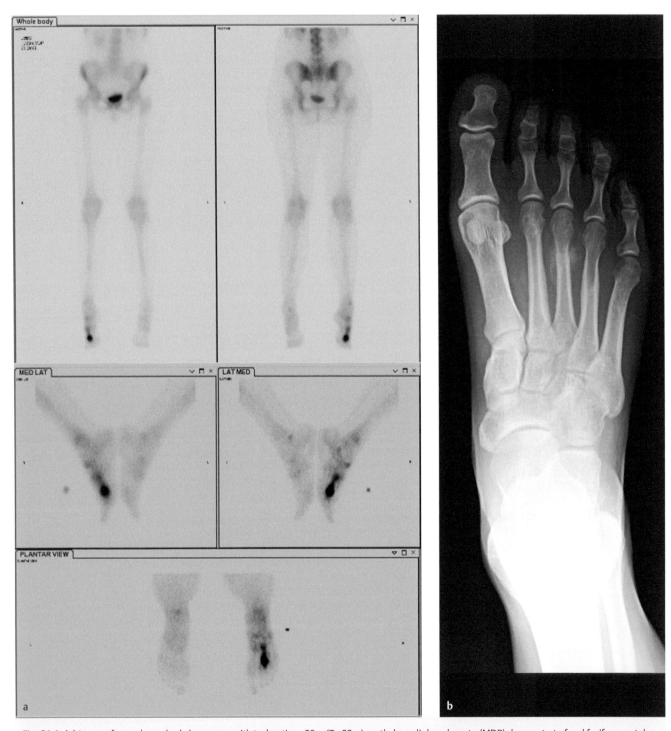

**Fig. 81.1** **(a)** Images from a lower body bone scan with technetium-99m (Tc-99m) methylene diphosphonate (MDP) demonstrate focal fusiform uptake extending completely across the mid left third metatarsal. **(b)** Correlative radiograph shows nondisplaced fracture with surrounding periosteal healing.

## ■ Clinical History

24-year-old female with right fourth metatarsal pain and tenderness (▶ Fig. 81.1).

■ **Key Finding**

Focal increased activity within an extremity on bone scan

■ **Top 3 Differential Diagnoses**

- **Stress fracture.** Tc-99m hydroxy diphosphonate (HDP) or methylene diphosphonate (MDP) localizes to areas of increased osteoblastic activity. Over 80% of fractures are detected within the first 24 hours and nearly 95% by 72 hours. Stress fractures are classified as either fatigue fractures, which are fractures in normal bone exposed to abnormal stress, or insufficiency fractures, which are fractures in abnormal bone exposed to normal stress. Repetitive stress can lead to microfractures which may progress to overt fracture if unrecognized. Typical sites for fatigue-type stress fractures include the tibia, fibula, medial femoral neck, inferior pubic ramus, metatarsals, and calcaneus. Stress fractures are seen as intense focal, fusiform activity on bone scan, typically greater in intensity than the anterior superior iliac spine on the anterior image or sacroiliac joints on the posterior image. Stress fractures within long bones can be graded based on their extent of corticomedullary involvement. Single-photon emission computed tomography (SPECT) should be performed if concern is for femoral neck stress fracture as up to 50% can be missed on planar images. Treatment includes rest and modification of activity.
- **Osteomyelitis.** This disease may occur due to extension from adjacent soft tissue cellulitis, direct inoculation from open wound, or by hematogenous spread. Three-phase bone scan (TPBS) has high negative predictive value for osteomyelitis. Cellulitis demonstrates hyperemia and soft-tissue uptake on early phases but no abnormal bone activity on delayed imaging. Osteomyelitis, in contrast, is positive on all three phases. Specificity for osteomyelitis is lower in the setting of recent trauma, surgery, or orthopedic hardware, necessitating correlation with indium-111-labeled white blood cells (In-111 WBC) and Tc-99m SC scans.
- **Neoplasm (benign and malignant).** Primary bone malignancies (e.g., osteosarcoma and Ewing's sarcoma) and osteoblastic metastases generally demonstrate avid uptake on bone scan. Sensitivity is lower for predominantly lytic lesions (multiple myeloma, renal cell carcinoma, and thyroid cancer). Benign bone tumors have a variable appearance on bone scan but generally do not demonstrate significant hyperemia with the exception of osteoid osteoma (OO). Osteoid osteoma has focal intense uptake within a central vascular nidus with comparatively less uptake in the surrounding reactive sclerosis, described as the "double-density" or "target" sign. Clinically, patients present with dull, achy night pain that is relieved by nonsteroidal anti-inflammatory drugs. Solitary bone cysts are generally photopenic, while bone islands and osseous hemangiomas rarely are detectable on bone scan. Benign, uncomplicated exostoses and enchondromas are usually warm on bone scan.

■ **Additional Diagnostic Consideration**

- **Fibrous dysplasia (FD):** It is a congenital, nonhereditary skeletal dysplasia that generally demonstrates intense uptake on bone scan. Common areas of involvement include the ribs, tibia, femur, and craniofacial bones. The skeletal lesions demonstrate the classic expanded ground glass matrix on plain film. Bone scan is helpful in detecting polyostotic involvement.

■ **Diagnosis**

Completed stress fracture.

✓ **Pearls**

- Stress fractures (fatigue or insufficiency) present as focal uptake in characteristic locations.
- OO is positive on all three phases of bone scan with a characteristic "target" sign.
- Multifocal uptake may be seen with metastases, osteomyelitis, insufficiency fractures, FD, or Paget's disease.
- Osseous metastases are generally seen within the axial rather than appendicular skeleton.

**Suggested Readings**

Bryant LR, Song WS, Banks KP, Bui-Mansfield LT, Bradley YC. Comparison of planar scintigraphy alone and with SPECT for the initial evaluation of femoral neck stress fracture. AJR Am J Roentgenol. 2008; 191(4):1010–1015

Love C, Din AS, Tomas MB, Kalapparambath TP, Palestro CJ. Radionuclide bone imaging: an illustrative review. Radiographics. 2003; 23(2):341–358

# Case 82

*Mickaila Johnston*

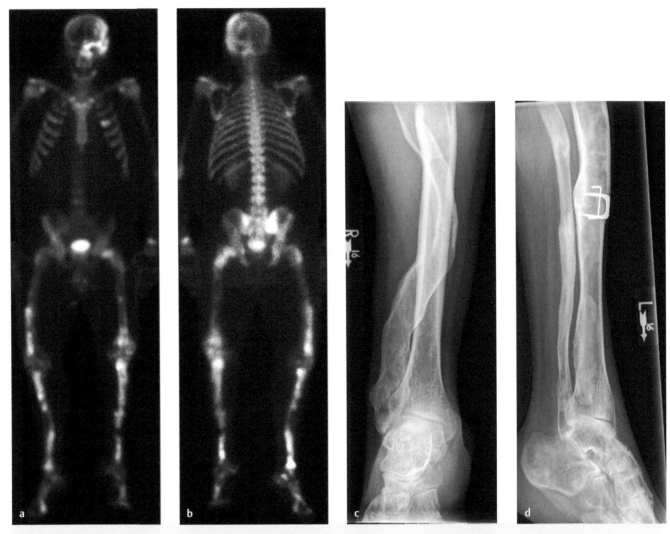

**Fig. 82.1** Anterior **(a)** and posterior **(b)** planar whole-body bone images with Tc-99m hydroxy diphosphonate (HDP) demonstrate multiple noncontiguously distributed long segment regions of heterogeneously increased uptake, predominantly in the bilateral lower extremities (both above and below the knee) and the left skull. Plain films through the right **(c)** and left **(d)** lower extremities reveal abnormal angulation or "bowing," predominantly lucent changes with ground glass type replacement and a few areas with well-defined borders of sclerosis. Moreover, there are multiple areas of cortical thinning and expansion with neither cortical disruption nor periosteal reaction.

■ **Clinical History**

43-year-old male with unilateral café-au-lait spots and multiple lytic fractures (▶ Fig. 82.1).

## ■ Key Finding

Regionally increased uptake on bone scintigraphy

## ■ Top 3 Differential Diagnoses

• **Fibrous dysplasia (FD).** One-fourth of FDs are polyostotic. Three-fourths are monostotic and most commonly involve the rib, proximal femur, tibia, and skull. Coxa vara angulation ("shepherd's crook") can be seen in the proximal femur as well as anterior bowing of the tibia ("saber shin"). Tc-99m medronic acid (MDP) bone scintigraphy demonstrates increased radiotracer deposition where there is increased osseous metabolism, not always contiguous. Classic radiographic findings include a well-circumscribed lucent lesion within the metaphysis or diaphysis, often with a ground glass matrix and fusiform enlargement. Bowing deformities may require surgical correction.

• **Paget's disease.** This disease evolves through three phases: early lytic, mixed, and sclerotic. A sharply demarcated line of osteolysis advances from the epiphysis toward the diaphysis in a contiguous manner. Bone scan will show increased uptake in all three phases, particularly in active disease.

• **Osteosarcoma.** This is a bone-forming malignant neoplasm that demonstrates increased radiotracer deposition on bone scintigraphy. Primary osteosarcoma usually presents in the metadiaphysis of long bones, secondary more frequently involving flat bones. Primary osteosarcoma is known to have "skip" lesions within the primary affected bone which can cause uptake similar to FD and Paget's disease on scintigraphy.

## ■ Additional Diagnostic Consideration

• **Complex regional pain syndrome:** CRPS most frequently presents as regional polyostotic periarticular increased radiotracer deposition on bone scintigraphy. It will involve most, if not all, of the osseous structures in the affected region. CRPS can be photopenic on bone scan, known as "cold CRPS," more commonly seen in pediatric patients.

## ■ Diagnosis

Polyostotic FD.

## ✓ Pearls

• FD rarely undergoes malignant change and often are not surgically corrected.
• Bone scan is better for staging of Paget's as radiography may underestimate disease.

• Osteosarcoma can present with "skip" lesions resulting in regional uptake on bone scan.
• Regional, polyostotic, and periarticular uptake is seen with CRPS which is hot on all three phases.

## Suggested Readings

Kwon HW, Paeng JC, Nahm FS, et al. Diagnostic performance of three-phase bone scan for complex regional pain syndrome type 1 with optimally modified image criteria. Nucl Med Mol Imaging. 2011; 45(4):261–267

Rubin AN, Byrns K, Zhou D, Freedman L. Fibrous dysplasia of the rib: AIRP best cases in radiologic-pathologic correlation. Radiographics. 2015; 35(7):2049–2052

Theodorou DJ, Theodorou SJ, Kakitsubata Y. Imaging of Paget disease of bone and its musculoskeletal complications: review. AJR Am J Roentgenol. 2011; 196(6, Suppl):S64–S75

# Case 83

*Mickaila Johnston*

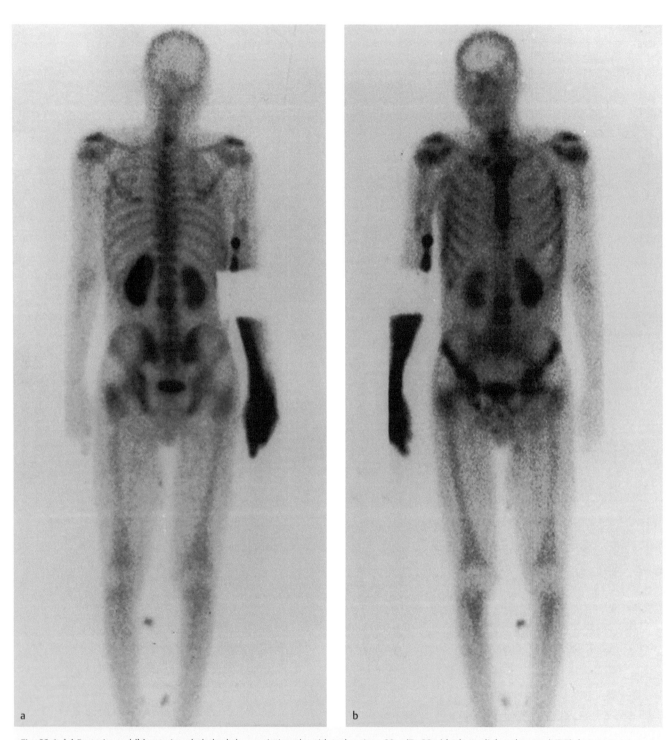

**Fig. 83.1** **(a)** Posterior and **(b)** anterior whole-body bone scintigraphy with technetium-99m (Tc-99m) hydroxy diphosphonate (HDP) demonstrates increased soft-tissue radiotracer deposition within the right forearm and hand.

■ **Clinical History**

Patient presents for whole-body bone scintigraphy (▶ Fig. 83.1).

■ Key Finding

Focal soft-tissue uptake on bone scintigraphy

■ Top 3 Differential Diagnoses

- **Heterotopic ossification (myositis ossificans).** Heterotopic ossification (HO), or bone formation where bone is not usually present, can be acquired or hereditary. Acquired HO is much more common and results from transformation of mesenchymal cells into osteogenic cells. It is usually seen after fracture, direct muscular trauma, surgery, closed head injury, or spinal cord injury. Clinical presentation is not specific and can include pain, fever, swelling, and erythema, with eventual loss of range of motion. If biopsied early, before the heterotopic bone has matured, pathology will show immature bone and fibrous proliferation and may be confused for osteosarcoma. Conventional radiography will initially show a nondescript calcific density that will evolve to mature bone on subsequent images. Three-phase bone scintigraphy is the most sensitive exam for early HO, with changes seen 4 to 6 weeks prior to the initial mineralization seen on radiographs. Initially, just the flow and blood pool images will be positive with delayed uptake seen around 1 week later. Bone scan will eventually show progressive decrease in deposition, with return to baseline after about 1 year.

- **Soft-tissue calcification.** The uptake mechanism for the phosphate analogue bone tracers, Tc-99m medronic acid (MDP) and Tc-99m HDP, involves chemisorption primarily into the hydroxyapatite phase of bone formation. However, some of the radiotracer will be taken up by amorphous calcification. Focal/regional extraosseous uptake can be seen due to altered biodistribution from changed vascularity, extraosseous calcification (dystrophic, metastatic, or tumoral), neoplasms, or an inflammatory process. Correlation with anatomic imaging and clinical history will be helpful. Metabolic abnormalities will result in more diffuse uptake.

- **Nonvenous injection.** Intra-arterial injection of radiotracer often produces a characteristic "glove" distribution pattern. Extravasation produces a focal area of radiotracer deposition at the injection site. With extravasation, there may also be focal radiotracer accumulation in the closest lymph node bed, often the axilla, mimicking focal soft-tissue uptake. Single-photon emission computed tomography (SPECT)/CT imaging can play an important role in establishing this as the etiology.

■ Additional Diagnostic Consideration

- **Breast tissue involvement:** There can be focal radiotracer uptake within the postpubertal, lactating, or nonlactating breast tissue. It can be a finding in the setting of mastitis. It can also be from metastases and primary breast malignancies.

■ Diagnosis

Nonvenous injection.

✓ Pearls

- Serial bone scans of HO demonstrate decreasing radiotracer deposition, paralleling injury resolution.
- Tumoral calcinosis is often associated with articular bursa along extensor surfaces.

- Nonvenous injection of radiotracer produces localized uptake often characteristic in nature.
- Clinical history and anatomic imaging are helpful in the setting of extraosseous bone scan uptake.

Suggested Readings

Olsen KM, Chew FS. Tumoral calcinosis: pearls, polemics, and alternative possibilities. Radiographics. 2006; 26(3):871–885

Shehab D, Elgazzar AH, Collier BD. Heterotopic ossification. J Nucl Med. 2002; 43(3):346–353

Wale DJ, Wong KK, Savas H, Kandathil A, Piert M, Brown RK. Extraosseous findings on bone scintigraphy using fusion SPECT/CT and correlative imaging. AJR Am J Roentgenol. 2015; 205(1):160–172

# Case 84

*Mickaila Johnston*

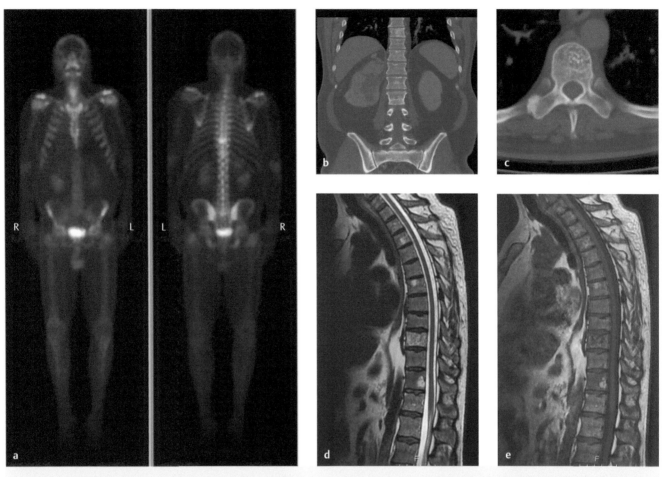

**Fig. 84.1** Anterior and posterior whole-body bone scintigraphy with technetium-99m (Tc-99m) hydroxy diphosphonate (HDP) demonstrates focally increased radiotracer deposition in the lower thoracic spine, seen best on the posterior image **(a)**. Select coronal CT image demonstrates "rainfall" or "corduroy" area of sclerosis in a lower thoracic vertebral body **(b)**. Select axial CT demonstrates "polka dot" pattern of sclerosis in the same vertebral body **(c)**. Fluid bright sequence (3-T) magnetic resonance image demonstrates increased fluid in a thoracic vertebral body **(d)**. Fluid dark sequence (3-T) magnetic resonance image demonstrates low signal in a vertebral body **(e)**.

■ Clinical History

58-year-old male with renal cell carcinoma (▶ Fig. 84.1).

## ■ Key Finding

Focal axial spine uptake on bone scintigraphy

## ■ Top 3 Differential Diagnoses

- **Degenerative joint disease.** Axial spine degenerative joint disease is pervasive in older generations. However, it most often presents with metabolic activity juxtaposed with the vertebral body in a periarticular distribution. Anatomic imaging facilitates interpretation and differentiation of osteophytes.
- **Metastatic disease.** Metastatic disease most often involves the vertebral body proper, the pedicle, and/or the posterior elements. It rarely involves the articular surfaces. While metastatic disease is most commonly multifocal, a single hot lesion in the spine on bone scan in a patient with a known malignancy is still likely to be a metastasis.

- **Spondylolysis.** It is often associated with focal low back pain that worsens with activity. It is often seen in athletic adolescents. Spondylolysis is the result of an ongoing stress reaction. As such, there can be bone scintigraphy findings before anatomic changes are noticed. Bone scan uptake indicates symptomatic spondylolysis with active healing that may benefit from immobilization. Bone scan may also show uptake in the contralateral pars interarticularis raising concern for impending fracture.

## ■ Additional Diagnostic Considerations

- **Discitis:** Bone scan can be used for initial nuclear medicine evaluation for discitis/osteomyelitis, and it should demonstrate uptake surrounding a disc space. Gallium-67 scintigraphy or flourine-18 FDG PET imaging is preferred over tagged WBC imaging for confirmation due to the high false-negative rate with WBC imaging in the spine.
- **Primary bone tumor:** Several primary bone lesions can be located within the axial spine and demonstrate increased

uptake on bone scan. These include OO, osteoblastoma, chondroblastoma (CB), malignant fibrous histiocytoma, Ewing's sarcoma, lymphoma, chordoma, giant cell tumor (GCT), and hemangioma among others. Hemangiomas are commonly encountered, usually incidentally discovered on anatomic imaging and indistinguishable on bone scan, but may present as focally increased or focally decreased radiotracer deposition.

## ■ Diagnosis

Vertebral hemangioma.

## ✓ Pearls

- Degenerative changes in the axial spine have periarticular hot spots.
- Metastatic disease is most often located eccentrically in the vertebral body or pedicle.

- Hemangiomas are usually "normal" on bone scintigraphy.
- Metabolic scintigraphy findings can precede anatomic changes in spondylolysis.

## Suggested Readings

Han BK, Ryu JS, Moon DH, Shin MJ, Kim YT, Lee HK. Bone SPECT imaging of vertebral hemangioma correlation with MR imaging and symptoms. Clin Nucl Med. 1995; 20(10):916–921

Park JS, Moon SK, Jin W, Ryu KN. Unilateral lumbar spondylolysis on radiography and MRI: emphasis on morphologic differences according to involved segment. AJR Am J Roentgenol. 2010; 194(1):207–215

Yang J, Servaes S, Edwards K, Zhuang H. Prevalence of stress reaction in the pars interarticularis in pediatric patients with new-onset lower back pain. Clin Nucl Med. 2013; 38(2):110–114

# Case 85

*Mickaila Johnston*

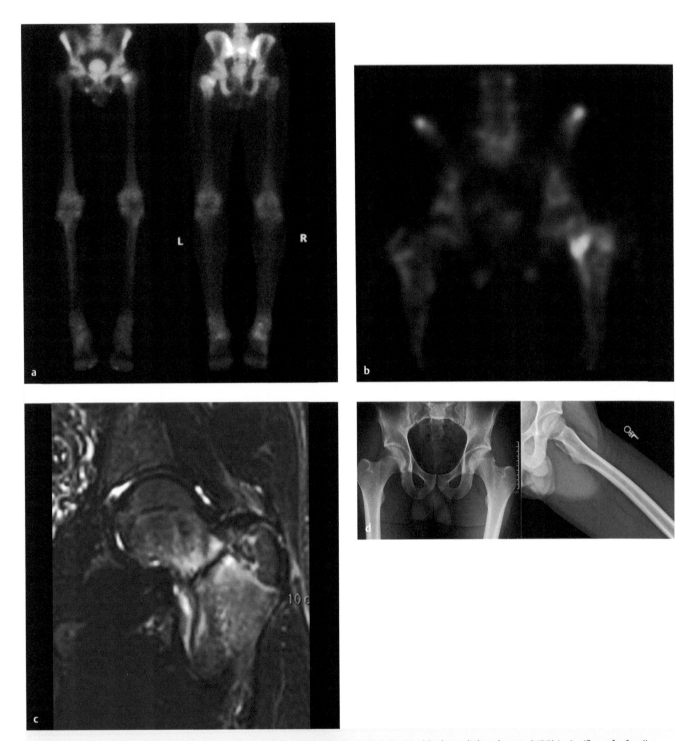

**Fig. 85.1** Anterior and posterior waist down bone scintigraphy with technetium-99m (Tc-99m) hydroxy diphosphonate (HDP) is significant for focally increased radiotracer deposition in the region of the left hip (a). Select coronal single-photon emission computed tomography image of the hips confirms focal radiotracer deposition in the left femoral neck (b). Select same day coronal left hip fluid bright sequence short tau inversion recovery (3-T) magnetic resonance image demonstrates a fatigue line, completely crossing the femoral neck with juxtaposed edema (c). The fracture was not evident on radiographs obtained one day prior (d).

■ **Clinical History**

21-year-old male with five days of left hip pain after completing an obstacle course (▶Fig. 85.1).

## ■ Key Finding

Focally increased uptake in the hip on bone scintigraphy

## ■ Top 3 Differential Diagnoses

- **Stress fracture.** Femoral neck stress fractures present with focal pain in the hip or groin, often in cases of athletes and runners. Plain film radiographs often fail to demonstrate significant changes, particularly early in the course. Untreated femoral neck stress fractures have complications including avascular necrosis (AVN), making diagnosis important. Single-photon emission computed tomography (SPECT) images are essential if bone scan is performed, as around half of femoral neck stress fractures will be missed on planar images. Magnetic resonance imaging is the gold standard in diagnosis showing edema and a fracture line. Stress fractures more commonly involve the compressive side of the femoral neck.

- Tension side femoral neck stress fractures must be made non-weight-bearing with immediate orthopedic referral.
- **Stress change without complete fracture.** Fracture is the result of ongoing stress change. With abatement of the causative factor, edema, subtotal fracture, and repair may occur. Bone scintigraphy will still demonstrate increased metabolic activity before anatomic imaging is abnormal.
- **Synovial herniation pit.** Also known as "Pitt's pit," it can present as a focal area of increased radiotracer distribution on bone scintigraphy. This is associated with a small round to oval lucency with surrounding thin sclerosis just distal to the femoral articular surface, in an anterior-superior location.

## ■ Additional Diagnostic Considerations

- **Degenerative changes:** Degenerative changes about the hip are seen frequently on bone scintigraphy, particularly in older patients usually being evaluated for metastatic disease. Like all degenerative type uptake, increased activity will be periarticular and is easily confirmed with comparison radiographs.

- **Tumor:** It is always important to consider primary and metastatic lesions with abnormal bone uptake, particularly in the axial and proximal appendicular skeleton.

## ■ Diagnosis

Femoral neck stress fracture.

## ✓ Pearls

- Stress injury starts with edema and stress change leading to complete fracture if stress continues.
- Synovial herniation pits can mimic tensile side femoral neck stress change, but are benign.
- Classically, stress changes start on the compressive side of the femoral neck.

- Tension side femoral neck stress fractures generally require immediate orthopedic consultation.
- Around half of femoral neck stress fractures seen on SPECT are missed on planar imaging.

## Suggested Readings

Bryant LR, Song WS, Banks KP, Bui-Mansfield LT, Bradley YC. Comparison of planar scintigraphy alone and with SPECT for the initial evaluation of femoral neck stress fracture. AJR Am J Roentgenol. 2008; 191(4):1010–1015

Pitt MJ, Graham AR, Shipman JH, Birkby W. Herniation pit of the femoral neck. AJR Am J Roentgenol. 1982; 138(6):1115–1121

# Case 86

*Victoria A. Campbell*

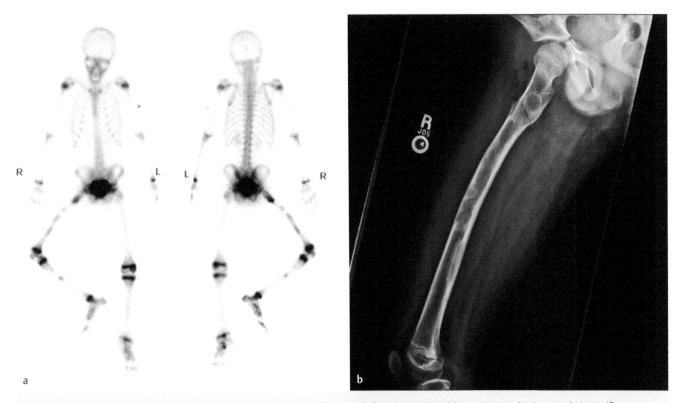

**Fig. 86.1** Anterior and posterior whole-body technetium-99m (Tc-99m) hydroxy diphosphonate (HDP) bone scintigraphy, in a youth, is significant for numerous focally increased areas of radiotracer deposition within the right lower extremity **(a)**. Plain radiography of the right femur demonstrates pathologic fracture through a mixed lytic and sclerotic lesion of the proximal femur **(b)**. Case reprinted with permission, originally published in: Campbell VA, Starsiak MD, Johnston MJ. Radiographically benign-appearing lesion in child with uptake on bone scan. J Am Osteopath Coll Radiol. 2016;5(3):24–26.

## ▪ Clinical History

8-year-old boy fell from monkey bars and could not bear weight on his right leg (▶Fig. 86.1).

## ■ Key Finding

Bone scan uptake associated with a radiographically benign lesion in a pediatric patient

## ■ Top 3 Differential Diagnoses

- **Fibrous dysplasia (FD).** FD lesions are not painful unless complicated by pathologic fracture. The radiographic appearance of FD lesions may be protean. Typically, FD lesions initially demonstrate a purely lytic appearance and then develop a hazy or "ground glass" appearance as the matrix calcifies and the bone scan becomes focally positive. Such lesions tend to occur centrally within bone, rather than cortically, and often have an expansile appearance. FD may present in monostotic (three-fourths) or polyostotic (one-fourth) patterns. When polyostotic, FD lesions are often unilateral.
- **Nonossifying fibroma.** Also known as fibroxanthoma. It is a common lesion in the pediatric population with incidences reported as high as 25%. Bone scintigraphy may reveal increased uptake during the "healing phase" of these lesions secondary to increased osteoblastic activity. Such lesions are typically seen within the metaphysis of long bones, often about the knee. Biopsy should be avoided as these lesions may reveal a more aggressive histopathological appearance resulting in unnecessary treatment-related morbidity.
- **Langerhans cell histiocytosis.** These lesions may or may not be associated with pain and are encountered nearly exclusively in the pediatric and young adult population. Langerhans cell histiocytosis is most commonly monostotic, but may be polyostotic.

## ■ Additional Diagnostic Consideration

- **Osteomyelitis:** Osteomyelitis can have a wide range of radiographic appearance, i.e., from aggressive to benign. Subacute or chronic osteomyelitis is more likely to present with a benign appearance. Uptake on bone scan is seen as the infection instigates an osteoblastic response, with uptake seen up to 14 days prior to radiographic findings. A negative three-phase bone scan (TPBS) essentially excludes osteomyelitis.

## ■ Diagnosis

Polyostotic FD.

## ✓ Pearls

- FD starts lytic and develops a "ground glass" matrix.
- Biopsy of nonossifying fibroma is not indicated and may lead to unnecessary treatment.
- Langerhans cell histiocytosis is most commonly monostotic.

## Suggested Readings

Fitzpatrick KA, Taljanovic MS, Speer DP, et al. Imaging findings of fibrous dysplasia with histopathologic and intraoperative correlation. AJR Am J Roentgenol. 2004; 182(6):1389–1398

Kilborn TN, Teh J, Goodman TR. Paediatric manifestations of Langerhans cell histiocytosis: a review of the clinical and radiological findings. Clin Radiol. 2003; 58(4):269–278

Machida K, Makita K, Nishikawa J, Ohtake T, Iio M. Scintigraphic manifestation of fibrous dysplasia. Clin Nucl Med. 1986; 11(6):426–429

# Case 87

*Mickaila Johnston*

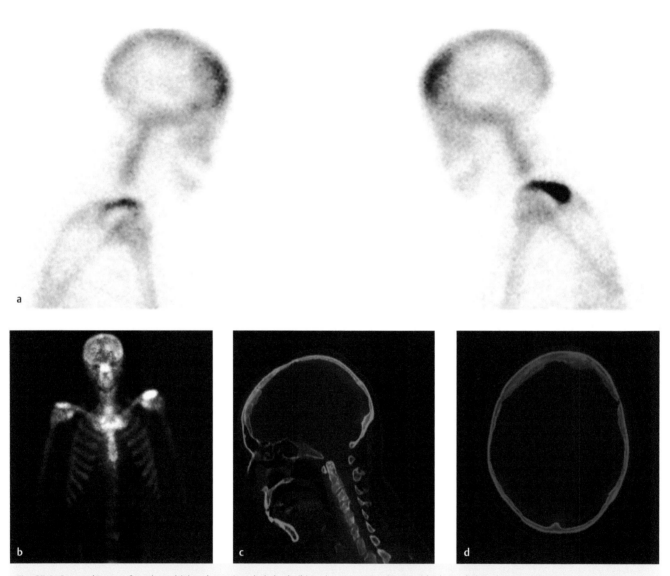

**Fig. 87.1** Cropped images from lateral **(a)** and anterior whole body **(b)** Technetium-99m (Tc-99m) hydroxy diphosphonate (HDP) bone scintigraphy demonstrate diffusely increased radiotracer deposition along the frontal skull as well as deposition within the left scapula. Same time, select sagittal **(c)** and axial **(d)** single-photon emission computed tomography/computed tomography (SPECT/CT) fused images demonstrate increased metabolic activity within frontal hyperostosis.

## ■ Clinical History

71-year-old male with known prostate cancer, metastatic to the left scapula (▶Fig. 87.1).

## ■ Key Finding

Calvarial uptake on bone scintigraphy

## ■ Top 3 Differential Diagnoses

- **Hyperostosis frontalis interna.** Isolated increased radiotracer deposition with bone seeking agents involving the frontal and parietal bones is characteristic for hyperostosis frontalis interna (HFI). CT will often demonstrate nodular thickening of the inner table of the frontal bone with extension to involve parietal bones. While there is no definitive etiology, prolonged estrogen exposure is a leading theory, as it is most often seen in postmenopausal women. HFI is a benign finding requiring no further work up.
- **Paget's disease.** Around three out of four patients with Paget's disease of bone are asymptomatic at presentation. Skull involvement may present with changing hat size. Osteoporosis circumscripta presents as a large cold skull lesion that is hypermetabolic peripherally. This is in contrast to the "tam o'shanter sign" which reveals hypermetabolic activity of the entire skull. Both are phases of Paget's disease of bone and thus represent excessive remodeling of osseous structures. Bone scintigraphy is useful for staging polyostotic disease. Calcitonin, second-generation bisphosphonates, and mithramycin are most commonly used to ameliorate the process.
- **Fibrous dysplasia (FD).** FD is a nonneoplastic process that results from dysfunctional differentiation of osteoblasts. It can affect any bone in the body. About one out of four cases of monostotic FD will involve the skull and facial bones, whereas in polyostotic disease the figures are three out of four cases. A single lesion often demonstrates variable metabolic activity.

## ■ Additional Diagnostic Considerations

- **Metastatic disease:** Skull metastases are common observed in approximately a quarter of all cancer patients. Primary tumors which most commonly metastasize to bone include prostate, breast, lung, thyroid, and kidney. Skull metastases will most frequently present as multiple foci of increased uptake on bone scan and are usually asymptomatic.
- **Metabolic bone disease:** Metabolic bone disease can result in a "superscan," meaning there is diffuse increased skeletal activity with suppressed renal and soft-tissue uptake. Intense calvarial uptake out of proportion to the remainder of the skeleton is another feature.
- **Sickle cell anemia:** Increased uptake in the calvarium with sickle cell anemia can be seen secondary to medullary expansion, resulting in expansion of the diploic spaces, as well as with healing bone infarcts.

## ■ Diagnosis

HFI.

## ✓ Pearls

- Isolated increased uptake on bone scan involving the frontal and parietal bones may be due HFI.
- Bone scan findings of Paget's disease of the skull is variable based on the phase of disease.
- The majority of patients with polyostotic FD will have skull and facial bone involvement.

## Suggested Readings

Ihde LL, Forrester DM, Gottsegen CJ, et al. Sclerosing bone dysplasias: review and differentiation from other causes of osteosclerosis. Radiographics. 2011; 31(7):1865–1882

Love C, Din AS, Tomas MB, Kalapparambath TP, Palestro CJ. Radionuclide bone imaging: an illustrative review. Radiographics. 2003; 23(2):341–358

O'Sullivan GJ, Carty FL, Cronin CG. Imaging of bone metastasis: An update. World J Radiol. 2015; 7(8):202–211

Theodorou DJ, Theodorou SJ, Kakitsubata Y. Imaging of Paget disease of bone and its musculoskeletal complications: review. AJR Am J Roentgenol. 2011; 196(6, Suppl):S64–S75

# Case 88

*Mickaila Johnston*

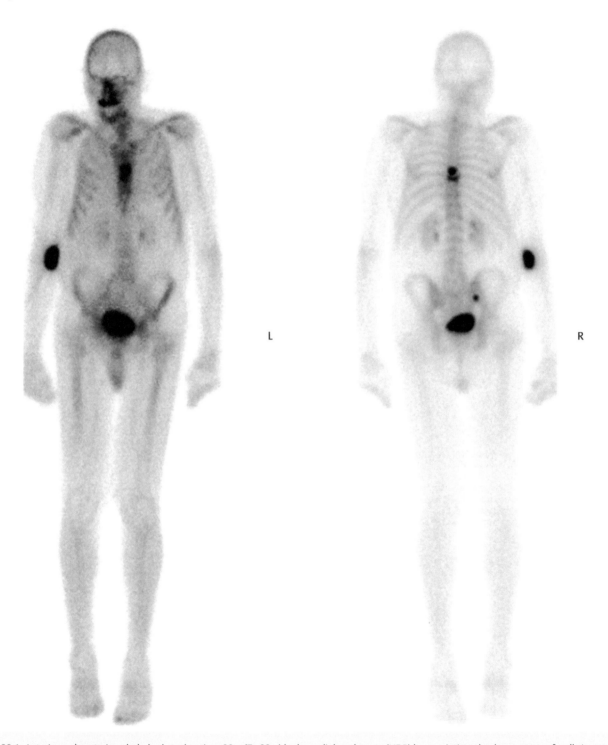

L    R

**Fig. 88.1** Anterior and posterior whole-body technetium-99m (Tc-99m) hydroxy diphosphonate (HDP) bone scintigraphy demonstrates focally increased radiotracer deposition within the mid thoracic vertebral column and adjacent to the right sacroiliac joint. Right antecubital fossa uptake is due to partial infiltration of the injection.

### ■ Clinical History

70-year-old male with metastatic prostate cancer and stable prostate-specific antigen (PSA) (▶ Fig. 88.1).

## ■ Key Finding

Sacral uptake on bone scintigraphy

## ■ Top 3 Differential Diagnoses

- **Benign tumors.** Benign processes include the usual list of osseous foci: GCTs, aneurysmal bone cysts (ABCs), OOs, osteoblastoma, hemangioma, and nerve sheath tumors. The differentiating features for each process are well defined and best evaluated with anatomic imaging instead of physiologic.
- **Insufficiency fracture.** On bone scintigraphy, an "H" or butterfly shape can be seen with sacral insufficiency fractures. Also described is a "linear dot" pattern of distribution. Outside of trauma, back pain is the most common presenting symptom. The risk for insufficiency fracture is higher when there is decreased mineralization, as seen with prior radiation therapy, steroids, osteoporosis, and rheumatoid arthritis.
- **Metastases.** Sacral metastases normally display a random distribution of involvement. Metastases are the most common malignant tumors of the sacrum, often from lung, breast, renal, and prostate primaries. The sacrum can accommodate a larger mass before symptoms arise, often leading to a delay in diagnosis. As a hematopoietic site, malignancies in the sacrum can include myeloma and lymphoma.

## ■ Additional Diagnostic Consideration

- **Primary neoplasm:** Chordomas are the most common primary sacral neoplasms, followed in incidence by chondrosarcoma, Ewing's sarcoma, and osteosarcoma. With the exception of Ewing's sarcoma, these neoplasms are predominantly found in the later half of life.

## ■ Diagnosis

Metastases to the right sacrum.

## ✓ Pearls

- Benign osseous foci can present in the sacrum; anatomic imaging helps differentiate etiologies.
- Sacral insufficiency fractures may have a classic "H" or butterfly shape on bone scintigraphy.
- Metastases are the most common sacral neoplasm.
- Primary sacral neoplasms are rare and most often hematopoietic based.

## Suggested Readings

Balseiro J, Brower AC, Ziessman HA. Scintigraphic diagnosis of sacral fractures. AJR Am J Roentgenol. 1987; 148(1):111–113

Diel J, Ortiz O, Losada RA, Price DB, Hayt MW, Katz DS. The sacrum: pathologic spectrum, multimodality imaging, and subspecialty approach. Radiographics. 2001; 21(1):83–104

Llauger J, Palmer J, Amores S, Bagué S, Camins A. Primary tumors of the sacrum: diagnostic imaging. AJR Am J Roentgenol. 2000; 174(2):417–424

Thornton E, Krajewski KM, O'Regan KN, Giardino AA, Jagannathan JP, Ramaiya N. Imaging features of primary and secondary malignant tumours of the sacrum. Br J Radiol. 2012; 85(1011):279–286

# Case 89

*Mickaila Johnston*

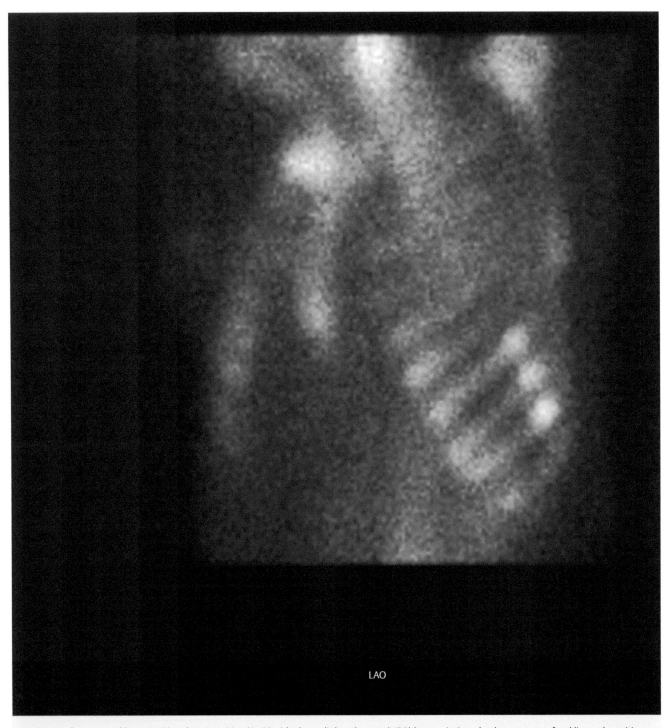

**Fig. 86.1** Left anterior oblique (LAO) technetium-99m (Tc-99m) hydroxy diphosphonate (HDP) bone scintigraphy demonstrates focal linear deposition of radiotracer along several left lateral ribs.

■ **Clinical History**

53-year-old male with a recent fall (▶ Fig. 89.1).

## ■ Key Finding

Rib uptake on bone scintigraphy

## ■ Top 3 Differential Diagnoses

- **Trauma.** Focal uptake on bone scintigraphy secondary to trauma is one of the "more common" abnormal findings, especially when there is a report of antecedent trauma. The pattern of distribution and clinical history are key to deciphering whether or not additional imaging is needed to explain the foci. Trauma presents as focal areas of increased radiotracer deposition which may be present within 24 hours of injury and persist for over 12 months. A linear distribution of radiotracer activity across multiple ribs is a frequently described pattern of distribution seen with thoracic trauma. Scintigraphy is well established in the unique setting of pediatric nonaccidental trauma, particularly when considering posterior rib fractures.
- **Metastases.** These are more common than primary malignancies involving the ribs. Osteoblastic metastases are more likely to have increased uptake on bone scintigraphy, although lytic metastases occasionally have increased activity due to reactive sclerosis or pathologic fracture. Rib metastases may appear to spread along the length of a rib in a linear pattern, morphologically different than traumatic uptake, and rarely involve contiguous ribs in a linear distribution. Metastatic disease is usually multifocal. A solitary rib lesion has around 10% chance of being metastatic in etiology in a patient with known malignancy. Ultrasound may be able to differentiate rib metastases from trauma.
- **Primary neoplasm.** Primary neoplasms of the ribs are rare. Chondroid processes are the more common and they most often occur at or near the costochondral junction. Anatomic imaging will show expansion with localized calcification. Chondrosarcoma, plasmacytoma, and lymphoma are the most common primary lesions involving ribs.

## ■ Diagnosis

Rib fractures (trauma).

## ✓ Pearls

- Multiple small, round foci in a linear pattern across multiple contiguous ribs suggest trauma.
- Metastases may appear to spread along the length of the involved rib, different than traumatic uptake.
- The most common malignancy involving the ribs is metastatic disease.
- Chondroid neoplasias occur at or near the costochondral junction.

## Suggested Readings

Guttentag AR, Salwen JK. Keep your eyes on the ribs: the spectrum of normal variants and diseases that involve the ribs. Radiographics. 1999; 19(5):1125–1142

Kleinman PK, Marks SC, Adams VI, Blackbourne BD. Factors affecting visualization of posterior rib fractures in abused infants. AJR Am J Roentgenol. 1988; 150(3):635–638

Paik SH, Chung MJ, Park JS, Goo JM, Im JG. High-resolution sonography of the rib: can fracture and metastasis be differentiated? AJR Am J Roentgenol. 2005; 184(3):969–974

# Case 90

*Mickaila Johnston*

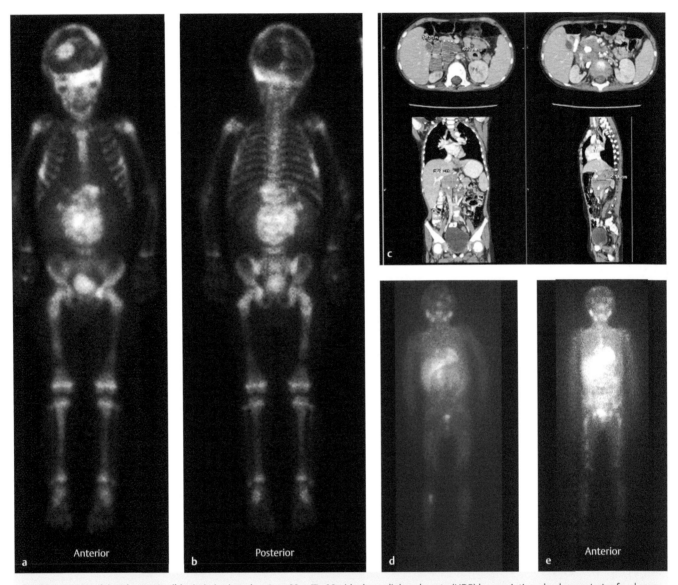

**Fig. 90.1** Anterior **(a)** and posterior **(b)** whole-body technetium-99m (Tc-99m) hydroxy diphosphonate (HDP) bone scintigraphy demonstrates focal areas of radiotracer deposition in the mid abdomen and in multiple osseous sites. One month prior contrast-enhanced CT select axial, coronal, and sagittal slices demonstrate a paramedian mass **(c)**. Four years prior **(d)** and current **(e)** 24-hour delayed anterior whole-body I-123 metaiodobenzylguanidine (MIBG) images demonstrate persistence of the abdominal mass with multiple osseous foci.

## ▪ Clinical History

8-year-old male with known abdominal malignancy (▶ Fig. 90.1).

## ■ Key Finding

Abdominal activity on bone scintigraphy

## ■ Top 3 Differential Diagnoses

- **Artifact.** Artifact from poor radiotracer preparation with the Tc-99m-labeled diphosphonates used for bone scintigraphy can result in uptake within the abdominal cavity. Free Tc-99m pertechnetate, if present, will demonstrate gastric uptake. This should have associated uptake in the salivary glands and thyroid. Liver uptake may occur if there is aluminum chemical impurity causing radiopharmaceutical colloid formation. A confirmatory finding is splenic activity and decreased osseous uptake.
- **Malignant ascites.** Bone scintigraphy findings can be positive in the abdomen anywhere there are malignant cells metabolizing calcium. Moreover, the diphosphonates may concentrate in extraosseous sites such as pleural effusions, pericardial effusions, and abdominal ascites. The exact etiology is unclear, but increased blood flow and vascular permeability are the likely causes.
- **Metastases.** The labeled diphosphonates used for bone scintigraphy are taken up via chemisorption into the formation of both hydroxyapatite and amorphous calcification. Distribution of uptake on the delayed image is primarily dependent on the calcium concentration of tissue. For this reason, calcifying metastatic lesions may show uptake on bone scan. Mucinous colorectal and ovarian adenocarcinoma are frequently responsible for calcifying metastatic lesions within the abdomen.

## ■ Additional Diagnostic Considerations

- **Neoplasm.** Several benign and malignant neoplasms have been shown to accumulate Tc-99m-labeled diphosphonates, including sarcomas and neuroblastoma, specific to abdominal uptake. Uptake may also be seen in any necrotic tumor likely due to neovascularity and hyperemia, as well as microscopic calcium deposition.
- **Dystrophic calcification/heterotopic ossification (HO).** Calcification in degenerating or necrotic tissue can cause extraosseous uptake anywhere in the body on bone scintigraphy.

Splenic autoinfartction and diffuse hepatic necrosis represent examples of such processes which occur in the abdomen. HO will also demonstrate bone tracer uptake, more frequently seen in lower extremity musculature than in the abdomen.
- **Soft-tissue calcification.** Soft-tissue uptake on bone scan can be seen with metastatic calcification due to hypercalcemia, often due to hyperparathyroidism, as well with inflammatory conditions such as dermatomyositis and in the setting of renal failure.

## ■ Diagnosis

Pediatric abdominal neuroblastoma with osseous metastases.

## ✓ Pearls

- Labeled diphosphonates may accumulate in extracellular fluid collections, such as malignant ascites.
- Uptake of bone tracers can be seen in any calcifying or ossifying process including neoplastic.
- Radiopharmaceutical colloid formation from aluminum breakthrough can result in liver uptake.

## Suggested Readings

Loutfi I, Collier BD, Mohammed AM. Nonosseous abnormalities on bone scans. J Nucl Med Technol. 2003; 31(3):149–153, quiz 154–156

Mahajan MS, Digamber NS, Sharma R. Technetium-99 m-methylene diphosphonate uptake in hepatic necrosis secondary to respiratory failure. World J Nucl Med. 2013; 12(3):116–119

Zuckier LS, Martineau P. Altered biodistribution of radiopharmaceuticals used in bone scintigraphy. Semin Nucl Med. 2015; 45(1):81–96

# Case 91

*Mickaila Johnston*

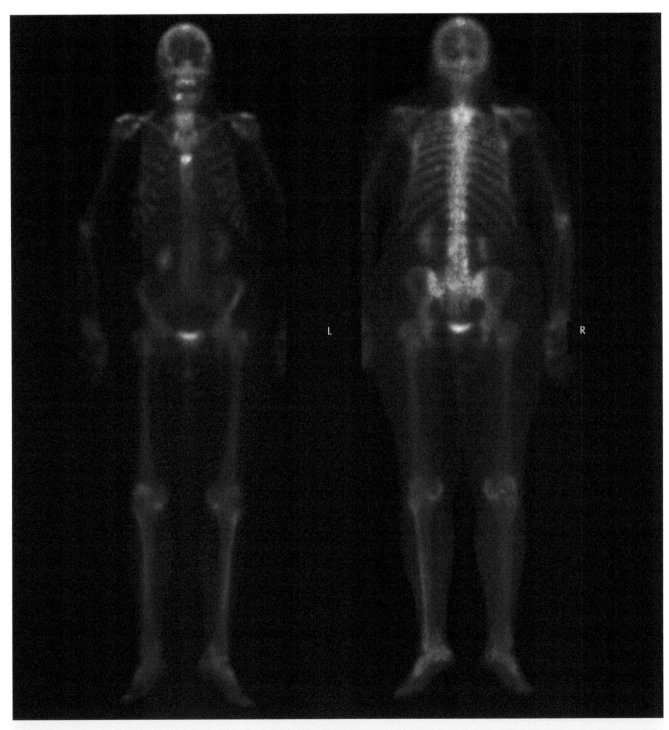

**Fig. 91.1** Anterior and posterior whole-body technetium-99m (Tc-99m) hydroxy diphosphonate (HDP) bone scintigraphy demonstrates focally increased radiotracer deposition within the sternum.

■ **Clinical History**

67-year-old female with breast cancer (▶ Fig. 91.1).

## ■ Key Finding

Focal sternal/manubrial activity on bone scintigraphy

## ■ Top 3 Differential Diagnoses

- **Degenerative change.** Degenerative changes at the manubrio-clavicular, sternomanubrial, costomanubrial, costochondral, and costosternal junctions are common findings in the elderly population. Degenerative change most often presents with focal uptake in a typically symmetric distribution juxtaposed with the sternum/manubrium.
- **Metastases.** As with any osseous structure, metastases may form in the sternum. However, differentiating arthritic changes from metastases can be difficult. The more central and asymmetric the change is in nature, the more suggestive

of a neoplastic process. The sternum is frequently the only site of metastatic disease in breast cancer; a solitary sternal lesion in a patient with known breast cancer has around an 80% chance of representing metastatic disease.
- **Iatrogenic/trauma.** After orthopedic trauma, such as midline sternotomy, there may be a linear deposition of radiotracer along the healing sternotomy, often in a craniocaudal orientation. Similarly, after cardiopulmonary resuscitation (CPR), there will often be symmetric rib fractures outlining the sternum.

## ■ Diagnosis

Breast cancer metastases to the sternum.

## ✓ Pearls

- Degenerative change often presents in a symmetric pattern outlining the sternum.
- Metastases are more likely with fewer number of more central and asymmetric foci of uptake.
- Midline sternotomy and CPR produce typical patterns of radiotracer deposition.
- A solitary sternal lesion in a patient with known breast cancer has more chances of being metastatic.

## Suggested Readings

Katz ME, Shier CK, Ellis BI, Leisen JC, Hardy DC, Jundt JW. A unified approach to symptomatic juxtasternal arthritis and enthesitis. AJR Am J Roentgenol. 1989; 153(2):327–333

Koizumi M, Yoshimoto M, Kasumi F, Ogata E. Comparison between solitary and multiple skeletal metastatic lesions of breast cancer patients. Ann Oncol. 2003; 14(8):1234–1240

Restrepo CS, Martinez S, Lemos DF, et al. Imaging appearances of the sternum and sternoclavicular joints. Radiographics. 2009; 29(3):839–859

Syed GM, Fielding HW, Collier BD. Sternal uptake on bone scintigraphy: age-related variants. Nucl Med Commun. 2005; 26(3):253–257

# Case 92

*John Dryden*

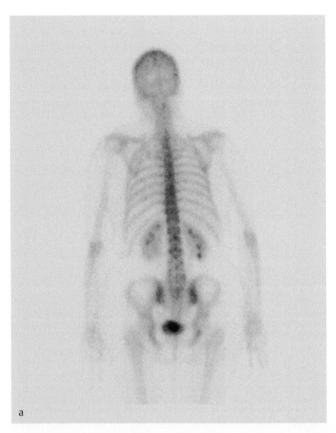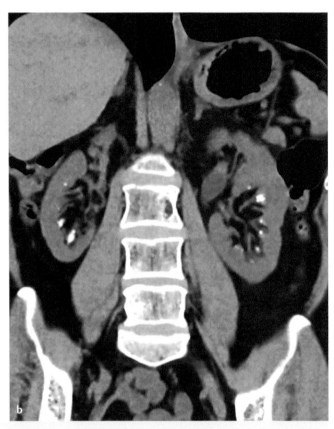

**Fig. 92.1** **(a)** Cropped posterior whole-body technetium-99m (Tc-99m) hydroxy diphosphonate (HDP) bone scintigraphy demonstrates multiple areas of punctate radiotracer deposition within the kidneys. **(b)** Select coronal noncontrast enhanced CT demonstrates medullary nephrocalcinosis.

## ■ Clinical History

60-year-old female with multiple falls (▶ Fig. 92.1). (Case courtesy of Ely Wolin, MD, David Grant USAF Medical Center.)

## ■ Key Finding

Increased bilateral renal activity on bone scintigraphy

## ■ Top 3 Differential Diagnoses

- **Acute kidney injury.** The Tc-99m-labeled diphosphonates are excreted by the kidneys. Therefore, anything that reduces renal secretory capabilities or glomerular filtration could result in increased renal activity on bone scan. Acute tubular necrosis (ATN) is the most common cause of intrinsic acute kidney injury (AKI). Hypovolemic states or drug toxicity causes injury and death of the tubular cells which results in decreased glomerular filtration. Bone scan may show temporarily increased renal uptake that normalizes with recovery of renal function. Laboratory findings in ATN include elevated creatinine and blood urea nitrogen, as well as the pathognomonic "muddy brown casts" on urinalysis. Implicated drugs in ATN include cyclooxygenase inhibitors, angiotensin-converting enzyme inhibitors, and amphotericin b, among others.

- **Metabolic abnormality.** Elevated calcium phosphate product is the proposed mechanism of action for increased diffuse renal uptake on bone scintigraphy. This can be seen with metastatic calcification, nephrocalcinosis, both cortical and medullary, as well as with hypercalcemia and hyperparathyroidism.
- **Iron overload.** The presence of excess iron alters the distribution of bone-seeking radiopharmaceuticals resulting in increased renal activity. This can be seen in the setting of sickle cell anemia, multiple blood transfusions, thalassemia major, hemochromatosis, and cirrhosis. The increased renal activity, in this setting, is usually accompanied by decreased bone uptake.

## ■ Additional Diagnostic Considerations

- **Chemotherapy:** Several chemotherapeutic agents, such as cyclophosphamide, vincristine, and doxorubicin, have been shown to result in increased renal uptake in bone scintigraphy. This is likely secondary to AKI; however, increased renal uptake has been seen in patients with no change in renal function.
- **High-grade obstruction:** Collecting system obstruction can lead to delayed clearance of the kidneys and therefore increased

renal activity on delayed images. Intense collecting system activity is often visualized leading to the level of obstruction. Obstruction is usually not bilateral and symmetric.
- **Renal artery stenosis/renal vein thrombosis:** Compromise in renal blood flow will result in delayed clearance of the radiopharmaceutical. This is more likely to be unilateral.

## ■ Diagnosis

Medullary nephrocalcinosis.

## ✓ Pearls

- Renal uptake on bone scan has many possible etiologies, correlative imaging is often helpful.
- Diphosphonates follow calcium ions; with increased calcium, there will be bone scan findings.

- Renal uptake greater than lumbar spine uptake on posterior imaging is generally considered increased.

## Suggested Readings

Love C, Din AS, Tomas MB, Kalapparambath TP, Palestro CJ. Radionuclide bone imaging: an illustrative review. Radiographics. 2003; 23(2):341–358

Ozdoğan O, Karahan NP, Sarıoğlu S, Durak H. Acute kidney injury secondary to NSAID diagnosed on 99 mTc MDP bone scan. Mol Imaging Radionucl Ther. 2013; 22(2):66–69

Zuckier LS, Martineau P. Altered biodistribution of radiopharmaceuticals used in bone scintigraphy. Semin Nucl Med. 2015; 45(1):81–96

# Case 93

*John Dryden*

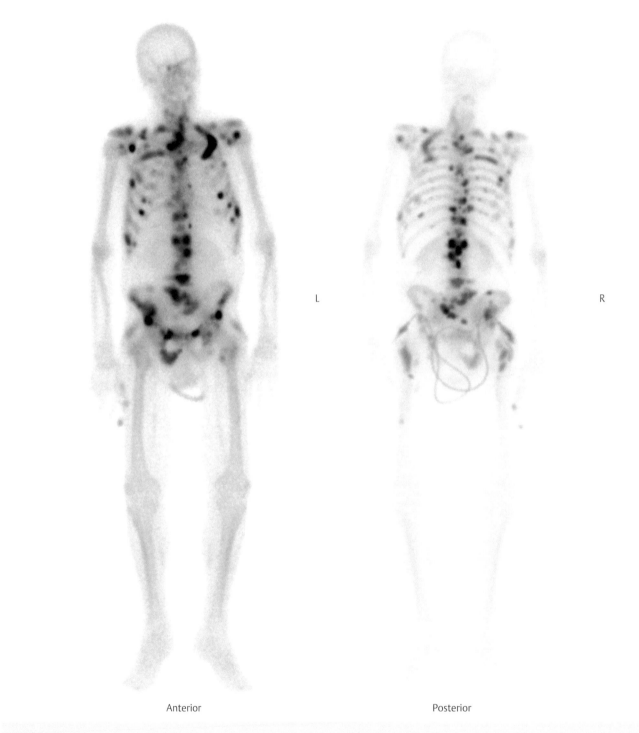

Anterior                                    Posterior

**Fig. 93.1** Anterior and posterior whole-body technetium-99m (Tc-99m) hydroxy diphosphonate (HDP) bone scintigraphy demonstrates multiple areas of focally increased radiotracer deposition predominantly involving the axial skeleton as well as decreased renal activity.

### ■ Clinical History

80-year-old male with prostate cancer (▶ Fig. 93.1).

■ **Key Finding**

Decreased renal uptake on bone scintigraphy

■ **Top 3 Differential Diagnoses**

• **Renal failure.** Chronic renal failure will result in decreased renal uptake of the Tc-99m diphosphonates which are renally cleared. This will also result in generalized increased soft-tissue activity throughout the soft tissues due to delayed clearance of radiopharmaceutical. Adding an 18- to 24-hour delayed image allows for increased target-to-background uptake and is occasionally beneficial in these patients. It should be noted that renal failure/dialysis patients can also have renal osteodystrophy that may result in a "metabolic superscan."

• **Superscan.** Diffuse increased skeletal uptake of either Tc-99m medronic acid (MDP) or HDP with decreased or absent renal and soft-tissue activity is known as a superscan. This can be due to diffuse osteoblastic metastatic disease, usually prostate cancer, or metabolic bone disease such as renal osteodystrophy. Bone deposition in a metastatic superscan is usually heterogeneous with multiple foci of increased uptake involving primarily the axial and proximal appendicular skeleton. Uptake on a metabolic superscan is usually more homogeneous and involves the entire skeleton.

• **Nephrectomy.** If the patient has undergone bilateral nephrectomy and has a functional transplant, then uptake of Tc-99m bone agent can be seen in the transplanted kidney, usually located within the pelvis.

■ **Additional Diagnostic Consideration**

• **Delayed imaging:** There will be relatively decreased renal activity if imaging is delayed in a patient with normal renal function. Normally, around half of the injected dose will be excreted by the kidneys in 24 hours with maximum bone uptake seen around 6 to 8 hours.

■ **Diagnosis**

Renal failure in a prostate cancer patient demonstrating a superscan.

✓ **Pearls**

• Decreased clearance of radiotracer with renal failure results in increased generalized soft-tissue uptake.

• Superscan results from marked increased osseous uptake from metastases or metabolic bone disease.

• An 18 to 24 hours delayed image can help in renal failure, allowing for improved target to background.

**Suggested Readings**

Love C, Din AS, Tomas MB, Kalapparambath TP, Palestro CJ. Radionuclide bone imaging: an illustrative review. Radiographics. 2003; 23(2):341–358

Weiner GM, Jenicke L, Muller V, et al. Artifacts and non-osseous uptake in bone scintigraphy. Imaging reports of 20 cases. Radiol Oncol. 2001; 35(3):185–191

# Case 94

*Mickaila Johnston*

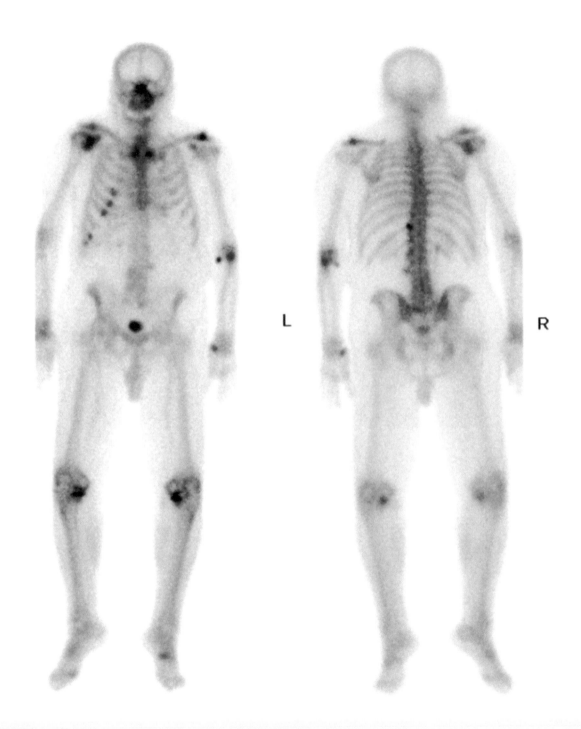

L    R

**Fig. 94.1** Anterior and posterior whole-body technetium-99m (Tc-99m) hydroxy diphosphonate (HDP) bone scintigraphy demonstrates multiple areas of focally increased radiotracer deposition in the anterior right rib cage suggestive of trauma.

## ■ Clinical History

97-year-old man with prostate cancer (▶ Fig. 94.1).

■ **Key Finding**

Multifocal uptake on bone scintigraphy

■ **Top 3 Differential Diagnoses**

• **Arthritis.** Bone scintigraphy frequently demonstrates periarticular uptake in a pattern consistent with degenerative change, particularly in the elderly population. At autopsy, there is almost universal presence of osteoarthritis in people aged 65 years and more. Frequently seen regions of degenerative type uptake include the acromioclavicular joints, sternoclavicular joints, elbows, wrists, knees, feet, and diffusely throughout the axial spine.

• **Metastases.** These may be solitary or multifocal and may present in similar locations to arthritic uptake but are usually not periarticular in distribution. Asymmetry and new-onset pain may elevate the concern for metastases. The majority of metastatic lesions occur in the axial and proximal appendicular spine, the distribution of red marrow. Prostate, breast, and lung cancers are most frequently seen with osteoblastic metastases. Kidney and thyroid malignancies are also known to commonly metastasize to bone, but are lytic metastases and will be missed on bone scan unless there is reactive sclerosis or associated injury.

• **Trauma.** This may present as multifocal uptake on bone scintigraphy. Correlation with clinical history is paramount. The majority of traumatic lesions will show uptake within 24 hours of injury. Uptake usually will resolve within 12 months, but occasionally can last for up to 3 years. A three-phase bone scan (TPBS) can help differentiate between acute and chronic traumatic injury. Bone scans may be useful if there is concern for nonaccidental trauma and if radiographs are negative.

■ **Additional Diagnostic Considerations**

• **Paget's disease:** It may be polyostotic and present with marked increased activity on bone scintigraphy in all three phases (lytic, mixed, and sclerotic). Progressive whole-bone involvement is seen as opposed to the random distribution seen in metastases. Activity will invariably involve the end of the long bone.

• **Bone dysplasia:** Several bone dysplasias can present with multifocal uptake on bone scintigraphy, fibrous dysplasia (FD) being the most frequently encountered. It may present with activity as intense as Paget's disease, but in a different distribution.

■ **Diagnosis**

Metastatic prostate cancer.

✓ **Pearls**

• Periarticular uptake in an elderly patient is common and suggestive of arthritic change.
• New-onset pain and nonperiarticular uptake both should increase suspicion for metastatic disease.
• Polyostotic long bone activity can be seen with Paget's disease and FD.
• Paget's disease will invariably involve at least one end of an involved long bone.

**Suggested Readings**

Guttentag AR, Salwen JK. Keep your eyes on the ribs: the spectrum of normal variants and diseases that involve the ribs. Radiographics. 1999; 19(5):1125–1142
Kim JY, Cho SK, Han M, Choi YY, Bae SC, Sung YK. The role of bone scintigraphy in the diagnosis of rheumatoid arthritis according to the 2010 ACR/EULAR classification criteria. J Korean Med Sci. 2014; 29(2):204–209
Love C, Din AS, Tomas MB, Kalapparambath TP, Palestro CJ. Radionuclide bone imaging: an illustrative review. Radiographics. 2003; 23(2):341–358

# Case 95

*Mickaila Johnston*

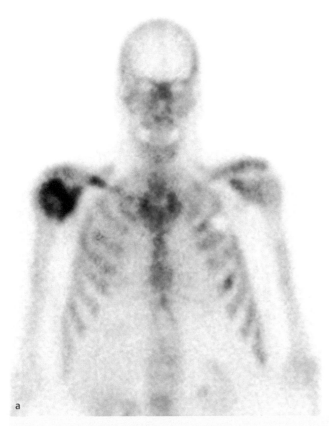
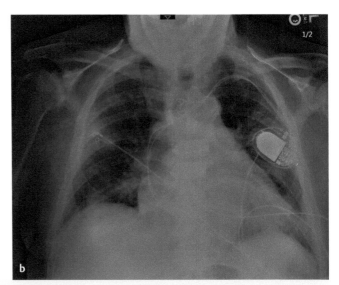

**Fig. 95.1** Anterior technetium-99m (Tc-99m) hydroxy diphosphonate (HDP) bone scintigraphy demonstrates a photopenic defect overlying the left chest, right shoulder periarticular uptake, and a focal area of radiotracer deposition within a left anterior rib (a). Plain film chest X-ray demonstrates a cardiac pacing device overlying the left hemithorax and cardiomegaly (b).

## ■ Clinical History

83-year-old male with prostate cancer and rising prostate-specific antigen (PSA) (▶ Fig. 95.1).

## ■ Key Finding

Photopenic defect on bone scintigraphy

## ■ Top 3 Differential Diagnoses

- **Attenuation.** Foreign bodies often cause focally decreased radiotracer deposition referred to as "cold" or photopenic defects. They are frequently seen with things such as cardiac pacing devices, implanted medication ports, belt buckles, and orthopedic hardware, among others, and present in characteristic locations. Soft-tissue attenuation may also cause apparent decreased radiotracer deposition. Comparison with anatomic imaging as well as imaging in different obliquities or with single-photon emission computed tomography (SPECT) is often helpful.
- **Post radiation change (XRT).** Antecedent external beam radiation frequently causes decreased radiotracer deposition

as a sequela of altered osseous calcium metabolism. This presentation is easily confirmed with history of radiation port locations. On scintigraphy, this also will usually appear as a regional area of decreased uptake with abrupt linear transitions to normal.
- **Early avascular necrosis (AVN).** In the early phases of AVN, there is decreased blood flow that results in decreased metabolism and radiotracer deposition. Confirmatory anatomic imaging is useful. Late AVN will show uptake on bone scan due to the sclerosis associated with repair.

## ■ Additional Differential Considerations

- **Osteolytic metastases:** Purely lytic bone metastases may present as focal areas of decreased uptake on bone scintigraphy. Lytic bone metastases are commonly seen with renal cell carcinoma and thyroid carcinoma, but can also be seen with breast carcinoma and lung carcinoma. Multiple myeloma is

the most common primary bone tumor in adults and may be photopenic on bone scan.
- **Marrow infiltrative process:** Any process that replaces bone marrow may have associated decreased uptake on bone scintigraphy, depending on the amount of reactive bone formation.

## ■ Diagnosis

Cardiac pacing device overlying left chest.

## ✓ Pearls

- Cold bone scan findings can include overlying metallic objects, soft tissues, and XRT changes.
- Early phases of AVN will be cold on bone scan due to decreased perfusion.

- True cold bone scan foci include osteolytic metastases, often myeloma, renal and thyroid carcinoma.

## Suggested Readings

Bhargava P, He G, Samarghandi A, Delpassand ES. Pictorial review of SPECT/CT imaging applications in clinical nuclear medicine. Am J Nucl Med Mol Imaging. 2012; 2(2):221–231

Gnanasegaran G, Cook G, Adamson K, Fogelman I. Patterns, variants, artifacts, and pitfalls in conventional radionuclide bone imaging and SPECT/CT. Semin Nucl Med. 2009; 39(6):380–395

Naddaf SY, Collier BD, Elgazzar AH, Khalil MM. Technical errors in planar bone scanning. J Nucl Med Technol. 2004; 32(3):148–153

# Case 96

*Mickaila Johnston*

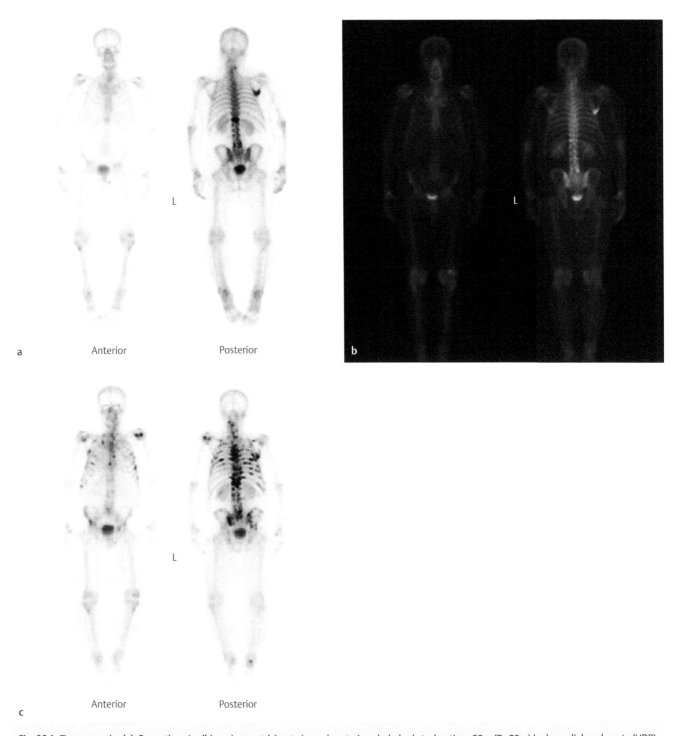

**Fig. 96.1** Five years prior **(a)**, 2 months prior **(b)**, and current **(c)** anterior and posterior whole-body technetium-99m (Tc-99m) hydroxy diphosphonate (HDP) bone scintigraphy demonstrates interval progression of osseous metastatic burden despite post radiation change (XRT) and enzalutamide, abiraterone, and zoladex. Initially, taxotere was effective **(b)**, but eventually disease progression was demonstrated despite the chemotherapeutic regimen **(c)**.

## ■ Clinical History

84-year-old female with breast cancer (▶ Fig. 96.1).

■ **Key Finding**

Increased uptake after chemotherapy on bone scintigraphy

■ **Top 3 Differential Diagnoses**

- **Flare phenomenon.** Bone scintigraphy performed within 6 months after chemotherapy may show an increase in both uptake and number of lesions in a patient with bone metastases who is actually showing a good response to therapy. This is likely due to osteoblastic activity associated with healing and remodeling. Bone scan performed after 6 months should show improvement from baseline. Early imaging after chemotherapy can utilize the flare phenomenon to provide a more accurate staging in patients at high risk for bone metastases but negative initial studies.

- **Interval disease progression.** Interval progression of malignancy or metastases is a common reason for new or increased radiotracer deposition after chemotherapy. This can be seen when the malignancy is not sensitive to the chemotherapeutic approach. Disease progression cannot be reliably diagnosed within 6 months of chemotherapy.
- **Pathologic fracture.** Fractures of any type yield increased radiotracer deposition. Chemotherapy may be given with coexistent large-volume bone-replacing masses. As the osseous structure is destroyed, there can be subsequent pathologic fracture.

■ **Additional Diagnostic Consideration**

- **Marrow stimulation:** Increased bone scan activity can be seen with marrow stimulation or reconversion. Diffuse increased activity within the axial and proximal appendicular spine, the areas containing hematopoietic marrow in adults, can be seen on both bone scan and fluorine-18 fluorodeoxyglucose positron-emission tomography (F-18 FDG PET)/CT due to

either pharmacologic or physiologic marrow stimulation. More focal uptake can be seen due to marrow reconversion associated with trauma/healing. Marrow reconversion can be difficult to differentiate from metastatic disease on routine bone scintigraphy. Tc-99m SC marrow imaging can be helpful.

■ **Diagnosis**

Prostate cancer demonstrating interval disease progression after chemotherapy failure.

✓ **Pearls**

- Flare phenomenon appears like paradoxical disease progression in a good response to chemotherapy.
- A worsening bone scan more than 6 months after chemotherapy is consistent with disease progression.

- Imaging of flare phenomenon can provide more accurate staging in high-risk patients.
- Tc-99m SC marrow imaging can be used to confirm marrow reconversion.

**Suggested Readings**

Agool A, Glaudemans AWJM, Boersma HH, Dierckx RA, Vellenga E, Slart RH. Radionuclide imaging of bone marrow disorders. Eur J Nucl Med Mol Imaging. 2011; 38(1):166–178

Cook GJ, Venkitaraman R, Sohaib AS, et al. The diagnostic utility of the flare phenomenon on bone scintigraphy in staging prostate cancer. Eur J Nucl Med Mol Imaging. 2011; 38(1):7–13

Messiou C, Cook G, deSouza NM. Imaging metastatic bone disease from carcinoma of the prostate. Br J Cancer. 2009; 101(8):1225–1232

# Case 97

*Mickaila Johnston*

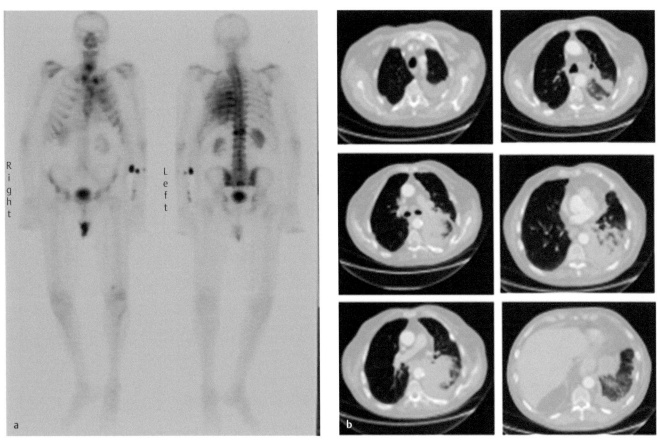

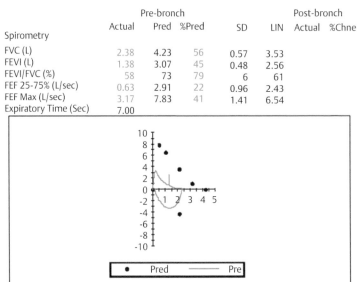

| Spirometry | Pre-bronch | | | | | Post-bronch | |
|---|---|---|---|---|---|---|---|
| | Actual | Pred | %Pred | SD | LIN | Actual | %Chne |
| FVC (L) | 2.38 | 4.23 | 56 | 0.57 | 3.53 | | |
| FEVI (L) | 1.38 | 3.07 | 45 | 0.48 | 2.56 | | |
| FEVI/FVC (%) | 58 | 73 | 79 | 6 | 61 | | |
| FEF 25-75% (L/sec) | 0.63 | 2.91 | 22 | 0.96 | 2.43 | | |
| FEF Max (L/sec) | 3.17 | 7.83 | 41 | 1.41 | 6.54 | | |
| Expiratory Time (Sec) | 7.00 | | | | | | |

**Fig. 97.1** Anterior and posterior whole-body technetium-99m (Tc-99m) hydroxy diphosphonate (HDP) bone scintigraphy demonstrates diffusely increased radiotracer deposition within the left hemithorax (a). Select contrast-enhanced axial CT slices demonstrate focal consolidation within the left lower lobe (b). Spirometry confirms findings (c).

■ **Clinical History**

76-year-old white male with shortness of air, nausea, and vomiting (▶ Fig. 97.1).

## ■ Key Finding

Increased intrathoracic uptake on bone scintigraphy

## ■ Top 3 Differential Diagnoses

- **Effusion.** Similar to ascites, pleural and pericardial effusions may show uptake with Tc-99m-labeled diphosphonates. Again, the mechanism is not completely understood but uptake is likely secondary to altered permeability due to tumor cells, in the case of malignant effusions, or passive diffusion with subsequent slow clearance.
- **Malignancy.** Both primary lung malignancy and pulmonary metastases may show uptake on bone scan. The uptake may be due to actual tumoral calcium metabolism or bone formation, such as with osteosarcoma and mucinous adenocarcinomas, or due to uptake within necrotic tissue.
- **Infection/inflammation.** Infection and inflammation result in hyperemia with associated increased capillary permeability which can present as increased uptake on bone scintigraphy. An example is radiation pneumonitis in which increased radiotracer deposition may be found in contrast to the decreased uptake within the juxtaposed osseous locations.

## ■ Additional Diagnostic Considerations

- **Myocardial uptake:** This has been described in myocardial infarction, amyloidosis, sarcoidosis, myocarditis, and pericarditis. If myocardial uptake is seen, it is important to exclude residual activity from recent myocardial perfusion scan.
- **Metastatic calcification:** Hyperparathyroidism and renal failure can result in microscopic calcium deposition in the lungs, as with all soft tissues, leading to uptake on bone scintigraphy.

## ■ Diagnosis

Small cell carcinoma of the left lower lobe.

## ✓ Pearls

- Like malignant ascites, malignant pleural and pericardial effusions can be positive on bone scan.
- There are multiple causes of myocardial uptake on bone scintigraphy, including infarction.
- Pulmonary infection/inflammation can result in bone scan uptake due to hyperemia and permeability.
- Several primary and metastatic lesions can have bone scan uptake associate with calcium or necrosis.

## Suggested Readings

Wale DJ, Wong KK, Savas H, Kandathil A, Piert M, Brown RK. Extraosseous findings on bone scintigraphy using fusion SPECT/CT and correlative imaging. AJR Am J Roentgenol. 2015; 205(1):160–172

Loutfi I, Collier BD, Mohammed AM. Nonosseous abnormalities on bone scans. J Nucl Med Technol. 2003; 31(3):149–153, quiz 154–156

Kosuda S, Yokoyama K, Nishiguchi I, Kunieda E, Kubo A, Hashimoto S. Bone scanning in patients with pleural effusion--experience in 76 cases. Ann Nucl Med. 1990; 4(2):55–58

# Case 98

*Mickaila Johnston*

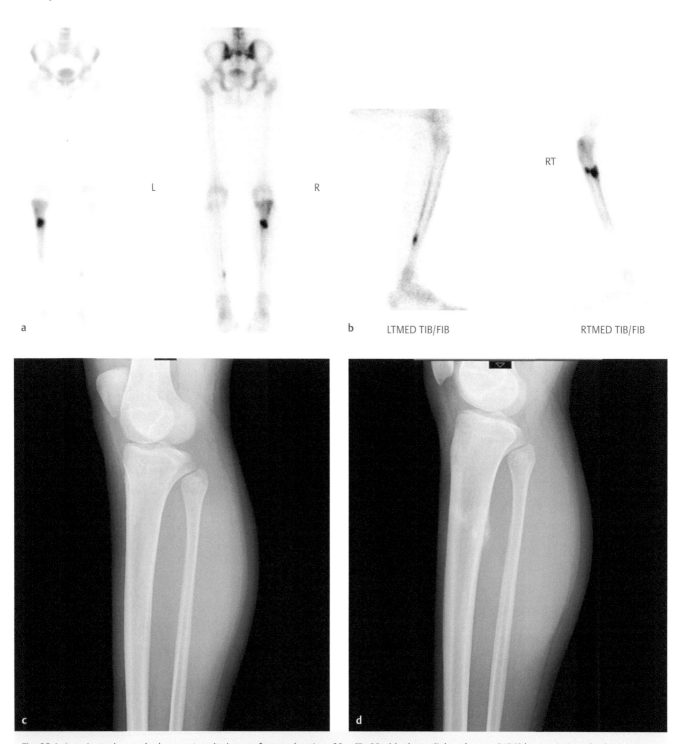

**Fig. 98.1** Anterior and posterior lower extremity images from technetium-99m (Tc-99m) hydroxy diphosphonate (HDP) bone scintigraphy demonstrate focally increased radiotracer within the right proximal tibia, right tibial plateau, and left distal tibia (a). Spot medial lower extremity views demonstrate similar findings (b). Plain film X-ray performed seven days prior to bone scintigraphy demonstrates smooth periosteal thickening (c). Plain film X-ray, performed four weeks after bone scintigraphy, demonstrates interval sclerosis in the proximal tibial diaphysis with adjacent periosteal reaction (d).

■ **Clinical History**

21-year-old male with right mid shin pain and tenderness to palpation (▶ Fig. 98.1).

## ■ Key Finding

Increased osseous activity in a distal extremity on bone scintigraphy

## ■ Top 3 Differential Diagnoses

- **Arthritis.** It is one of the most frequently seen sources of metabolic activity on a bone scan. However, the pattern of distribution, history, and anatomic imaging (if needed) often account for the bone scintigraphy findings. Arthritic uptake is most often periarticular involving multiple joints.
- **Trauma.** Both soft tissue and osseous trauma can result in bone scan uptake. Bleeding, tissue damage, and subsequent calcification results in uptake in soft-tissue injuries, as seen with both dystrophic calcification and myositis ossificans. Osseous trauma will be hot on bone scan within 24 hours of injury, with uptake resolving after about 12 months in the majority. Stress fracture will show uptake earlier than radiographic changes. An acute lower extremity stress fracture

will show more intense uptake than the anterior superior iliac spine on anterior imaging, and the sacroiliac joints on posterior imaging.
- **Metastases.** While osseous metastases most commonly occur within the axial and proximal appendicular spine, the sites of hematopoietic marrow in adults, metastatic lesions are infrequently seen within the distal appendicular skeleton. Small cell carcinoma (SCC) of the lung is the most likely primary malignancy to present with metastatic lesions distal to the elbow or knee, with breast, prostate, and renal cell carcinoma as additional possibilities. Multiple myeloma can also present with lesions in the distal extremities.

## ■ Additional Diagnostic Considerations

- **Bone dysplasia/metabolic bone disease:** Many of the known bone dysplasia, such as fibrous dysplasia (FD) and melorheostosis, and metabolic bone diseases, such as Paget's disease, may result in increased distal extremity uptake on bone scintigraphy.

- **"Tram-track" uptake:** Uptake in the long bones resulting in a "tram-track" appearance can be seen with hypertrophic pulmonary osteoarthropathy, shin splints, and venous insufficiency. This is discussed in a separate case.
- **Osteomyelitis:** It can occur anywhere, especially when secondary to direct extension from soft-tissue infection.

## ■ Diagnosis

Stress fracture with evolving radiographic findings.

## ✓ Pearls

- Osseous trauma will result in increased bone scan uptake within 24 hours, usually resolving in 1 year.
- Osseous metastases distal to the knee or elbow is rare, most commonly seen with SCC of lung.

- Degenerative uptake is very common on bone scans. It is usually periarticular involving multiple joints.

## Suggested readings

Kim JY, Cho SK, Han M, Choi YY, Bae SC, Sung YK. The role of bone scintigraphy in the diagnosis of rheumatoid arthritis according to the 2010 ACR/EULAR classification criteria. J Korean Med Sci. 2014; 29(2):204–209

Kumar K. Three phase bone scan interpretation based upon vascular endothelial response. Indian J Nucl Med. 2015; 30(2):104–110

Love C, Din AS, Tomas MB, Kalapparambath TP, Palestro CJ. Radionuclide bone imaging: an illustrative review. Radiographics. 2003; 23(2):341–358

# Case 99

*John Dryden*

a

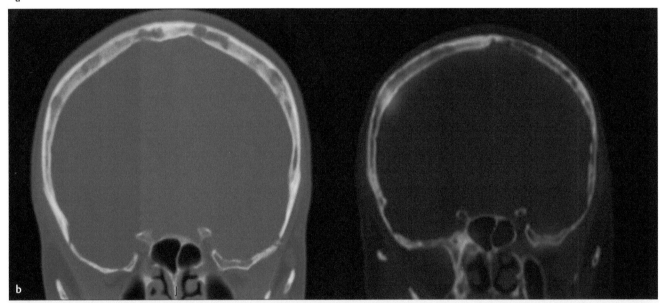

b

**Fig. 99.1** (a) Right and left lateral images of the skull from technetium-99m (Tc-99m) hydroxy diphosphonate (HDP) bone scintigraphy demonstrate multiple areas of increased radiotracer deposition within the skull as well as focally decreased left parietal uptake. (b) Select coronal CT and fused single-photon emission computed tomography (SPECT)/CT images demonstrate multiple areas of ground glass density and lucency with variable levels of uptake.

### ■ Clinical History

50-year-old female with unexplained lytic foci in skull (▶Fig. 99.1).

# ■ Key Finding

Focal photopenic defect in the skull, on bone scintigraphy

# ■ Top 3 Differential Diagnoses

- **Postsurgical/trauma.** Changes can result in a photopenic defect through one of two ways: loss of the native bone and addition of an attenuating material. Postsurgical or traumatic changes, where a portion of the cranium is removed, would mean there is no native bone to uptake the Tc-99m bone agent. Attenuating materials, which remove photons from radiation flux via absorption, could likewise result in a focal defect on bone scintigraphy within the skull. These materials include metal, calcium, and barium. A metal plate overlying the cranium would have to be between the skull and the detector, and would not be obvious on every view.

- **Metastatic disease.** Photopenic metastases are usually due to osteolytic, aggressive tumors. Common metastatic lesions producing photopenic defects include kidney, lung, thyroid, and breast tumors.
- **Multiple myeloma.** It is a malignant neoplasm of plasma cells in bone marrow. Lesions may demonstrate either increased or decreased focal uptake on bone scintigraphy. Tc-99m-labeled diphosphonate bone scan has a sensitivity of around 75% for lesion detection. Fluorine-18 fluorodeoxyglucose positron-emission tomography (F-18 FDG PET)/CT is superior for initial staging and restaging of the disease.

# ■ Additional Diagnostic Considerations

- **Osteoporosis circumscripta:** Large areas of circumscribe radiolucency in the skull can be seen in the early phase of Paget's disease of bone, as well as with hyperparathyroidism. There may be decreased bone scan uptake associated with the lucent region, but generally intense uptake at the margins, particularly in the case of Paget's disease.

- **Gorham's disease:** This disease is also known as disappearing or vanishing bone disease. It is a rare disease of uncertain etiology that results in massive osteolysis from progressive intraosseous hemangiomatous tissue proliferation. It most often involves the shoulders and pelvis.

# ■ Diagnosis

Multiple stages of Paget's disease.

# ✓ Pearls

- Both loss of the native bone and addition of an attenuating material can cause cold foci on bone scan.
- Common cold metastases on bone scan are: kidney, lung, thyroid, and breast tumors.

- FDG PET/CT is more sensitive than bone scintigraphy for multiple myeloma.
- Osteoporosis circumscripta will usually have intense uptake at the margins of the lesion on bone scan.

## Suggested Readings

Lo CP, Chen CY, Chin SC, Juan CJ, Hsueh CJ, Chen A. Disappearing calvarium in Gorham disease: MR imaging characteristics with pathologic correlation. AJNR Am J Neuroradiol. 2004; 25(3):415–418

Love C, Din AS, Tomas MB, Kalapparambath TP, Palestro CJ. Radionuclide bone imaging: an illustrative review. Radiographics. 2003; 23(2):341–358

Mitsuya K, Nakasu Y, Horiguchi S, et al. Metastatic skull tumors: MRI features and a new conventional classification. J Neurooncol. 2011; 104(1):239–245

Smith SE, Murphey MD, Motamedi K, Mulligan ME, Resnik CS, Gannon FH. From the archives of the AFIP. Radiologic spectrum of Paget disease of bone and its complications with pathologic correlation. Radiographics. 2002; 22(5): 1191–1216

# Case 100

*Mickaila Johnston*

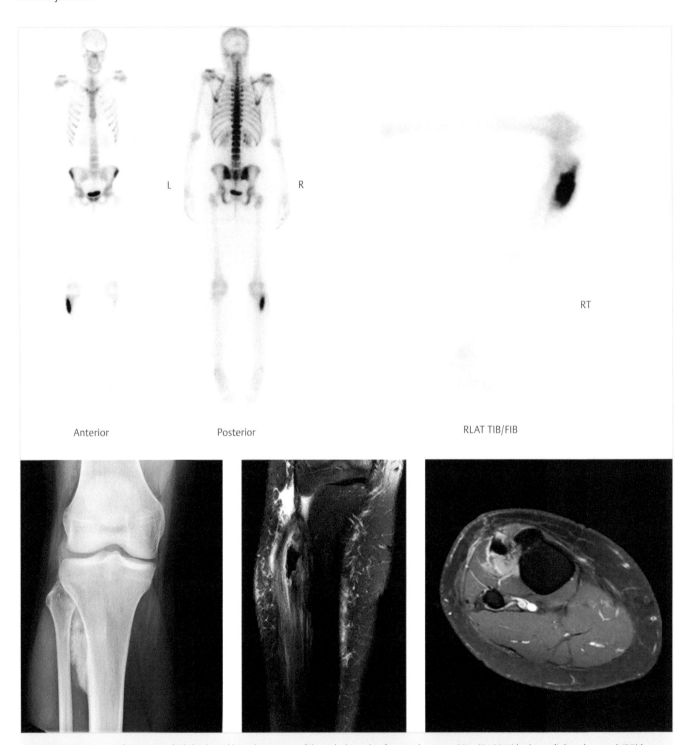

**Fig. 100.1** Anterior and posterior whole body and lateral spot view of the right lower leg from technetium-99m (Tc-99m) hydroxy diphosphonate (HDP) bone scintigraphy demonstrates focally increased radiotracer deposition within the right proximal tibia. Anterior plain film radiograph of the right knee demonstrates a calcified soft-tissue mass lateral to the proximal right tibia. Sagittal fluid bright turbo spin echo fat saturated and axial T1 fat saturation contrast-enhanced MR images demonstrate an enhancing mass along the anterolateral aspect of the right proximal tibia with cortical involvement and thinning.

### ■ Clinical History

24-year-old male with a known pathology of the proximal right tibia (▶ Fig. 100.1).

## ■ Key Finding

Increased uptake at the end of a long bone on bone scintigraphy

## ■ Top 3 Differential Diagnoses

- **Osteosarcoma.** It is the most common primary malignant tumor of bone, excluding plasma cell myeloma, and presents as an aggressive process. Osteosarcoma has eight subtypes, largely determined by anatomic imaging findings. "Conventional" osteosarcoma is the most common, presenting as an intramedullary mass with cloudlike bone formation in the metaphyses. Osteosarcoma starts as a small mass penetrating the osseous cortex and locally advances. Bone scan findings often grow in a contiguous pattern, yet skip lesions do occur.
- **Ewing's sarcoma.** In the pediatric setting, Ewing's sarcoma is second only to osteosarcoma. It arises from the medul-lary cavity and invades the Haversian system. Half of the presentations are of the lower limbs. Three-phase bone scan (TPBS) will be positive on all three phases. Like osteosarcoma, chemotherapy followed by local surgical resection is the treatment of choice.
- **Chondrosarcoma.** It is the third most common primary bone malignant tumor. It is an excessive production of cartilage matrix, often lobular in presentation. Pain is the most common clinical symptom. It is insidious, progressive, and worse at night. Anatomic imaging is useful for classification of this bony process.

## ■ Additional Differential Diagnoses

- **Neuroblastoma metastases:** Neuroblastoma is the most common solid malignancy in children to metastasize to bone. Metastatic lesions tend to occur at metaphyses, making diagnosis on bone scan difficult at times due to the normal physeal uptake on bone scintigraphy in the skeletally immature.
- **Avascular necrosis (AVN):** Some of the most common locations for AVN include the femoral head, the humeral head, and the femoral and tibial metadiaphysis, among others. On bone scintigraphy, AVN will be photopenic early due to decreased perfusion but demonstrate increased uptake in the healing phases. Uptake may be in a "donut" pattern with reparative uptake surrounding the central photopenic area of necrosis.
- **Trauma:** Traumatic injuries can of course occur at the end of long bones, usually obvious from history and correlative anatomic imaging.

## ■ Diagnosis

Osteosarcoma of the right tibia.

## ✓ Pearls

- Increased long bone uptake on bone scan in the absence of trauma requires consideration for tumor.
- Osteosarcoma, Ewing's sarcoma, and chondrosarcoma present in that order of prevalence.
- Metaphyseal neuroblastoma metastases may be obscured by physeal uptake in pediatric patients.

## Suggested Readings

Murphey MD, Foreman KL, Klassen-Fischer MK, Fox MG, Chung EM, Kransdorf MJ. From the radiologic pathology archives imaging of osteonecrosis: radiologic-pathologic correlation. Radiographics. 2014; 34(4):1003–1028

Stacy GS, Mahal RS, Peabody TD. Staging of bone tumors: a review with illustrative examples. AJR Am J Roentgenol. 2006; 186(4):967–976

Yarmish G, Klein MJ, Landa J, Lefkowitz RA, Hwang S. Imaging characteristics of primary osteosarcoma: nonconventional subtypes. Radiographics. 2010; 30(6):1653–1672

# Case 101

*Joseph M. Yetto, Jr.*

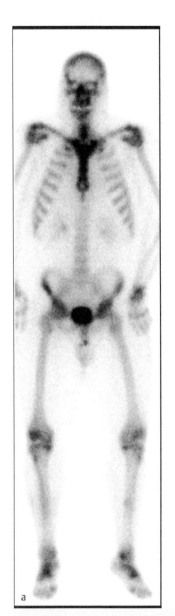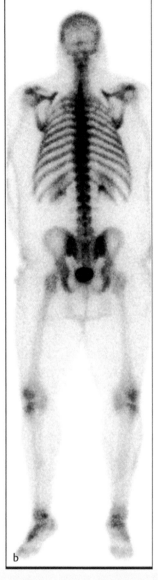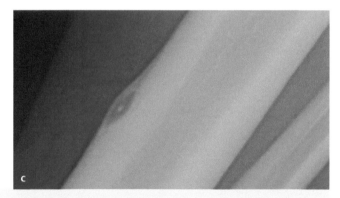

Fig. 101.1 (a and b) Anterior and posterior whole-body images from technetium-99m (Tc-99m) hydroxy diphosphonate (HDP) bone scintigraphy demonstrate focally increased radiotracer deposition in the left diaphyseal tibia (intentionally increased intensity). (c) Cropped radiographs of the left lower extremity demonstrate a cortical lucency with central nidus.

## ■ Clinical History

25-year-old male with a 6-month history of left lower extremity pain, without trauma, and with occasional tenderness to palpation (▶Fig. 101.1).

## ■ Key Finding

Intense radiotracer deposition in a benign bone lesion

## ■ Top 3 Differential Diagnoses

- **Osteoid osteoma.** OO is a benign bone-forming tumor that classically presents in adolescents with night pain that is relieved by salicylates. The tumor has a central osteoblastic nidus surrounded by reactive sclerosis. Pain is secondary to release of prostaglandins from the nidus. They usually occur in long bones, most commonly in the proximal femur, but can be seen in the phalanges and spine. When in the spine, OO may cause painful scoliosis. Ablation or resection are commonly used for treatment; conservative management is an option as they will spontaneously resolve. OO will typically show intense central uptake with surrounding less intense uptake on bone scan. A good percentage can be missed on radiographs, particularly in the spine; radionuclide bone scintigraphy is useful in this setting. Pinhole collimators may be helpful as the lesions may be small.
- **Giant cell tumor (GCT).** GCT of bone contains a diffuse osteoclastic giant cell component and presents radiographically as a large, eccentric, lytic, meta-epiphyseal lesion extending to the subchondral bone. Most common sites include around the knee, the distal radius, sacrum, and proximal humerus. The majority will show increased uptake of Tc-99m-labeled diphosphonates, occasionally with uptake in adjacent bones secondary to associated hyperemia.
- **Fibrous dysplasia (FD).** It is a nonneoplastic process that results from dysfunctional differentiation of osteoblasts, resulting in replacement of normal bone/marrow with immature bone and fibrous stroma. Monostotic FD most commonly affects the femur and tibia. The imaging appearance is variable, but generally is seen as a lucent, intramedullary, well-defined lesion. On bone scan, FD can range from no metabolic activity to markedly increased metabolic activity.

## ■ Additional Differential Diagnosis

- **Aneurysmal bone cyst (ABC):** ABC is an expansile, lucent lesion with blood-filled spaces and septations, most commonly located in the tibia and then femur. On bone scan, ABCs demonstrate peripheral uptake with decreased central uptake, the so-called donut sign pattern.
- **Chondroblastoma (CB):** CBs are well-defined lucent lesions that form in epiphyseal equivalents, most commonly in long bones. There is frequently periosteal reaction in the metaphysis adjacent to a CB. Uptake is seen on bone scan on all phases, with uptake in adjacent bones due to hyperemia.

## ■ Diagnosis

Osteoid osteoma of the left tibia.

## ✓ Pearls

- Intense bone scan uptake in a bone tumor is a sign of malignancy, but can be seen in benign lesions also.
- Other benign bone lesions (bone island, enchondroma, non-ossifying fibroma (NOF), osteochondroma) may show mild uptake.
- Bones adjacent to a lesion may show uptake due to hyperemia, mimicking a joint centered process.

## Suggested Readings

Focacci C, Lattanzi R, Iadeluca ML, Campioni P. Nuclear medicine in primary bone tumors. Eur J Radiol. 1998; 27(Suppl 1):S123–S131

Murphey MD, Nomikos GC, Flemming DJ, Gannon FH, Temple HT, Kransdorf MJ. From the archives of AFIP. Imaging of giant cell tumor and giant cell reparative granuloma of bone: radiologic-pathologic correlation. Radiographics. 2001; 21(5):1283–1309

Park JH, Pahk K, Kim S, Lee SH, Song SH, Choe JG. Radionuclide imaging in the diagnosis of osteoid osteoma. Oncol Lett. 2015; 10(2):1131–1134

Steffner R. Benign bone tumors. Cancer Treat Res. 2014; 162:31–63

# Case 102

*Joseph M. Yetto, Jr.*

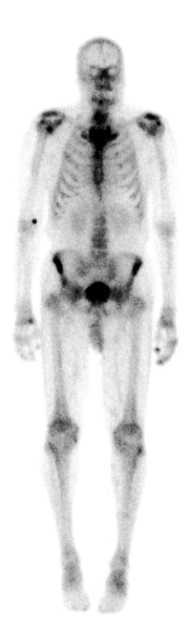

**Fig. 102.1** Anterior whole-body technetium-99m (Tc-99m) hydroxy diphosphonate (HDP) bone scintigraphy demonstrates focally increased radiotracer deposition within the shoulders, sternoclavicular region, right wrist, and left fingers.

■ Clinical History

86-year-old male with prostate cancer and shoulder pain (▶Fig. 102.1).

## ■ Key Finding

Periarticular radiotracer deposition on bone scintigraphy

## ■ Top 3 Differential Diagnoses

- **Osteoarthritis.** Osteoarthritis, specifically secondary osteoarthritis, is the most common form of arthritis and is characterized radiographically by osteophytosis, subchondral sclerosis, subchondral cystic changes, and joint space narrowing. On bone scintigraphy, osteoarthritis demonstrates periarticular uptake of variable intensity depending on level of active inflammation and bone formation. Degenerative type uptake is often seen involving the shoulders, wrist (first carpometacarpal joint), hand (distal interphalangeal joints), medial compartment of the knee, and feet.
- **Inflammatory arthritis.** This is a generic term which applies to any cause of arthritis that results secondary to inflammation instead of cartilage degeneration or trauma. Common radiographic findings of inflammatory arthritis include joint space narrowing, periarticular osteopenia, and erosions. Rheumatoid arthritis classically does not present with any bone formation (i.e., osteophytes), unless secondary osteoarthritis is present. Infectious/septic arthritis must be excluded if only one joint is involved, as this is not usual for the other inflammatory arthropathies which are often musculoskeletal manifestations of systemic disease. Common differentials for an erosive arthritis include rheumatoid, psoriatic arthritis, reactive arthritis, erosive osteoarthritis, and gout. Inflammation within and around the joint shows increased metabolic activity on bone scintigraphy.
- **Complex regional pain syndrome.** CRPS, formerly known as reflex sympathetic dystrophy (RSD), is a chronic pain condition that has associated autonomic nervous dysfunction. Type I CRPS occurs in the absence of a nerve injury. Patients present with severe pain, swelling, warmth, erythema, and hypersensitivity of the involved limbs. The process may progress, occasionally even ending in contractures. Trauma and surgery are often inciting events. Radiographs may show osteopenia. Three-phase bone scan (TPBS) is nearly 100% sensitivity for CRPS. TPBS will show increased blood flow and blood pool activity in the affected region along with intense periarticular uptake on delayed images. Alternatively, decreased uptake may be seen in the affected region, known as "cold CRPS" and more common in the pediatric population.

## ■ Diagnosis

Prostate cancer patient with polyarticular osteoarthritis.

## ✓ Pearls

- Septic arthritis must be considered with focally increased uptake surrounding a single joint.
- Variable intensity periarticular and synovial uptake is associated with osteoarthritis.
- TPBS is useful for diagnostic confirmation of CRPS in a patient with pain and autonomic dysfunction.

## Suggested Readings

Jacobson JA, Girish G, Jiang Y, Resnick D. Radiographic evaluation of arthritis: inflammatory conditions. Radiology. 2008; 248(2):378–389

Van den Wyngaert T, Strobel K, Kampen WU, et al. EANM Bone & Joint Committee and the Oncology Committee. The EANM practice guidelines for bone scintigraphy. Eur J Nucl Med Mol Imaging. 2016; 43(9):1723–1738

Wüppenhorst N, Maier C, Frettlöh J, Pennekamp W, Nicolas V. Sensitivity and specificity of 3-phase bone scintigraphy in the diagnosis of complex regional pain syndrome of the upper extremity. Clin J Pain. 2010; 26(3):182–189

Zeman MN, Scott PJH. Current imaging strategies in rheumatoid arthritis. Am J Nucl Med Mol Imaging. 2012; 2(2):174–220

# Case 103

*Joseph M. Yetto, Jr.*

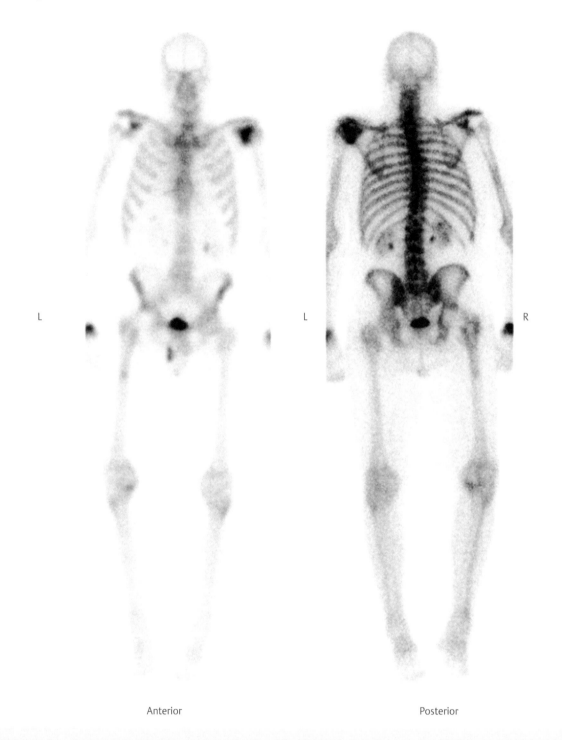

Anterior                                                    Posterior

**Fig. 103.1** Anterior and posterior whole-body images from technetium-99m (Tc-99m) hydroxy diphosphonate (HDP) bone scintigraphy demonstrate focally decreased radiotracer deposition in the right proximal humerus and right proximal femur consistent with orthopedic hardware. Additionally, there is focally increased radiotracer deposition at the tip of the right femoral prosthetic.

■ **Clinical History**

88-year-old male with multiple orthopedic implants and pain in the right hip (▶ Fig. 103.1).

## ■ Key Finding

Periprosthetic increased metabolic activity on bone scintigraphy

## ■ Top 3 Differential Diagnoses

• **Mechanical loosening/small particle disease (osteolysis).** Aseptic loosening is seen within one-half of prostheses by 10 years after joint replacement surgery and with up to one-third cases requiring revision. Aseptic loosening generally presents with pain and is multifactorial. Nevertheless, a significant number of cases are due to a robust inflammatory immune reaction as phagocytes repeatedly attempt to breakdown particulate debris from prosthetic fragmentation. Ultimately, this results in osteolysis around the prosthesis. The most common radiographic findings are perihardware lucencies which are nonspecific and can be seen in both aseptic loosening and in, its primary differential, periprosthetic infection. The lucency is usually more focal with small particle disease. Bone scintigraphy demonstrates periprosthetic uptake. With a cemented hip prosthesis, increased uptake at the tip of the femoral component is suggestive of loosening, but not 100% specific.

• **Periprosthetic infection.** Periprosthetic infection generally presents with pain. The rate of infection increases somewhat significantly after revision surgeries. The most common etiologies are *Staphylococcus epidermis* and *S. aureus* infections. Approximately one-third of infections develop within 3 months, another one-third within 1 year, and the final one-third after 1 year. Histopathologically, periprosthetic infection is identical to aseptic loosening with one major exception: the presence of neutrophils within infected joints. Bone scintigraphy usually demonstrates diffuse periprosthetic delayed uptake with increased uptake on both blood flow and blood pool imaging; but the pattern of uptake is not diagnostic. Both tagged WBC scan and fluorine-18 fluorodeoxyglucose positron-emission tomography (F-18 FDG PET) may provide more diagnostic accuracy, but bone scan remains a good screening exam as a negative exam can essentially exclude loosening and infection.

• **Postsurgical changes.** Metabolic activity can persist for up to 2 years after a joint replacement.

## ■ Diagnosis

Right hip arthroplasty with loosening of the femoral component.

## ✓ Pearls

• Aseptic loosening versus infection differentiation is difficult as scintigraphic findings can be similar.
• Focal uptake at the femoral component tip suggests loosening in the setting of a cemented prosthesis.

• Tagged WBC imaging can be used to differentiate periprosthetic infection from mechanical loosening.

## Suggested Readings

Love C, Tomas MB, Marwin SE, Pugliese PV, Palestro CJ. Role of nuclear medicine in diagnosis of the infected joint replacement. Radiographics. 2001; 21(5): 1229–1238

Kumar K. Three phase bone scan interpretation based upon vascular endothelial response. Indian J Nucl Med. 2015; 30(2):104–110

Reinartz P, Mumme T, Hermanns B, et al. Radionuclide imaging of the painful hip arthroplasty: positron-emission tomography versus triple-phase bone scanning. J Bone Joint Surg Br. 2005; 87(4):465–470

White ML, Johnson GB, Howe BM, Peller PJ, Broski SM. Spectrum of benign articular findings at FDG PET/CT. Radiographics. 2016; 36(3):824–839

# Part 9

## Infection and Inflammation

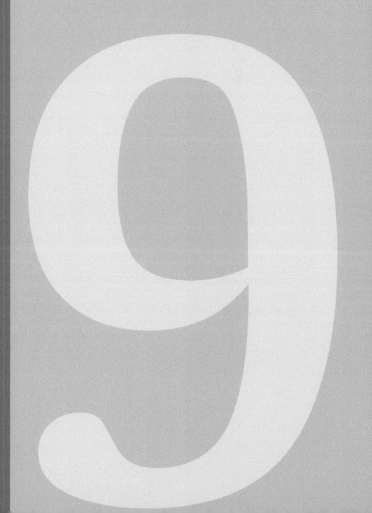

# Case 104

*Ely A. Wolin*

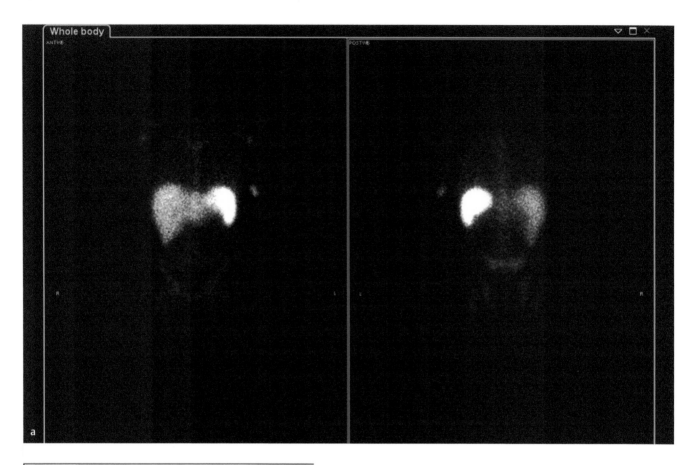

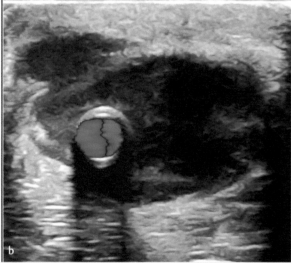

**Fig. 104.1** (a) Anterior and posterior Indium-111 (In-111) white blood cell whole-body images show focal abnormal uptake in the medial left upper arm. (b) Representative image from correlative ultrasound performed the following day shows hematoma surrounding a left upper arm arteriovenous graft.

■ **Clinical History**

27-year-old male with end-stage renal disease secondary to focal segmental glomerulonephritis presented with fevers and was found to have methicillin-susceptible *Staphylococcus aureus* bacteremia without known source (▶Fig. 104.1).

## ■ Key Finding

Focal abnormal uptake on tagged white blood cell (WBC) scintigraphy

## ■ Top 3 Differential Diagnoses

- **Infection.** WBCs can be removed from the patient and tagged with either In-111 oxine or technetium-99m (Tc-99m) hexamethylpropyleneamine oxime (HMPAO) for use with whole-body imaging. Tagging can be done in vivo, in vitro, or with a mixed technique. The in vitro technique is most commonly used as it is most efficient. In-111 oxine has the advantage of a long half-life and no hepatobiliary, genito-urinary, or intestinal clearance. Tc-99m HMPAO provides better imaging statistics and less radiation dose to the patient. Both are useful for many indications, many of which have been replaced by CT and magnetic resonance imaging (MRI). In-111 oxine WBC imaging is most useful for renal infection, chronic osteomyelitis, and fever of unknown origin (FUO). Tc-99m HMPAO WBC imaging is most useful for acute osteomyelitis of the appendicular skeleton, vascular graft infection, and soft-tissue infection. Both can be used for inflammatory bowel disease (IBD), with some studies showing improved sensitivity with early imaging with Tc-99m HMPAO, before hepatobiliary clearance interferes, due to the improved imaging statistics. Mucosal uptake may be sloughed limiting the utility of In-111 oxine. Abnormal uptake of either one of the tagged WBC imaging agents results from a combination of hyperemia, vascular permeability, and chemotaxis. Focal uptake is worrisome for pyogenic infection. Infectious uptake is generally as intense as physiologic liver uptake, with more intense uptake raising suspicion for abscess. Single-photon emission computed tomography (SPECT)/CT imaging can provide additional characterization.
- **Inflammation.** As WBC uptake is not the only uptake mechanism for radiolabeled WBCs, increased uptake is not specific for pyogenic infection. Any inflammation can result in hyperemia and increased vascular permeability, and therefore, result in increased uptake of either In-111 oxine WBC or Tc-99m HMPAO WBC. In general, inflammatory uptake may be less intense than infectious uptake, more along the level of physiologic bone marrow activity.
- **Healing.** Both postsurgical and traumatic healing will demonstrate increased radiolabeled WBC activity. Correlation with clinical history is important.

## ■ Additional Diagnostic Consideration

- **Bleed:** While radiolabeled WBC distribute in the reticuloendothelial system (spleen, liver, and bone marrow), they also circulate within the blood pool. It is therefore possible for abnormal activity to be seen with active bleeding. Gastrointestinal (GI) bleeding has been seen on tagged WBC imaging.

## ■ Diagnosis

Left upper arm arteriovenous graft hematoma.

## ✓ Pearls

- Tagged WBC uptake can be seen with infection, inflammation, healing, and bleeding.
- As a general guideline, uptake in abscess may be greater than infection and inflammation.
- Fluorine-18 fluorodeoxyglucose positron-emission tomography (F-18 FDG PET) imaging has proved equally or more useful than tagged WBC imaging for many indications.

## Suggested Readings

Becker W, Meller J. The role of nuclear medicine in infection and inflammation. Lancet Infect Dis. 2001; 1(5):326–333

Cortés J, Villaverde J, Garrido M, Pombo M, Ruibal A. Incidental detection of gastrointestinal bleeding from an aortoenteric fistula on 99 mTc leukocyte scintigraphy. Clin Nucl Med. 2012; 37(11):1123–1125

Gotthardt M, Bleeker-Rovers CP, Boerman OC, Oyen WJ. Imaging of inflammation by PET, conventional scintigraphy, and other imaging techniques. J Nucl Med Technol. 2013; 41(3):157–169

# Case 105

*Ely A. Wolin*

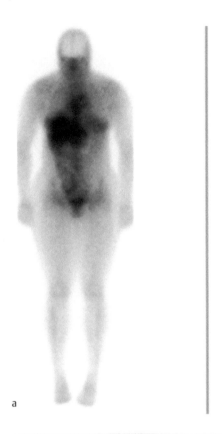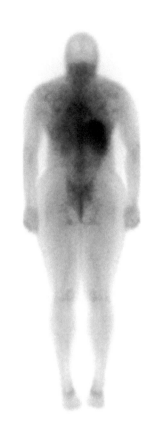

a

**Fig. 105.1** In addition to the sarcoidosis-related mediastinal and hilar lymph node uptake, 24-hour anterior and posterior whole-body Gallium (Ga)-67 citrate images show mild bilateral breast activity, confirmed on single-photon emission computed tomography (SPECT).

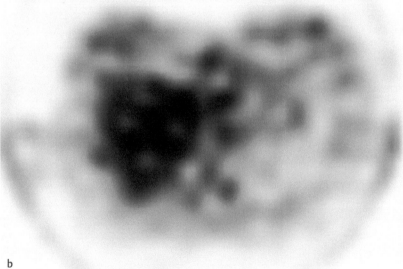

b

## ■ Clinical History

48-year-old female with sarcoidosis, lung and lymph node involvement (▶ Fig. 105.1).

## ■ Key Finding

Increased breast uptake on Ga-67 citrate scintigraphy

## ■ Top 3 Differential Diagnoses

- **Hormone stimulation.** Both prolactin and estrogen can stimulate breast uptake of Ga-67 citrate. Hyperprolactinemia results in intense, symmetric, increased bilateral breast uptake; most intense when seen in the immediate postpartum state. There may be relative photopenia in the subareolar region resulting in a "doughnut" configuration, likely due to peripheral lobular development stimulated by prolactin. The "doughnut" pattern can help differentiate from estrogen therapy which generally results in a more subareolar or diffuse pattern of uptake. Hyperprolactinemia can be seen with renal failure as well as a side effect of several medications, in addition to normal postpartum lactation.

- **Infection.** Ga-67 citrate is primarily used as an infection/inflammation imaging agent due to its avidity for bacterial infections as well as acute and chronic inflammatory pathology. Asymmetric increased breast activity can be seen with mastitis. More focal uptake may suggest an abscess.
- **Lymphoma.** Ga-67 citrate has been used extensively for lymphoma evaluation, most prominently to help assess response to therapy, but now it has largely been replaced by fluorine-18 fluorodeoxyglucose positron-emission tomography (F-18 FDG PET) imaging. However, Ga-67 citrate scintigraphy does have good sensitivity for extranodal lymphoma. Secondary breast involvement is more common than primary breast lymphoma.

## ■ Additional Diagnostic Consideration

**Primary breast pathology:** Ga-67 citrate scintigraphy is not routinely used for evaluation of breast pathology, as uptake in primary breast malignancies is variable. However, Ga-67 citrate uptake has been seen in primary breast pathology, including invasive ductal carcinoma, fibroadenoma, and fibrocystic change.

## ■ Diagnosis

Physiologic breast uptake.

## ✓ Pearls

- Symmetric increased Ga-67 citrate breast uptake is almost always due to hormonal stimulation.
- Symmetric increased breast uptake may be seen in renal failure due to associated hyperprolactinemia.

- Asymmetric or focal Ga-67 citrate breast uptake is more concerning, but not always pathologic.

## Suggested Readings

Kim YC, Brown ML, Thrall JH. Scintigraphic patterns of gallium-67 uptake in the breast. Radiology. 1977; 124(1):169–175

Moralidis E, Mandala E, Venizelos I, et al. A breast fibroadenoma mimicking an extranodal deposit of Hodgkin's lymphoma in 67Ga imaging. Br J Radiol. 2009; 82(975):e58–e62

Taher MA, Navalkissoor S, Hilson AJ, Buscombe JR. Gallium citrate uptake is a marker of breast malignancy: true or false? Nucl Med Rev Cent East Eur. 2007; 10(1):21–22

# Case 106

*Ely A. Wolin*

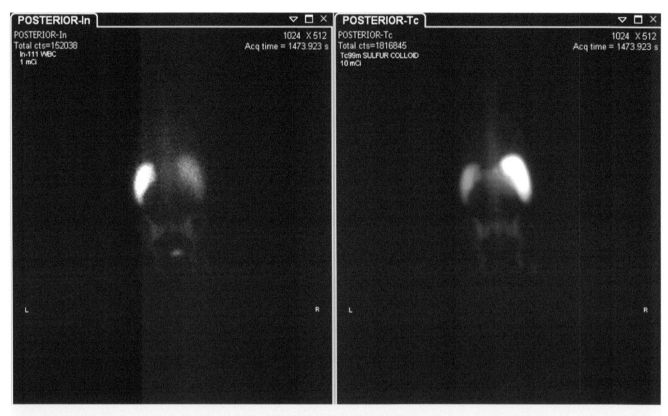

**Fig. 106.1** Posterior images from a dual isotope study, obtained 24 hours after the administration of indium-111-labeled white blood cells (In-111 WBC) and 15 minutes after the administration of technetium-99m sulfur colloid (Tc-99m SC), show uptake in the urinary bladder on the In-111 image only.

## ■ Clinical History

73-year-old female referred for left knee pain 5 years after total knee arthroplasty, concern for infection and/or loosening (▶ Fig. 106.1).

## ■ Key Finding

Genitourinary tract uptake on In-111-labeled WBC scan

## ■ Top 3 Differential Diagnoses

- **Infection.** In-111 is cyclotron produced, decays by electron capture releasing 173 and 247 keV gamma photons, with a physical half-life of 67 hours. In-111 oxine-labeled WBC scintigraphy is frequently used for infection imaging. Labeling is most commonly done in vitro which allows for the best efficiency and results in irreversible binding of the radionuclide to intracellular components primarily within neutrophils. Uptake mechanism is via chemotaxis of WBC. Imaging is generally performed around 24 hours after injection of the radiolabeled WBC. Normal distribution entails higher uptake within the spleen than liver and bone marrow. There is no hepatobiliary, intestinal, or genitourinary clearance. It is important to remember that there is no normal physiologic renal activity seen with In-111 WBC, since renal activity is so frequently seen on other nuclear medicine exams, including Tc-99m hexamethylpropyleneamine (HMPAO)-labeled WBC which has both hepatobiliary and genitourinary clearance. Urinary tract infection may present as activity within the genitourinary collecting system on In-111 WBC scintigraphy. Parenchymal renal uptake suggests pyelonephritis.
- **Transplant complications.** In-111 WBC uptake in a transplant kidney is not specific. Uptake can be seen with rejection, acute tubular necrosis (ATN), and infection. Immunosuppressive therapy may limit the effectiveness of tagged WBC scintigraphy.
- **Other radiopharmaceutical.** In-111 WBC scintigraphy is often performed in conjunction with other nuclear medicine exams, such as Tc-99m medronic acid (MDP) bone scan and Tc-99m SC bone marrow imaging for osteomyelitis evaluation. Genitourinary uptake, in this setting, may be due to normal renal clearance of one of the Tc-99m based radiopharmaceuticals.

## ■ Diagnosis

Urinary tract infection.

## ✓ Pearls

- In-111-tagged leukocytes demonstrate no hepatobiliary, intestinal, or genitourinary clearance.
- Genitourinary uptake on an In-111 WBC scan is abnormal and concerning for infection.
- In-111 WBC uptake in a renal transplant is not specific and can be seen with ATN, rejection, and infection.

## Suggested Readings

Hughes DK. Nuclear medicine and infection detection: the relative effectiveness of imaging with 111 In-oxine-, 99 mTc-HMPAO-, and 99 mTc-stannous fluoride colloid-labeled leukocytes and with 67Ga-citrate. J Nucl Med Technol. 2003; 31(4):196–201, quiz 203–204

Love C, Palestro CJ. Radionuclide imaging of infection. J Nucl Med Technol. 2004; 32(2):47–57, quiz 58–59

# Case 107

*Ely A. Wolin*

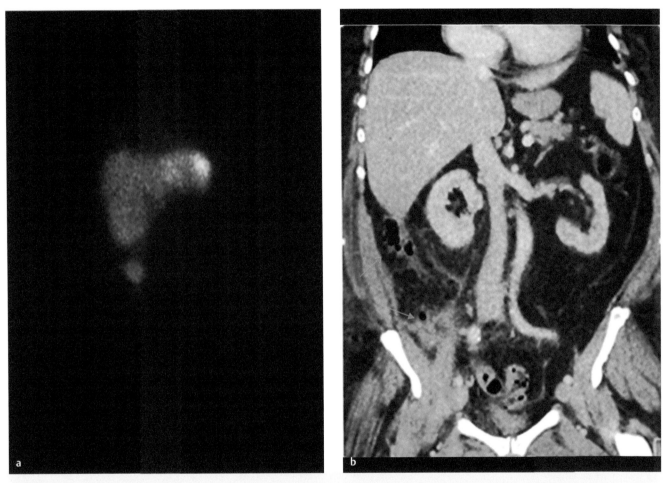

**Fig. 107.1** (a) Anterior image from indium-111 (In-111) white blood cell scan shows abnormal radiotracer uptake in the right mid to low abdomen. (b) Representative coronal image from correlative CT scan shows a right retroperitoneal air and fluid collection (*red arrows*), incompletely depicted.

## ■ Clinical History

63-year-old female with fever, elevated inflammatory markers, and low back with new neurologic deficits, concern for epidural abscess. Too obese for MRI (▶ Fig. 107.1).

## ■ Key Finding

Abnormal intra-abdominal uptake on tagged leukocyte scintigraphy

## ■ Top 3 Differential Diagnoses

- **Infection.** Either In-111 oxine or Tc-99m hexamethylpropyleneamine (HMPAO)-tagged WBC scintigraphy remains useful tool for localization of infection. Sensitivity for abdominal abscess is greater than both ultrasound (US) and CT, although CT does have higher specificity. Leukocyte scintigraphy generally involves 24-hour imaging, making it less useful if immediate diagnosis is needed. Tagged WBC scan is most useful in a patient with presumed abdominal infection without localizing signs and negative anatomic imaging. Utilizing single-photon emission computed tomography (SPECT)/CT imaging allows for immediate anatomic localization and procedure planning, if the associated anatomic imaging is of high enough quality. In-111 oxine WBC scan is preferred for abdominal infection imaging as there is no hepatobiliary, intestinal, or genitourinary clearance.
- **Inflammation.** One of the main limitations of leukocyte scintigraphy is difficulty in distinguishing infection from inflammation. Although as a general rule, infection will have uptake equal to or greater than the liver, and inflammation less than the liver, these patterns are not 100% specific. The uptake mechanism in inflammation includes hyperemia and vascular permeability, and less so WBC chemotaxis. Leukocyte scintigraphy can be useful for imaging IBD, as it is noninvasive, allows for imaging of the entire bowel, may distinguish between Crohn's disease and ulcerative colitis, and does not require bowel preparation. While In-111 oxine WBC is generally preferred for intra-abdominal imaging, Tc-99m HMPAO WBC is preferred for IBD. This is due to early imaging and improved statistics, as late imaging with In-111 oxine WBC may be falsely negative due to sloughing mucosa.
- **Accessory spleen.** Physiologic distribution of labeled leukocytes involves the reticuloendothelial system, more uptake in spleen than liver and bone marrow. Focal uptake in an accessory spleen in a patient with prior splenectomy can be confusing and mimic intra-abdominal infection. Correlation with anatomic imaging, or a Tc-99m SC liver spleen scan, can be confirmatory.

## ■ Additional Diagnostic Considerations

- **Gastrointestinal bleed/hematoma:** Radiolabeled leukocyte activity may be seen with ongoing gastrointestinal (GI) bleed, or in a hematoma, if bleeding occurred after injection.
- **Aneurysm:** Focal blood pool activity within an aneurysm, particularly saccular, may mimic infection.

## ■ Diagnosis

Retroperitoneal abscess.

## ✓ Pearls

- Radiolabeled leukocyte uptake is not specific for pyogenic infection.
- Leukocyte scintigraphy is noninvasive, images the whole bowel, and does not require bowel preparation.
- Main limitation of tagged WBC scan is difficulty in distinguishing infection from inflammation.

## Suggested Readings

Almer S, Granerus G, Ström M, et al. Leukocyte scintigraphy compared to intra-operative small bowel enteroscopy and laparotomy findings in Crohn's disease. Inflamm Bowel Dis. 2007; 13(2):164–174

Coleman RE, Welch D. Possible pitfalls with clinical imaging of indium-111 leukocytes: concise communication. J Nucl Med. 1980; 21(2):122–125

Liberatore M, Calandri E, Ciccariello G, et al. The labeled-leukocyte scan in the study of abdominal abscesses. Mol Imaging Biol. 2010; 12(6):563–569

# Case 108

*Ely A. Wolin*

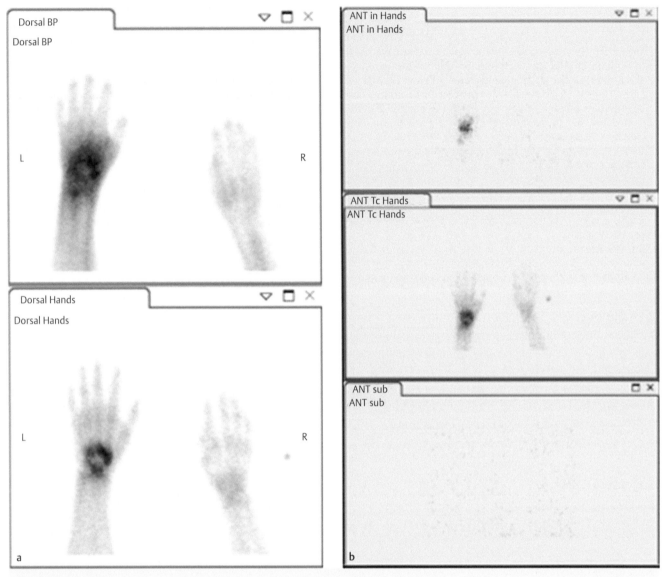

**Fig. 108.1** Dorsal blood pool and delayed images of the hands from Tc-99m methyl diphosphonate bone scintigraphy (**a**) show increased radiotracer activity throughout the left carpus. In-111 white blood cell and Tc-99m SC dual isotope imaging was subsequently performed with matched uptake seen in the left carpus (**b**, subtraction image on bottom).

## ■ Clinical History

68-year-old male with left hand cellulitis, slow to respond to intravenous antibiotics, referred for osteomyelitis evaluation (▶Fig. 108.1).

## ■ Key Finding

Focal increased osseous uptake on leukocyte scintigraphy

## ■ Top 2 Differential Diagnoses

- **Osteomyelitis.** Tagged WBC scintigraphy, when coupled with a three-phase bone scan, provides high sensitivity and specificity for osteomyelitis outside of the spine. Focal osseous uptake on leukocyte scintigraphy that matches an area of three-phase positivity on bone scan is suggestive of osteomyelitis. The bone scan is used for sensitivity, as a normal bone scan essentially excludes osteomyelitis. The tagged WBC scan then adds specificity as degenerative disease, trauma, and postsurgical changes can result in similar bone scan findings. In-111-labeled WBC imaging is often advantageous due to radiopharmaceutical stability, less variability in physiologic distribution, and the ability to perform dual isotope bone marrow imaging. Tc-99m-labeled WBC imaging allows for earlier imaging and better imaging statistics. With either agent, a WBC count of at least 2,000 per microliter is recommended to ensure adequate imaging. Leukocyte scintigraphy is much less sensitive for vertebral osteomyelitis/discitis, possibly secondary to increased pressure preventing WBC migration, and Ga-67 citrate or F-18 FDG are primarily used in this setting.

- **Altered marrow distribution/reactive marrow.** Labeled leukocyte activity will normally be seen in hematopoietic bone marrow in addition to infection. In adults, the hematopoietic marrow is usually located within the axial and proximal appendicular spine. This distribution can be altered, however, in multiple conditions including trauma, surgery, anemia, and tumors, among others. Tc-99m SC bone marrow scintigraphy can be used to compliment the tagged WBC images, as Tc-99m SC activity will be seen in reactive marrow but not infection. This can be performed simultaneously with In-111-labeled WBCs or after at least a 2-day delay if Tc-99m WBCs are used. Infection is confirmed in a location with bone scan uptake, matched leukocyte activity, and no SC uptake. A reasonable approach to radionuclide imaging of suspected osteomyelitis, outside of the spine and not confirmed with anatomic imaging, includes a three-phase bone scan, followed by labeled leukocyte and bone marrow scintigraphy, if positive. This approach should provide greater than 90% sensitivity and specificity.

## ■ Diagnosis

Reactive marrow.

## ✓ Pearls

- Bone scan followed by labeled leukocyte and bone marrow scintigraphy is great for osteomyelitis imaging.
- Tc-99m SC imaging helps to distinguish between infection and hematopoietic marrow.

- Bone scan alone has high specificity for osteomyelitis if there is no abnormality (arthropathy, trauma, hardware).
- Labeled leukocyte scintigraphy has poor sensitivity for spinal osteomyelitis/discitis.

## Suggested Readings

Love C, Palestro CJ. Radionuclide imaging of inflammation and infection in the acute care setting. Semin Nucl Med. 2013; 43(2):102–113

Palestro CJ. Radionuclide imaging of osteomyelitis. Semin Nucl Med. 2015; 45(1):32–46

Termaat MF, Raijmakers PG, Scholten HJ, Bakker FC, Patka P, Haarman HJ. The accuracy of diagnostic imaging for the assessment of chronic osteomyelitis: a systematic review and meta-analysis. J Bone Joint Surg Am. 2005; 87(11):2464–2471

# Case 109

*Ely A. Wolin*

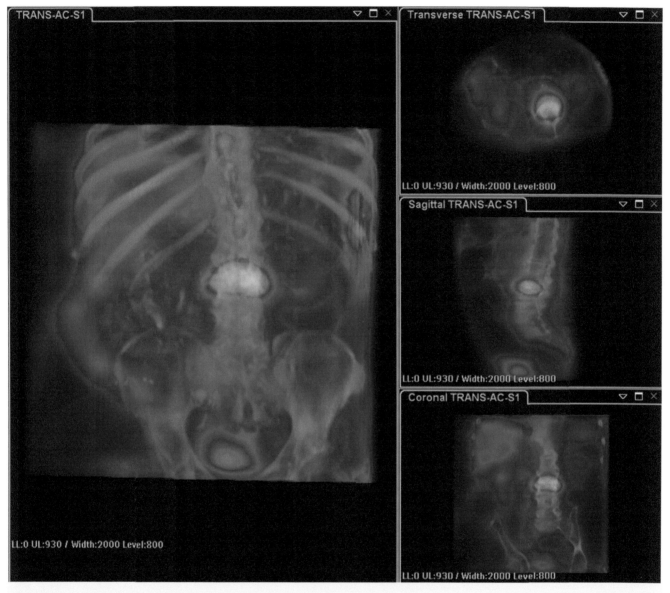

**Fig. 109.1** Fused single-photon emission computed tomography/CT images from Gallium (Ga)-67 citrate scan show increased focal uptake at the L2–3 level.

## ■ Clinical History

74-year-old male with sever low back pain with L3–5 inflammatory changes on MRI, referred to evaluate for evidence of discitis/osteomyelitis (▶ Fig. 109.1).

## ■ Key Finding

Focal spinal uptake on Ga-67 citrate scintigraphy

## ■ Top 3 Differential Diagnoses

- **Discitis/osteomyelitis.** Ga-67 citrate is a nonspecific imaging agent for infection, inflammation, and tumor. While fluorine-18 fluorodeoxyglucose (F-18 FDG) is the imaging agent of choice for radionuclide evaluation of spinal osteomyelitis/discitis, in the absence of fixation hardware, Ga-67 citrate is preferred over radiolabeled leukocytes as the sensitivity of labeled leukocyte imaging is known to be very low. As with imaging of appendicular osteomyelitis, correlation with bone scan is essential as it provides an accurate mapping of affected osseous structures. Discitis/osteomyelitis is suspected when Ga-67 citrate uptake exceeds Tc-99m MDP/HDP uptake in size and/or intensity. Uptake similar in intensity and distribution to the bone scan abnormality is equivocal for infection.

- **Degenerative disc disease.** Ga-67 citrate is not a specific radiotracer for infection. Uptake can be seen due to inflammation associated with degenerative changes. In this setting uptake on bone scan is usually more centered on the endplates surrounding a disc space, and Ga-67 citrate uptake will not exceed the bone scan uptake.
- **Postsurgical changes.** Ga-67 citrate is preferred over F-18 FDG imaging for discitis/osteomyelitis in the presence of spinal hardware. However, it is important to remember that healing is an inflammatory process and will result in Ga-67 citrate uptake for several months.

## ■ Additional Diagnostic Consideration

- **Malignancy:** Ga-67 citrate is a nonspecific tumor imaging agent. Uptake within the spine could possibly be due to primary or metastatic malignancy.

## ■ Diagnosis

Degenerative disc disease. Subsequent CT-guided biopsy with culture revealed no microorganism growth.

## ✓ Pearls

- Ga-67 citrate is a nonspecific infection, inflammation, and tumor imaging agent.
- Imaging of discitis/osteomyelitis is one of the few remaining indications for Ga-67 citrate scintigraphy.

- F-18 FDG imaging is preferable to Ga-67 citrate for discitis/osteomyelitis but can be limited with hardware.
- Ga-67 citrate uptake more intense than bone scan, or discordant in distribution, suggests spondylodiscitis.

## Suggested Readings

As T, Abele JT. Bone and gallium single-photon emission computed tomography is equivalent to magnetic resonance imaging in the diagnosis of infectious spondylodiscitis: a retrospective study. Can Assoc Radiol J. 2016

Gemmel F, Dumarey N, Palestro CJ. Radionuclide imaging of spinal infections. Eur J Nucl Med Mol Imaging. 2006; 33(10):1226–1237

Mazzie JP, Brooks MK, Gnerre J. Imaging and management of postoperative spine infection. Neuroimaging Clin N Am. 2014; 24(2):365–374

# Case 110

*Ely A. Wolin*

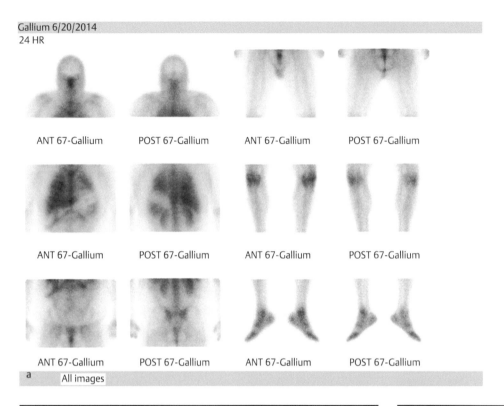

Gallium 6/20/2014
24 HR

ANT 67-Gallium    POST 67-Gallium    ANT 67-Gallium    POST 67-Gallium

ANT 67-Gallium    POST 67-Gallium    ANT 67-Gallium    POST 67-Gallium

ANT 67-Gallium    POST 67-Gallium    ANT 67-Gallium    POST 67-Gallium

a    All images

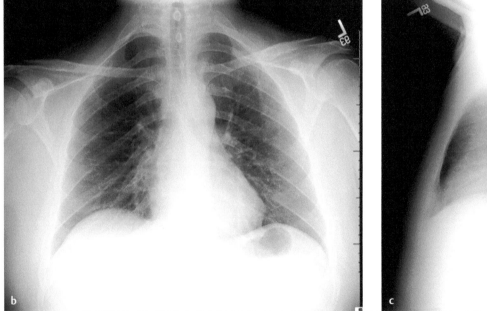

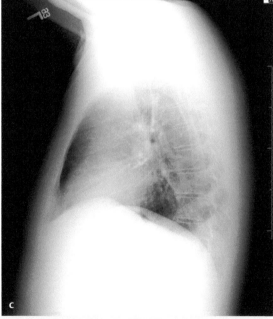

**Fig. 110.1** Delayed imaging at 120 hours following Gallium (Ga)-67 citrate administration demonstrates diffuse uptake within the lung bilaterally. Corresponding PA and lateral chest radiograph are normal.

## ■ Clinical History

54-year-old male liver transplant recipient on immunosuppressive therapy (▶Fig. 110.1). (Case courtesy of Joseph S. Fotos, MD, Penn State Hershey Medical Center.)

■ Key Finding

Pulmonary uptake on Ga-67 citrate scintigraphy

■ Top 3 Differential Diagnoses

- **Sarcoidosis.** Ga-67 citrate will demonstrate uptake in multiple granulomatous diseases of the lung, including tuberculosis and sarcoidosis. Ga-67 citrate scintigraphy is very sensitive for active sarcoidosis and can help distinguish active granulomatous disease and alveolitis from inactive disease and fibrosis. Findings on Ga-67 citrate scan may be present before any sarcoid related radiographic abnormality is evident. Due to its ability to distinguish active from inactive disease and detect sites of disease in the absence of clinical symptoms, Ga-67 citrate can be useful to monitor response to therapy.
- **Infection.** Ga-67 citrate will bind to both lactoferrin released from destroyed macrophages as well as bacterial siderophores, making it a useful infection imaging agent occasionally used for evaluation of FUO. Pulmonary uptake in this setting is concerning for infection. While bacterial pneumonia will likely demonstrate more focal uptake associated with the consolidated injection, atypical infections, including viral pneumonia and *Pneumocystis jiroveci* pneumonia (PJP), may show diffuse pulmonary uptake. Ga-67 citrate scintigraphy is highly sensitive for PJP, with a negative scan essentially excluding the diagnosis. Uptake will usually be diffuse and may be heterogeneous. When used in conjunction with thallium-201, it can help differentiate from lymphoma: PJP should only show uptake with Ga-67 citrate, lymphoma will show uptake with both. Ga-67 citrate scintigraphy can also be used to monitor treatment. Kaposi's sarcoma will also not demonstrate Ga-67 citrate uptake.
- **Hypersensitivity pneumonitis.** Many pharmacologic therapies used routinely in clinical medicine are known to cause lung injury, including methotrexate, amiodarone, nitrofurantoin, among others. Ga-67 citrate scintigraphy is highly sensitive for pulmonary inflammation and can show findings of drug-induced hypersensitivity pneumonitis before any radiographic abnormality.

■ Additional Diagnostic Considerations

- **Idiopathic interstitial pulmonary fibrosis:** Diffuse pulmonary uptake of Ga-67 citrate can be seen with idiopathic interstitial pulmonary fibrosis with relatively high sensitivity.
- **Malignancy:** Pulmonary uptake of Ga-67 citrate can be seen with malignancy, including primary lung neoplasms and lymphoma, both of which are among the most Ga-67 avid neoplasms.

■ Diagnosis

Findings are suspicious for an atypical pneumonia, such as *P. jiroveci*, in this immunocompromised patient.

✓ Pearls

- Ga-67 citrate lung uptake, like uptake elsewhere, can be seen with infection, inflammation, or malignancy.
- Ga-67 citrate scan in sarcoidosis can distinguish active from inactive disease and monitor treatment response.
- Ga-67 citrate scintigraphy has been replaced by fluorine-18 fluorodeoxyglucose (F-18 FDG) imaging, where available, for the majority of indications.

## Suggested Readings

Abdel-Dayem HM, Bag R, DiFabrizio L, et al. Evaluation of sequential thallium and gallium scans of the chest in AIDS patients. J Nucl Med. 1996; 37(10):1662–1667

Basu S, Zhuang H, Torigian DA, Rosenbaum J, Chen W, Alavi A. Functional imaging of inflammatory diseases using nuclear medicine techniques. Semin Nucl Med. 2009; 39(2):124–145

Rosso J, Guillon JM, Parrot A, et al. Technetium-99 m-DTPA aerosol and gallium-67 scanning in pulmonary complications of human immunodeficiency virus infection. J Nucl Med. 1992; 33(1):81–87

Schuster DM, Alazraki N. Gallium and other agents in diseases of the lung. Semin Nucl Med. 2002; 32(3):193–211

# Case 111

*Ely A. Wolin*

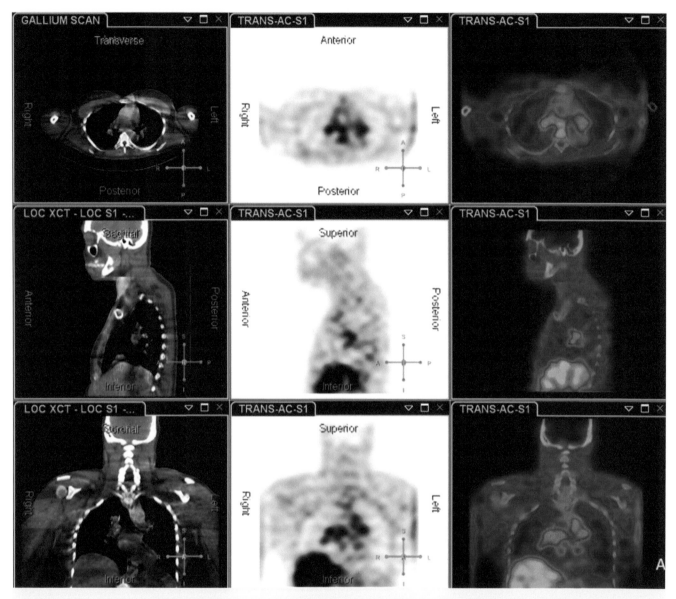

**Fig. 111.1** Axial, sagittal, and coronal CT, single-photon emission computed tomography (SPECT), and fused images from Gallium (Ga)-67 citrate scintigraphy show increased radiotracer uptake in bilateral hilar and mediastinal lymph nodes.

■ **Clinical History**

48-year-old female with presumed sarcoidosis (▶ Fig. 111.1).

■ Key Finding

Ga-67 citrate uptake in mediastinal and/or hilar lymph nodes

■ Top 3 Differential Diagnoses

- **Sarcoidosis.** While mostly replaced by fluorine-18 fluorode-oxyglucose positron-emission tomography (F-18 FDG PET)/CT, Ga-67 citrate scan remains a useful imaging modality for sarcoidosis. The scan can be used for confirmation of a diagnosis as well as to monitor therapy, as uptake is seen with active inflammation and not with chronic fibrosis or inactive granulomata. The "lambda" sign is a classic finding of sarcoidosis on Ga-67 citrate scintigraphy, so called due to the appearance of uptake within right paratracheal and bilateral hilar lymph nodes appearing to be in the shape of the Greek letter "λ." Grading of uptake is usually based on subjective comparison to global soft tissue and hepatic uptake.
- **Lymphoma.** Ga-67 citrate is a nonspecific tumor imaging agent, a characteristic making it useful for whole-body imaging in the evaluation of FUO. Uptake in mediastinal and hilar lymph nodes can therefore be seen with malignancy, most commonly lymphoma.
- **Infection.** Mediastinal and hilar adenopathy due to infection can show increased activity on Ga-67 citrate scintigraphy. Ga-67 citrate is most useful for difficult cases, but has proven value particularly with mycobacterial infections, including mycobacterial tuberculosis (TB). The main utility of Ga-67 citrate scintigraphy, in this regard, is the high sensitivity and negative predictive value, as uptake is not specific. Ga-67 citrate scan may also help distinguish between active TB and nontuberculous mycobacterial infection. Active TB is generally more inflammatory and rapidly progressive with correlative higher uptake of Ga-67 citrate.

■ Diagnosis

Sarcoidosis.

✓ Pearls

- The "lambda" sign from active right paratracheal and hilar nodes on Ga-67 citrate scan suggests sarcoidosis.
- Ga-67 citrate uptake is not specific, regardless of location, and seen with infection, inflammation, and malignancy.
- A negative Ga-67 citrate scan essentially excludes active *Mycobacterium tuberculosis* infection.
- Ga-67 citrate may help differentiate between tuberculous and nontuberculous mycobacterial infection.

Suggested Readings

Schuster DM, Alazraki N. Gallium and other agents in diseases of the lung. Semin Nucl Med. 2002; 32(3):193–211

Yeh JJ, Huang YC, Teng WB, Huang YF, Chuang YW, Hsu CC. The role of gallium-67 scintigraphy in comparing inflammatory activity between tuberculous and nontuberculous mycobacterial pulmonary diseases. Nucl Med Commun. 2011; 32(5):392–401

# Case 112

*Kamal D. Singh*

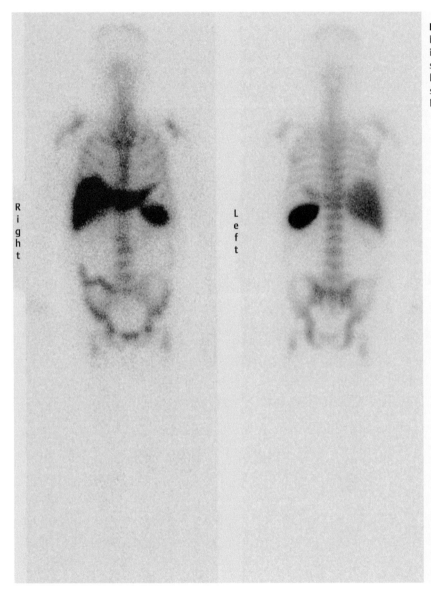

**Fig. 112.1** Whole-body indium-111-labeled white blood cells (In-111 WBC) scan 24 hours post injection in anterior and posterior projections demonstrates segmental tubular uptake within the anterior right lower quadrant of abdomen. Physiologic uptake is seen within the spleen greater than liver, as well as bone marrow.

■ **Clinical History**

39-year-old male with vague abdominal pain, fever, and elevated WBCs (▶ Fig. 112.1).

## ■ Key Finding

Focal bowel uptake on In-111-labeled WBC scan

## ■ Top 3 Differential Diagnoses

- **Infectious enteritis/colitis.** Indications for In-111-labeled WBC scan include detection and localization of abdominopelvic abscesses, acute osteomyelitis (including orthopedic hardware), infected vascular grafts, and work up for an FUO. Approximately 50 mL of blood is drawn from the patient and In-111 oxine is labeled to leukocytes (predominantly neutrophils). Imaging is generally performed starting 24 hours after injection. In-111-labeled WBCs localize to sites of infection by chemotaxis and increased vascular permeability. Donor WBCs (ABO matched) may be used in neutropenic patients with WBC < 2,000 cells/mL. Physiologic activity is seen within spleen, liver, and bone marrow. Early, transient, nonfocal pulmonary activity is physiologic and normally decreases over time. The lack of significant gastrointestinal (GI) uptake or hepatobiliary/renal excretion makes In-111-labeled WBCs preferable over gallium for abdominopelvic infectious processes, such as abscesses, enteritis/colitis, and appendicitis. There is lower sensitivity for detection of chronic nonpyogenic processes. False-positive studies may be secondary to an accessory spleen, or abdominal wall inflammation from surgical wounds, percutaneous tubes, or catheters.
- **Inflammatory bowel disease (IBD).** Segmental bowel activity may be seen in active IBD due to WBCs within sloughed mucosa at the site of inflammation. Localization and extent of active disease is best depicted on early imaging (1–6 hour post injection) before migration of activity distal to site of origin due to peristalsis. Tc-99m hexamethylpropyleneamine (HMPAO)-labeled WBCs are typically used in pediatric patients instead of indium to reduce radiation dose to the spleen. When Tc-99m HMPAO is used, early imaging (before 4 hours) is paramount to avoid interfering physiologic colonic activity.
- **Gastrointestinal bleed.** Active GI bleeding causes passage of WBCs (along with red blood cells [RBCs] and platelets) into the bowel lumen, resulting in activity which may simulate active intestinal infection or inflammation. Careful patient history and correlation with Tc-99m-labeled RBCs (more sensitive and specific for active GI bleeding) can aid in establishing the correct diagnosis. Acute hematomas can also accumulate labeled WBCs.

## ■ Additional Diagnostic Consideration

- **Swallowed activity from sinusitis/pharyngitis:** Focal infection from a more proximal source, such as sinusitis, pharyngitis, or esophagitis, may have mucosal shedding of WBCs, resulting in poorly localized transient bowel activity. This can also be seen in the setting of inflammation around indwelling endotracheal or nasogastric tubes.

## ■ Diagnosis

Inflammatory bowel disease (IBD; Crohn's disease).

## ✓ Pearls

- In-111-labeled WBC scan is more specific than bone scan and gallium scan for acute pyogenic infection.
- Sensitivity of the In-111 WBC scan is generally not affected by antibiotic therapy for acute infection.
- False-negative scans are seen in chronic nonpyogenic infections and vertebral osteomyelitis.
- False-positive scans are seen in operative wounds, GI bleeding, focal inflammation, and reactive marrow.

## Suggested Readings

Becker W, Meller J. The role of nuclear medicine in infection and inflammation. Lancet Infect Dis. 2001; 1(5):326–333

Hughes DK. Nuclear medicine and infection detection: the relative effectiveness of imaging with 111In-oxine-, 99 mTc-HMPAO-, and 99 mTc-stannous fluoride colloid-labeled leukocytes and with 67Ga-citrate. J Nucl Med Technol. 2003; 31(4):196–201, quiz 203–204

Navab F, Boyd CM. Clinical utility of In-111 leukocyte imaging in Crohn's disease. Clin Nucl Med. 1995; 20(12):1065–1069

renal transplant recipients, in identifying an localizing supsepcted infection? World J Nucl Med. 2015; 14(3):184–188

# Case 113

*Ely A. Wolin*

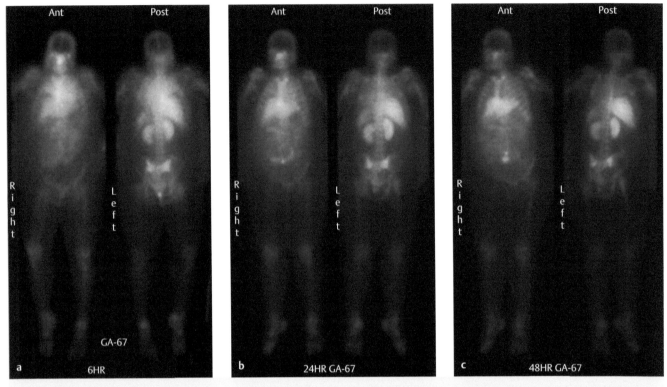

**Fig. 113.1** (a) 6-, (b) 24-, and (c) 48-hour anterior and posterior whole-body images from Gallium-67 (Ga-67) citrate scintigraphy show persistent bilateral renal activity.

## ■ Clinical History

▶ Fig. 113.1

## ■ Key Finding

Renal activity beyond 24 hours on Ga-67 citrate scintigraphy

## ■ Top 2 Differential Diagnoses

• **Renal disease.** Ga-67 citrate, originally designed as a bone imaging agent, was the first radiopharmaceutical used clinically for infection imaging. Ga-67 is produced by cyclotron, decays via electron capture emitting 93, 185, 300, and 394 keV gammas, and has a physical half-life of 78 hours. Ga-67 citrate circulates in the body bound to transferrin. Uptake in infectious and inflammatory processes is likely due in part to hyperemia and increased capillary permeability, along with binding to lactoferrin released from leukocytes and bacterial siderophores. Ga-67 citrate is also a nonspecific tumor imaging agent, making it useful in the evaluation of fever of unknown origin. Normal distribution shows greatest uptake in the liver, bone marrow and spleen. Lacrimal gland activity is often used as a discriminating factor to identify a Ga-67 citrate scan. Renal clearance is seen during the first 24 hours, but should not be seen after that, with subsequent excretion primarily through bowel. Visualization of renal activity beyond 24 hours is abnormal. This may signify renal disease, such as

infection, interstitial nephritis or abscess, but is not specific. Renal Ga-67 citrate activity on delayed image warrants further biochemical and imaging analysis to evaluate for the presence of renal disease.

• **Altered biodistribution.** Several things are known to cause an alteration in the biodistribution of Ga-67 citrate resulting frequently in increased renal activity on delayed images. This can be seen with iron overload (such as with multiple blood transfusions), chemotherapy/radiotherapy and gadolinium administration. Excess iron saturates transferring, preventing Ga-67 binding with resultant change in distribution. Chemotherapy/ granulocyte stimulating factors or whole body irradiation can result in marrow stimulation and altered serum binding. Altered biodistribution of Ga-67 citrate has been reported after the intravenous administration of gadolinium-base MRI contrast agents, possibly due to a carrier effect, but this has not been confirmed.

## ■ Diagnosis

Acute interstitial nephritis.

## ✓ Pearls

• Ga-67 citrate is cleared through the kidneys for the first 24 hours, then through the intestines.
• Renal activity on Ga-67 citrate scan beyond 24 hours is abnormal and requires investigation.

• Delayed renal Ga-67 citrate activity suggests renal disease, but can be seen with altered biodistribution.

## Suggested Readings

Graham F, Lord M, Froment D, Cardinal H, Bollée G. The use of gallium-67 scintigraphy in the diagnosis of acute interstitial nephritis. Clin Kidney J. 2016; 9(1):76–81

Nowosinska E, Navalkissoor S, Quigley AM, Buscombe JR. Is there a role for Gallium-67 citrate SPECT/CT, in patients with renal impairment or who are renal transplant recipients, in identifying an localizing suspected infection? World J Nucl Med. 2015; 14(3):184–188

# Part 10

## Fluorine-18 Fluorodeoxyglucose Positron-Emission Tomography

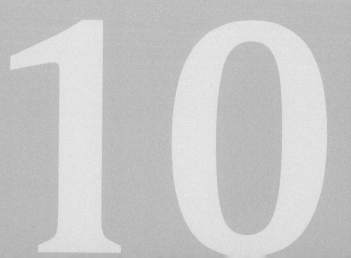

# Case 114

*Ely A. Wolin*

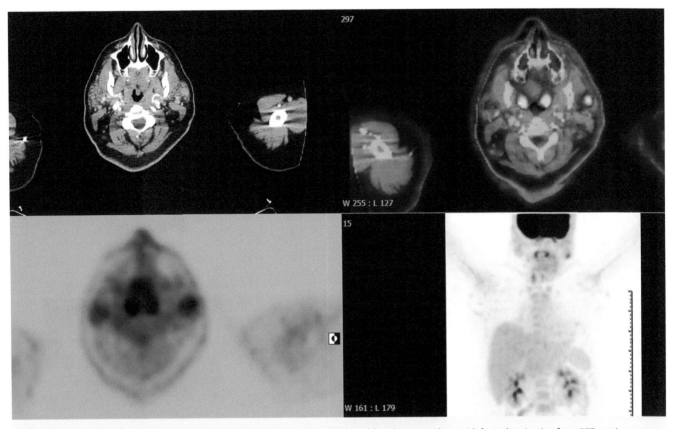

**Fig. 114.1** Axial CT, attenuation corrected positron emission tomography (PET), and fused images, along with frontal projection from PET maximum intensity projection, show focal increased fluorodeoxyglucose avidity associated with soft-tissue nodularity in the left parotid gland.

■ Clinical History

47-year-old female with marginal zone lymphoma of the left parotid gland (▶ Fig. 114.1).

## ■ Key Finding

Focal fluorine-18 fluorodeoxyglucose (F-18 FDG) uptake in the parotid gland

## ■ Top 2 Differential Diagnoses

- **Primary parotid neoplasm.** Physiologic activity on F-18 FDG positron emission tomography/computed tomography (PET/CT) can complicate interpretation of the head and neck. Physiologic uptake is commonly seen within the brain, extraocular muscles, soft and hard palate mucosa, Waldeyer's ring, neck, pharyngeal and laryngeal muscles, and thyroid. Uptake can also be seen in brown adipose tissue. Physiologic parotid uptake is variable, as F-18 FDG is taken up by the salivary glands and secreted in saliva, but it is typically diffuse and symmetric. Several benign entities can result in increased, asymmetric, salivary gland uptake, including sarcoidosis, infection, and radiation-induced sialadenitis. Any focal increased FDG avidity within the parotid requires scrutiny of the associated anatomic imaging, and often further evaluation with magnetic resonance imaging (MRI) and/or biopsy. Several benign and malignant primary parotid neoplasms

can show focal increased FDG avidity, including Warthin's tumor, pleomorphic adenoma, primary parotid lymphoma, mucoepidermoid, salivary duct, and adenoid cystic carcinomas. High-grade malignant parotid lesions tend to have higher uptake, but no statistically significant standardized uptake value (SUV) cutoff has been defined to differentiate. Some low-grade lesions, such as adenoid cystic carcinomas and low-grade mucoepidermoid carcinomas, may result in false-negative F-18 FDG PET/CT.

- **Metastatic disease.** Focal F-18 FDG uptake in the parotid gland may represent either a parotid parenchymal or intraparotid lymph node metastasis. While head and neck squamous cell carcinomas and melanoma are the most likely malignancies to metastasize to the parotid gland, parotid metastases have been also seen with lung, breast, renal, prostate, and gastrointestinal malignancies.

## ■ Diagnosis

Marginal zone lymphoma of the parotid gland.

## ✓ Pearls

- Focal parotid gland uptake on F-18 FDG PET/CT can be seen with benign and malignant lesions.
- High-grade primary parotid neoplasms typically show higher uptake values, but uptake is not diagnostic.

- Parotid mets can be from multiple malignancies, most commonly head and neck cancers and melanoma.
- Further evaluation of focal parotid uptake on PET is usually with MRI.

## Suggested Readings

Nakamoto Y, Tatsumi M, Hammoud D, Cohade C, Osman MM, Wahl RL. Normal FDG distribution patterns in the head and neck: PET/CT evaluation. Radiology. 2005; 234(3):879–885

Purohit BS, Ailianou A, Dulguerov N, Becker CD, Ratib O, Becker M. FDG-PET/CT pitfalls in oncological head and neck imaging. Insights Imaging. 2014; 5(5):585–602

Roh JL, Ryu CH, Choi SH, et al. Clinical utility of 18F-FDG PET for patients with salivary gland malignancies. J Nucl Med. 2007; 48(2):240–246

# Case 115

*Jonathan Muldermans*

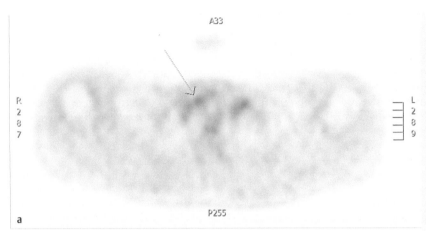

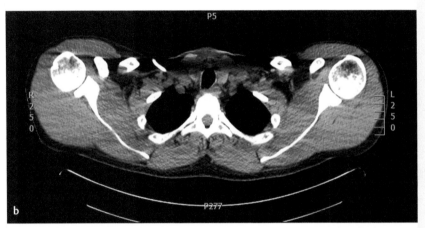

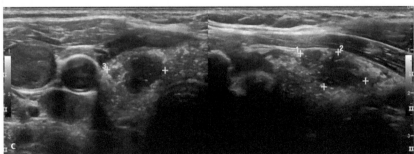

**Fig. 115.1** Axial positron emission tomography (PET) image **(a)** shows focal increased metabolic activity in the right lobe of the thyroid gland. CT acquired at the same time **(b)** shows no definite anatomic correlate, with evaluation limited by attenuation. Correlative transverse and longitudinal ultrasound images **(c)** of the right lobe of the thyroid gland show a heterogeneous, primarily hypoechoic lesion. Ultrasound-guided biopsy was subsequently performed.

## ■ Clinical History

46-year-old male with history of chronic lymphocytic leukemia (CLL) status post allogeneic hematopoietic stem cell transplant with new bilateral cervical lymphadenopathy (▶ Fig. 115.1).

## ■ Key Finding

F-18 FDG uptake in the thyroid

## ■ Top 3 Differential Diagnoses

- **Thyroiditis.** F-18 FDG is a radiolabeled glucose analogue that competes with glucose for intracellular transport via the GLUT 1 and 3 transporters. F-18 is cyclotron produced, has a physical half-life of 110 minutes, and undergoes positron emission resulting in two directly opposed 511-KeV gamma photons after an annihilation reaction. FDG is phosphorylated by hexokinase but does not undergo glycolysis. As the thyroid is not unique in its affinity for glucose, FDG is not an ideal radiotracer for dedicated thyroid imaging. However, thyroid uptake on FDG studies employed for other reasons is common. Diffusely increased uptake within the thyroid gland is nonspecific, but is most often seen in the setting of thyroiditis (approximately 80% of cases), including both Hashimoto's and subacute forms. Reactive lymphocytes and inflammatory cells uptake the FDG, with increased uptake present early in the disease which may be diffuse or patchy. The gland itself is usually normal in size. As the disease progresses, the thyroid gland becomes "burned out," and will demonstrate decreased or absent uptake.
- **Normal thyroid.** The thyroid gland normally has mild to moderate symmetric FDG uptake. One study reported that the average standardized uptake value (SUV) in the thyroid is $1.39 \pm 0.31$ for men, and $1.23 \pm 0.27$ for women. Alternatively, decreased or near absent FDG uptake within the thyroid could be a normal finding, but may also be seen in the setting of ectopic thyroid, after radioactive iodine ablation or post thyroidectomy. No thyroid uptake in a woman should prompt evaluation of the pelvis to exclude struma ovarii. Correlating the functional PET images with the anatomic CT images, in conjunction with lab analysis, should help narrow the differential.
- **Malignancy.** Interestingly, thyroid cancers often demonstrate an inverse relationship between radioiodine and FDG uptake; higher-grade/less well-differentiated tumors tend to have increased FDG and decreased radioiodine avidity. This is the reason F-18 FDG PET/CT is used for a thyroid cancer patient with new elevated thyroglobulin levels on follow up and a negative whole-body radioiodine scan. Focal FDG uptake within thyroid is malignant in about one out of five cases, and should be considered malignant until proven otherwise. Malignant nodules usually demonstrate uptake twice the background level. Ultrasound and biopsy are recommended in most cases. Thyroid lymphoma, alternatively, will show diffuse increased FDG uptake, usually significantly higher than seen with thyroiditis.

## ■ Additional Diagnostic Considerations

- **Grave's disease:** In this disease, the autonomously hyperfunctioning thyroid gland is responsible for the increased FDG uptake, as opposed to reactive lymphocytes and inflammatory cells in thyroiditis. The gland is generally enlarged and FDG avid throughout the disease course.
- **Multinodular goiter:** A multinodular goiter may demonstrate a variety of uptake patterns, from focal to patchy to symmetrically increased uptake, depending on the activity level of the individual nodules. Anatomic imaging is likely to demonstrate an enlarged, heterogeneous thyroid gland in this setting.

## ■ Diagnosis

Papillary thyroid carcinoma.

## ✓ Pearls

- A diffusely hyperactive thyroid gland on FDG PET/CT is more often thyroiditis than lymphoma.
- Focal FDG uptake within the thyroid should be considered malignant until proven otherwise.
- Thyroid cancers are often FDG avid but not iodine avid; well-differentiated tumors may be negative on FDG PET.

## Suggested Readings

Barrio M, Czernin J, Yeh MW, et al. The incidence of thyroid cancer in focal hypermetabolic thyroid lesions: an 18F-FDG PET/CT study in more than 6000 patients. Nucl Med Commun. 2016; 37(12):1290–1296

Blodgett TM, Fukui MB, Snyderman CH, et al. Combined PET-CT in the head and neck: part 1. Physiologic, altered physiologic, and artifactual FDG uptake. Radiographics. 2005; 25(4):897–912

Nakamoto Y, Tatsumi M, Hammoud D, Cohade C, Osman MM, Wahl RL. Normal FDG distribution patterns in the head and neck: PET/CT evaluation. Radiology. 2005; 234(3):879–885

# Case 116

*Kamal D. Singh*

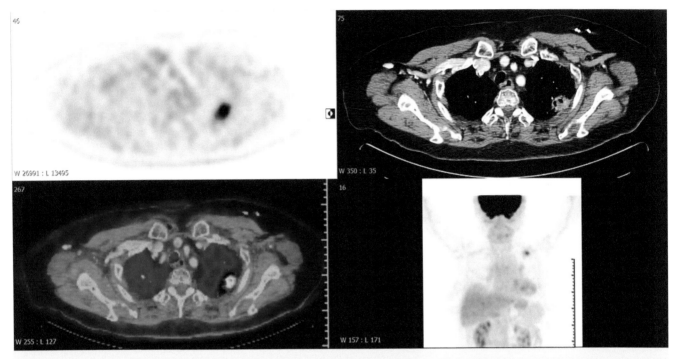

**Fig. 116.1** Positron emission tomography scan with fluorine-18 fluorodeoxyglucose demonstrates a hypermetabolic left upper lobe cavitary lesion.

## ■ Clinical History

84-year-old female with left upper lobe cavitary lesion (▶ Fig. 116.1).

■ **Key Finding**

Solitary hypermetabolic pulmonary lesion on PET scan

■ **Top 3 Differential Diagnoses**

• **Malignancy.** Standard PET imaging is performed from the skull base to proximal thighs 45 to 90 minutes after injection of around 10 to 15 mCi of F-18 FDG. Corresponding low-dose CT is performed for attenuation correction and anatomic localization. Malignant cells have increased metabolic activity and generally have upregulated glucose transporters along with downregulated glucose-6-phosphatase. Positron emission tomography/computed tomography (PET/CT) is indicated for detection and staging of malignancies, including posttherapy response. PET/CT has sensitivity of about 95% and specificity of about 80% for determining whether a solitary pulmonary nodule greater than 1 cm in size is benign or malignant. Negative findings on PET are less helpful in the setting of high pretest likelihood of malignancy. Standardized uptake value (SUV) is a semiquantitative index for tumor metabolism and a maximum SUV ($SUV_{max}$) of 2.5 is generally regarded as a cutoff for malignancy. However, any uptake within a pulmonary nodule is suspicious. False negatives may occur due to the partial volume effect in subcentimeter nodules and low-grade or well-differentiated malignancies.

• **Active granulomatous disease.** FDG uptake is nonspecific and can be seen within active nonneoplastic processes, including granulomatous diseases such as sarcoidosis, fungal infection, and tuberculosis. Increased glycolysis within activated macrophages is likely responsible for FDG uptake. SUV may be high (>2.5) within these benign lesions. A biopsy or close follow-up may be the next appropriate step for definitive diagnosis. Dual-time point imaging in some instances may improve accuracy since nonneoplastic lesions generally do not demonstrate increasing FDG accumulation on delayed scan.

• **Pulmonary infection/inflammation.** Increased activity is also seen within sites of active infection or inflammation, likely due to inflammatory cell metabolism and mediators. Focal pulmonary infection, abscesses, radiation pneumonitis, active fibrosis, and postsurgical changes can demonstrate high FDG uptake simulating malignancy. Correlation with the patient's history and corresponding anatomic imaging (i.e., CT scan) can aid in making appropriate diagnosis.

■ **Diagnosis**

Airway centered acute or chronic inflammation and fibrosis; no evidence of malignancy.

✓ **Pearls**

• Patient preparation prior to PET includes 4-hour fasting, no recent regular insulin, and serum glucose < 200 mg/dL.
• FDG uptake is nonspecific and is seen in the setting of neoplasm and active infection or inflammation.

• An SUV ≥ 2.5 is generally considered as the cutoff for malignancy, but is not reliable in small lesions.
• Bronchoalveolar carcinoma (BAC) or mucinous metastases to the lung may be falsely negative on PET scan.

**Suggested Readings**

Bunyaviroch T, Coleman RE. PET evaluation of lung cancer. J Nucl Med. 2006; 47(3):451–469

Choromańska A, Macura KJ. Evaluation of solitary pulmonary nodule detected during computed tomography examination. Pol J Radiol. 2012; 77(2):22–34

Truong MT, Ko JP, Rossi SE, et al. Update in the evaluation of the solitary pulmonary nodule. Radiographics. 2014; 34(6):1658–1679

# Case 117

*Ely A. Wolin*

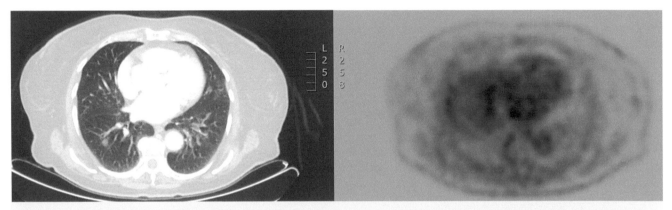

**Fig. 117.1** Representative axial images from simultaneously acquired F-18 fluorodeoxyglucose (FDG) positron emission tomography/computed tomography (PET/CT) show a right lower lobe subsolid nodule without associated increased FDG avidity. CT-guided biopsy was subsequently performed.

## ■ Clinical History

79-year-old female with right lower lobe enlarging ground glass nodule on chest CT (▶ Fig. 117.1).

## ■ Key Finding

Solitary hypometabolic pulmonary lesion on PET scan

## ■ Top 3 Differential Diagnoses

- **Granuloma.** PET/CT is a useful tool for the evaluation of solitary pulmonary nodules. The main advantage of PET/CT is the negative predictive value (NPV), meaning a lesion without uptake is unlikely to be malignant (NPV around 97%). Using PET/CT for evaluation can thus prevent some unnecessary biopsies of benign lesions. Pulmonary granulomas are frequently encountered lesions. While characteristic calcifications (central, diffuse, or laminated) are frequently seen allowing for accurate morphologic diagnosis, calcifications are not always present. An active granuloma will still have F-18 FDG uptake and may be a false positive. When present, the uptake should usually be less than a 2.5 standardized uptake value $(SUV)_{max}$

- (and less than the mediastinal blood pool), but further evaluation would still be required to exclude malignancy.
- **Adenocarcinoma in situ (AIS).** Formerly known as bronchoalveolar carcinoma (BAC). These well-differentiated tumors are known to be hypometabolic on F-18 FDG PET/CT. Around half of these will not demonstrate increased FDG uptake, particularly the mucinous variety.
- **Carcinoid.** These low-grade malignancies account for a very small portion of lung neoplasms, around 1 to 2%. The majority of these occur within central bronchi. They do have the ability to invade and metastasize, but are generally slow growing with low metabolic rates.

## ■ Additional Considerations

- **Hamartoma:** Imaging features are often characteristic, including popcorn chondroid calcifications and intranodular fat.
- **Small bronchogenic carcinoma:** Spatial resolution for PET is around 7 to 8 mm. For this reason, small metabolically active lesions may appear photopenic secondary to volume averaging.

- **Metastasis:** A solitary lesion makes metastatic disease less likely, although it is still possible. Metastases from some primary malignancies, such as renal cell carcinoma and mucinous neoplasms, are often hypometabolic.

## ■ Diagnosis

Invasive adenocarcinoma.

## ✓ Pearls

- Size and morphologic features must be evaluated before confidently calling a non-FDG avid nodule benign.
- Carcinoma in situ and carcinoid are two known malignancies which are frequently cold on F-18 FDG PET.

- Mucinous neoplasms often demonstrate less uptake on F-18 FDG PET due to the low cellularity.
- A granuloma can be hypermetabolic.

## Suggested Readings

Bunyaviroch T, Coleman RE. PET evaluation of lung cancer. J Nucl Med. 2006; 47(3):451–469

Sim YT, Poon FW. Imaging of solitary pulmonary nodule-a clinical review. Quant Imaging Med Surg. 2013; 3(6):316–326

Truong MT, Ko JP, Rossi SE, et al. Update in the evaluation of the solitary pulmonary nodule. Radiographics. 2014; 34(6):1658–1679

# Case 118

*Jonathan Muldermans*

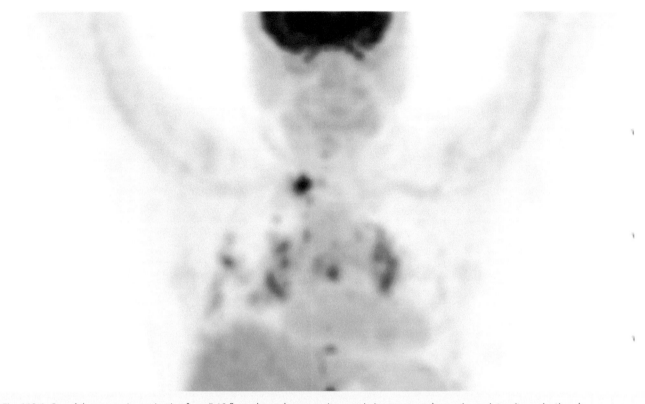

**Fig. 118.1** Coned down anterior projection from F-18 fluorodeoxyglucose positron emission tomography maximum intensity projection shows hypermetabolic bilateral pulmonary nodules, mediastinal, and hilar lymph nodes. Mediastinal adenopathy was biopsied.

■ **Clinical History**

63-year-old female with pulmonary nodules (▶ Fig. 118.1).

## ■ Key Finding

Hypermetabolic mediastinal adenopathy

## ■ Top 3 Differential Diagnoses

- **Metastatic disease.** Size criteria for CT evaluation of the mediastinal lymph nodes are not sensitive as metastatic nodes may not be enlarged. F-18 FDG positron emission tomography/computed tomography (PET/CT) provides the ability to identify hypermetabolic nodes, particularly important in staging lung cancers. Increased mediastinal nodal uptake compared to mediastinal blood pool, or increased compared to normal nodes, should be regarded as suspicious. It is important to remember that small lymph nodes may produce a partial-volume effect, with 7 to 8 mm generally considered the size threshold for PET resolution. Low-grade and well-differentiated malignancies may by hypometabolic, and thus may be missed on FDG PET studies. For posttreatment scans, waiting 1 to 2 weeks after the last cycle of chemotherapy is advised to avoid transient fluctuations in tumor metabolism that can decrease diagnostic accuracy.
- **Lymphoma.** FDG avidity in lymphoma tends to correspond to tumor grade. Comparing nodal FDG avidity to mediastinal blood pool and liver background activity is the basis for the Deauville Criteria, an international scale for staging and restaging of Hodgkin's disease (HD) and certain types of non-Hodgkin's lymphomas (NHL). Low-grade lesions, such as gastrointestinal mucosa-associated lymphoid tissue (MALT) lymphoma, may produce false negatives. PET imaging has improved sensitivity and specificity over CT and Gallium (Ga)-67 citrate scan for detecting nodal disease. NHL is much more common than HD overall, but HD is more likely to involve the thoracic cavity. About 98% of cases of HD involve the superior mediastinal nodes, and if these nodes are spared HD should be lower on the differential. While it is the histopathologic classification of NHL that determines prognosis, anatomic extent of disease is prognostic in HD.
- **Granulomatous disease.** Increased FDG uptake is also seen in active granulomatous disease, including sarcoidosis, tuberculosis, or fungal infection. The reactive macrophages are the hypermetabolic cells. The distribution of uptake may suggest a diagnosis, such as bilateral hilar and right paratracheal nodes in sarcoidosis (equivalent to the "Lambda" or "1–2–3" signs). Uptake values may be similar to malignant nodes often requiring short-term follow up or biopsy. Dual-time point imaging may improve diagnostic accuracy as nonmalignant uptake should decrease on delayed images.

## ■ Additional Diagnostic Considerations

- **Reactive adenopathy:** Lymph nodes appropriately responding to active infection/inflammation may be hypermetabolic. This is also seen in the postsurgical/therapy setting, during active pulmonary fibrosis and secondary to radiation pneumonitis.
- **Sarcoid-like reaction:** Some patients with underlying malignancies and no signs or symptoms of systemic sarcoidosis will develop noncaseating granulomas in the tumor itself, in lymph nodes draining the tumor(s), and even in nonregional tissues.

## ■ Diagnosis

Sarcoidosis.

## ✓ Pearls

- The Deauville Criteria are used in HD and certain types of NHL for staging and restaging purposes.
- In the setting of suspected lymphoma, hypermetabolic superior mediastinal lymph nodes are suspicious for HD.
- Metabolic information from lymph nodes smaller than around 8 mm is not reliable due to partial volume effect.

## Suggested Readings

Barrington SF, Mikhaeel NG, Kostakoglu L, et al. Role of imaging in the staging and response assessment of lymphoma: consensus of the International Conference on Malignant Lymphomas Imaging Working Group. J Clin Oncol. 2014; 32(27):3048–3058

Craun JB, Banks KP, Clemenshaw MN, Moren RW. Sarcoidlike reaction of neoplasia causing hypermetabolic thoracic adenopathy in setting of extrathoracic malignancy: report of two cases and a review of the differential diagnostic considerations. J Nucl Med Technol. 2012; 40(4):231–235

Schmidt-Hansen M, Baldwin DR, Hasler E, Zamora J, Abraira V, Roqué I Figuls M. PET-CT for assessing mediastinal lymph node involvement in patients with suspected resectable non-small cell lung cancer. Cochrane Database Syst Rev. 2014; 13(11):CD009519

# Case 119

*Ely A. Wolin*

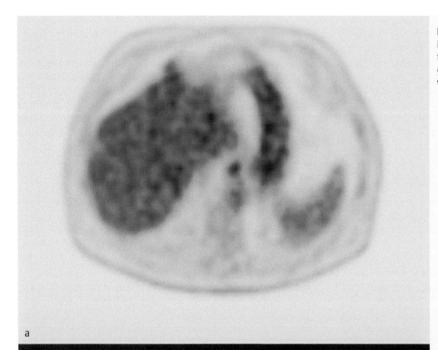

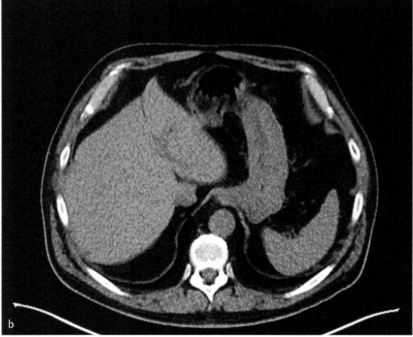

**Fig. 119.1** (a) Axial positron emission tomography image shows moderate heterogeneous increased fluorodeoxyglucose avidity associated with the gastric wall. (b) Correlative CT image shows gastric wall thickening.

■ Clinical History

66-year-old male with pulmonary nodules referred for positron emission tomography/computed tomography (PET/CT) prior to biopsy (▶ Fig. 119.1).

■ Key Finding

Gastric uptake on F-18 FDG PET/CT

■ Top 3 Differential Diagnoses

- **Gastritis.** Physiologic gastric uptake of F-18 FDG is likely secondary to smooth muscle activity, metabolically active mucosa, or swallowed secretions. Physiologic activity is typically low level. While quantitative data has limited accuracy due to multiple variables which contribute to the amount of FDG uptake at any given time, physiologic activity has been shown, by some studies, to generally have an standardized uptake value $(SUV)_{max}$ of less than 4. Gastritis may present with diffuse increased uptake, possibly with associated wall thickening. While this appearance is suggestive of an infectious or inflammatory gastritis, it is difficult to differentiate from an infiltrative gastric neoplasm.
- **Gastric neoplasm.** Any focal increased FDG avidity in the stomach raises concern for a gastric neoplasm, such as adenocarcinoma or a gastrointestinal stromal tumor (GIST). Gastric cancer is very common worldwide, although less common in Western countries. Interestingly, in the West gastric cancer is typically seen in the lesser curvature, gastric cardia, or near the gastroesophageal junction, as opposed to the more common distal distribution seen in Eastern countries. While complete surgical resection is really the only chance of cure, the surgery has high morbidity requiring accurate staging prior to therapy planning. GIST tumors are almost always hot on F-18 FGT PET/CT; however, gastric cancer uptake will vary

based on histology. Mucinous, signet ring cell, and poorly differentiated adenocarcinoma tend to have less uptake. PET is not helpful in terms of staging the primary tumor itself, as the ability to delineate invasion into the muscularis mucosa, muscularis propria, subserosal tissue, or beyond, is limited by volume averaging. However, PET is very helpful for identification of distant metastases, including para-aortic lymph nodes, possibly preventing an unnecessarily risky surgery. PET may also help with prognosis as decreased uptake after initiation of chemotherapy has been shown to predict responders.
- **Lymphoma.** The stomach is the most common site for extranodal lymphoma. Gastric lymphoma is usually either low-grade mucosa-associated lymphoid tissue (MALT) lymphoma or diffuse large B-cell lymphoma. F-18 FDG PET has nearly 100% sensitivity for diffuse large B-cell lymphoma, beneficial even over endoscopy as submucosal disease can be missed with direct visualization. The addition of F-18 FDG PET/CT in the workup of gastric lymphoma has been shown to accurately both upstage or downstage a decent percent of cases. In terms of lymphoma, higher FDG avidity tends to correspond to more advanced disease. The FDG avidity also is not reliant on wall thickening, versus nonlymphomatous gastric cancers which show a more linear relationship between maximum wall thickness and $SUV_{max}$.

■ Diagnosis

Presumed gastritis.

✓ Pearls

- Diffuse gastric wall FDG avidity suggests infectious or inflammatory gastritis, but is not diagnostic.
- Infiltrative neoplasm can be difficult to differentiate from gastritis on imaging requiring endoscopy.

- F18-FDG PET/CT has near 100% sensitivity for diffuse large B-cell lymphoma of the stomach.

Suggested Readings

Hopkins S, Yang GY. FDG PET imaging in the staging and management of gastric cancer. J Gastrointest Oncol. 2011; 2(1):39–44

Salaun PY, Grewal RK, Dodamane I, Yeung HW, Larson SM, Strauss HW. An analysis of the 18F-FDG uptake pattern in the stomach. J Nucl Med. 2005; 46(1):48–51

Wu J, Zhu H, Li K, Wang XG, Gui Y, Lu GM. 18F-fluorodeoxyglucose positron emission tomography/computed tomography findings of gastric lymphoma: Comparisons with gastric cancer. Oncol Lett. 2014; 8(4):1757–1764

# Case 120

*Ely A. Wolin*

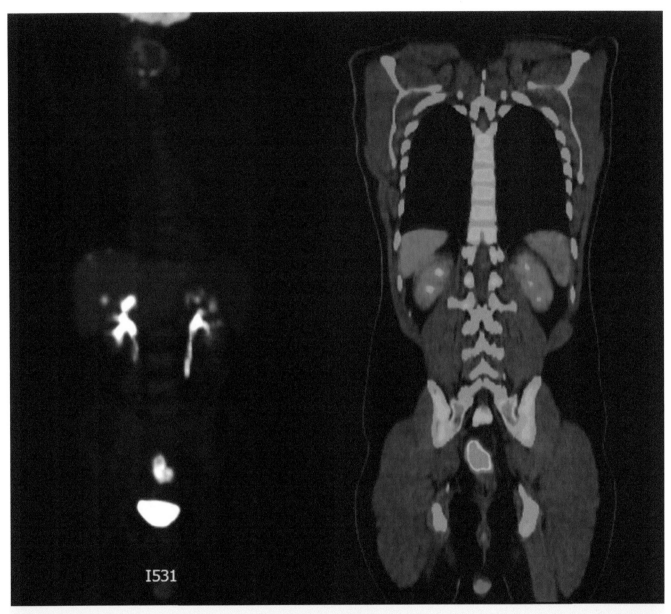

**Fig. 120.1** Positron emission tomography (PET) maximum intensity projection (MIP) and fused coronal images from F-18 fluorodeoxyglucose (FDG) PET/CT show focal hypermetabolism in the rectum. Small foci of increased FDG uptake are also noted in the liver (on MIP) consistent with metastatic disease.

## ■ Clinical History

33-year-old male with new diagnosis of rectal cancer (▶Fig. 120.1).

■ Key Finding

Intestinal uptake on F-18 FDG PET/CT

■ Top 3 Differential Diagnoses

- **Physiologic.** As with the stomach, physiologic small and large bowel FDG uptake is likely in part due to smooth muscle, metabolically active mucosa, and swallowed secretions. However, there also may be contribution from microbial uptake. Normal uptake has significant variability, limiting accuracy. There is often increased activity in the region of the cecum, possibly secondary to a high concentration of lymphocytes.
- **Infection/inflammation.** Infectious or inflammatory enteritis or colitis will result in increased uptake of F-18 FDG. Typically, the uptake will be segmental. Inflammatory changes such as wall thickening and fat stranding may be evident on corresponding CT. F-18 FDG PET is very sensitive for active bowel inflammation, and may have a role for noninvasive monitoring of patients with inflammatory bowel disease.
- **Malignancy.** Focal increased uptake in either the small bowel or colon raises concern for malignancy, particularly if associated with focal mural thickening. FDG PET has very high sensitivity for colorectal cancer, but specificity is limited. Findings on anatomic imaging can help delineate some of the nonneoplastic causes of focal increased FDG avidity, such as appendicitis and diverticulitis. However, in the absence of explanatory imaging and clinical findings, any focal areas of increased activity within bowel should be further evaluated with endoscopy, if possible. Small bowel neoplasms can be difficult to diagnose and often present at a more advanced stage due to absence of symptoms. PET/CT can be helpful in the diagnosis, staging, and follow up of small bowel neoplasms, including adenocarcinoma, lymphoma, and sarcoma. Metastatic involvement of the small bowel is seen as often as primary small bowel neoplasia, with involvement via direct extension from gastric, colonic, uterine and ovarian tumors, and via hematogenous spread of melanoma, and lung and breast tumors.

■ Additional Diagnostic Consideration

- **Metformin:** Diabetic patients who use the antihyperglycemic drug metformin for maintenance can show intense, diffuse, increased uptake of F-18 FDG in bowel. This uptake may mask neoplastic activity, or mimic an inflammatory or infectious process. Consideration should be given to discontinuing metformin for 48 hours prior to PET/CT, if the patient can tolerate.

■ Diagnosis

Rectal cancer.

✓ Pearls

- Physiologic intestinal uptake of F-18 FDG is highly variable, but usually heterogenous and mild.
- Focal increased FDG uptake in bowel raises concern for malignancy and should be further evaluated.
- Infectious or inflammatory intestinal FDG uptake is usually segmental in distribution.
- Diabetic patients taking metformin can show intense increased large and small bowel FDG uptake.

Suggested Readings

Bybel B, Greenberg ID, Paterson J, Ducharme J, Leslie WD. Increased F-18 FDG intestinal uptake in diabetic patients on metformin: a matched case-control analysis. Clin Nucl Med. 2011; 36(6):452–456

Cronin CG, Scott J, Kambadakone A, et al. Utility of positron emission tomography/CT in the evaluation of small bowel pathology. Br J Radiol. 2012; 85(1017):1211–1221

Prabhakar HB, Sahani DV, Fischman AJ, Mueller PR, Blake MA. Bowel hot spots at PET-CT. Radiographics. 2007; 27(1):145–159

# Case 121

*Ely A. Wolin*

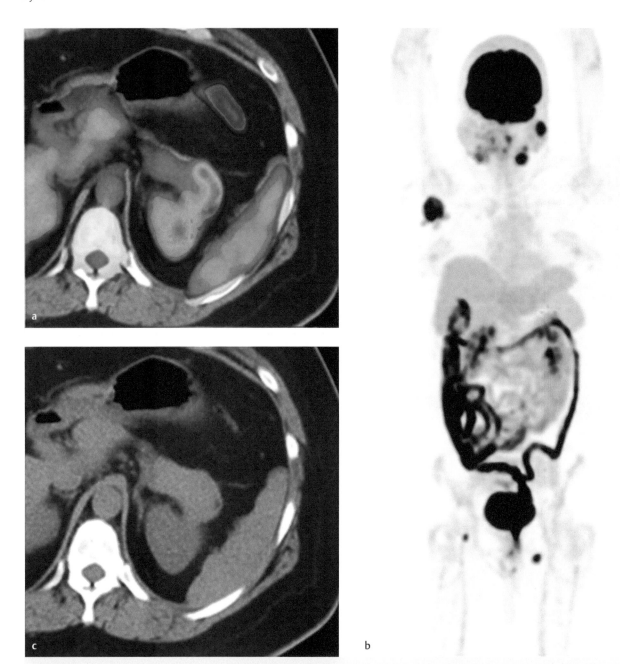

**Fig. 121.1** Axial fused positron emission tomography/computed tomography (PET/CT) and CT images from F-18 fluorodeoxyglucose (FDG) PET/CT show abnormal increased FDG avidity in an area of mass-like enlargement of the pancreatic tail. Maximum intensity projection image shows additional abnormal areas of radiotracer uptake in the salivary glands, right axilla, and bilateral inguinal region.

### ■ Clinical History

38-year-old female with IgG4 related disease (▶Fig. 121.1).

## ■ Key Finding

Increased F-18 FDG uptake in the pancreas

## ■ Top 3 Differential Diagnoses

• **Pancreatic malignancy.** FDG PET/CT can be useful for evaluation of pancreatic masses, especially in the setting of indeterminate imaging characteristics or a nondiagnostic biopsy. Pancreatic adenocarcinoma will usually appear as a focal area of increased metabolic activity within the pancreas. Level of FDG uptake within the mass is determined by tumor biology and the amount of desmoplastic response, meaning some pancreatic adenocarcinomas will have low level uptake. Despite this, some studies have shown the sensitivity of PET/CT for pancreatic adenocarcinoma to approach 100%, even for small lesions. As is true with other malignancies, one of the main benefits of F-18 FDG PET in pancreatic adenocarcinoma is more accurate staging through identification of metastatic disease which could help direct management and prevent patients from unnecessarily undergoing surgery with high morbidity rates. In terms of cystic neoplasms, FDG PET may provide some help differentiating between benign and malignant lesions; however, PET-negative lesions may be benign, borderline, or malignant. Invasive lesions are almost always FDG positive.

• **Pancreatitis.** Pancreatitis can result in increased FDG avidity mimicking malignancy, particularly in the case of mass-forming pancreatitis. In general, malignancy shows higher rates of avidity, but there is some overlap. F-18 FDG PET may be helpful in determining the cause of pancreatitis, if unclear. Around one-third of patients with autoimmune pancreatitis (AIP) will show FDG avidity in other organs such as the salivary/lacrimal glands and lymph nodes. This can be particularly helpful in cases of AIP that manifest as a focal pancreatic mass. PET/CT can also be used to assess response to therapy for AIP.

• **Lymphoma.** Primary pancreatic lymphoma is rare. Hypermetabolism may involve the entire pancreas or be seen at various levels within multiple foci throughout the gland.

## ■ Additional Diagnostic Considerations

• **Neuroendocrine tumor:** These make up a very small percentage of pancreatic neoplasms. They can be functioning, with insulinoma and gastrinoma being the most common, or nonfunctioning. Nonfunctioning tumors are often diagnosed later due to the lack of clinical symptoms. Well-differentiated tumors often demonstrate little to no FDG uptake. Poorly differentiated tumors are more likely to uptake FDG and may be falsely negative on indium-111 (In-111) pentetreotide imaging due to decreased somatostatin receptor expression.

• **Metastatic disease:** Pancreatic metastases can be seen with lung, breast, gastric, renal, colorectal, and ovarian primaries, as well as with melanoma. Lesions are usually not solitary.

## ■ Diagnosis

Autoimmune pancreatitis/IgG4 related disease.

## ✓ Pearls

• Focal increased FDG avidity in the pancreas is concerning for malignancy.
• FDG uptake will often be seen in additional organ systems in the setting of AIP.

• Poorly differentiated pancreatic neuroendocrine tumors may be more evident on PET than octreoscan.

## Suggested Readings

Dong A, Dong H, Zhang L, Zuo C. Hypermetabolic lesions of the pancreas on FDG PET/CT. Clin Nucl Med. 2013; 38(9):e354–e366

Sahani DV, Bonaffini PA, Catalano OA, Guimaraes AR, Blake MA. State-of-the-art PET/CT of the pancreas: current role and emerging indications. Radiographics. 2012; 32(4):1133–1158, discussion 1158–1160

Santhosh S, Mittal BR, Rana SS, et al. Metabolic signatures of malignant and non-malignant mass-forming lesions in the periampulla and pancreas in FDG PET/CT scan: an atlas with pathologic correlation. Abdom Imaging. 2015; 40(5):1285–1315

# Case 122

*Ely A. Wolin*

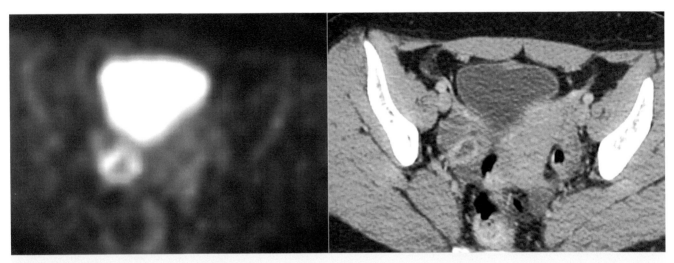

**Fig. 122.1** Axial positron emission tomography (PET) and CT images show circumferential increased fluorodeoxyglucose avidity associated with a cystic right ovarian lesion.

■ **Clinical History**

27-year-old female with history of non-Hodgkin's lymphoma (NHL) referred for PET/CT due to a mediastinal mass on CT (▶Fig. 122.1).

## ■ Key Finding

Ovarian uptake on F-18 FDG PET/CT

## ■ Top 3 Differential Diagnoses

- **Physiologic.** Physiologic ovarian uptake of F-18 FDG occurs in premenopausal women only. It is usually seen during the late follicular to early luteal phase of the menstrual cycle. The uptake may be secondary to increased metabolic demand associated with dominant follicle growth and corpus luteum formation. There is also likely an inflammatory reaction associated with ovulation, with uptake due to induced macrophages.
- **Primary ovarian neoplasm.** The majority of malignant ovarian tumors are epithelial tumors and occur in postmenopausal patients. Most malignant ovarian neoplasms will show increased FDG avidity. A standardized uptake value $(SUV)_{max}$ of 2.9 or greater has been shown by some studies to have good positive predictive value and negative predictive value (NPV) for detecting malignancy, although clear cell and mucinous adenocarcinoma may show less uptake. Differentiating between benign and borderline malignant neoplasms based on FDG avidity is not possible. PET/CT is useful for staging and assessing response to therapy for primary ovarian lymphoma, which is rare. Ovarian cancer is unfortunately often diagnosed at advanced stage as there are no specific symptoms or effective screening tests. PET/CT may play a role in screening and diagnosis as it has high sensitivity and specificity for malignancy in the setting of elevated cancer antigen 125 (CA 125) and an ovarian mass on ultrasound. However, the role of PET has not been clearly delineated. Ovarian cancer will usually metastasize to the peritoneum, less frequently through hematogenous or lymphatic spread.
- **Metastatic disease.** Uptake in ovarian metastases is based on histology, but metastases often show less FDG avidity than primary ovarian malignancy. Ovarian metastases can be seen with gastrointestinal, breast, lung, and endometrial primaries, as well as with melanoma, lymphoma, and other neoplasms.

## ■ Additional Diagnostic Considerations

- **Torsion:** Vascular congestion and hemorrhage from ovarian torsion can result in increased focal F-18 FDG activity on PET/CT. This can be confused for an ovarian neoplasm, especially if painless.
- **Tubo-ovarian abscess:** The nonspecific nature of F-18 FDG PET imaging is always a limitation; Infectious uptake can mimic malignancy. Abscesses usually show peripherally increased activity with central hypometabolism, but activity can also be more homogeneous.

## ■ Diagnosis

Physiologic uptake in a corpus luteal cyst.

## ✓ Pearls

- Ovarian F-18 FDG uptake in a postmenopausal woman is always abnormal and requires evaluation.
- An $SUV_{max}$ over 2.9 is a good cutoff for ovarian malignancy but can miss borderline lesions.
- Ovarian torsion can demonstrate increased uptake on PET/CT, often confused for tumor if painless.

## Suggested Readings

Nishizawa S, Inubushi M, Okada H. Physiological 18F-FDG uptake in the ovaries and uterus of healthy female volunteers. Eur J Nucl Med Mol Imaging. 2005; 32(5):549–556

Tanizaki Y, Kobayashi A, Shiro M, et al. Diagnostic value of preoperative SUV$_{max}$ on FDG-PET/CT for the detection of ovarian cancer. Int J Gynecol Cancer. 2014; 24(3):454–460

Fenchel S, Grab D, Nuessle K, et al. Asymptomatic adnexal masses: correlation of FDG PET and histopathologic findings. Radiology. 2002; 223(3):780–788

Rakheja R, Makis W, Hickeson M. Bilateral tubo-ovarian abscess mimics ovarian cancer on MRI and 18F-FDG PET/CT. Nucl Med Mol Imaging. 2011; 45(3):223–228

# Case 123

*Ely A. Wolin*

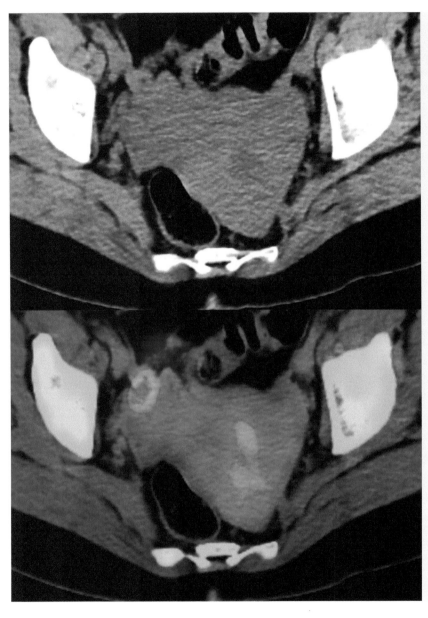

**Fig. 123.1** Axial CT and fused positron emission tomography/computed tomography (PET/CT) images show mild fluorodeoxyglucose avidity associated with fluid density within the endometrial canal.

■ **Clinical History**

44-year-old female with breast cancer post surgery and chemotherapy referred for PET/CT for evaluation of a pulmonary nodule (▶ Fig. 123.1).

## ▪ Key Finding

Uterine uptake on F-18 FDG PET/CT

## ▪ Top 3 Differential Diagnoses

- **Physiologic.** Physiologic F-18 FDG uptake can be seen in premenopausal women. Intense endometrial uptake is usually seen during the first 3 days of the menstrual cycle, thought to be secondary to either bleeding in degenerating endometrium or subendometrial myometrium peristalsis. Less intense uptake may also be seen around the ovulatory phase of the menstrual cycle. No physiologic activity is seen in postmenopausal women, even when on hormone therapy.
- **Primary neoplasm.** Benign uterine lesions, including leiomyoma, adenomyosis, and endometrial hyperplasia, can show mild uptake. Uptake in fibroids is more common in premenopausal women and varies throughout the menstrual cycle, rarely higher than the liver. Leiomyosarcomas generally show higher uptake than leiomyomas, but there is no accurate cutoff value for differentiation, particularly since degenerating fibroids may also show higher uptake. PET/CT has good sensitivity for endometrial cancer, which generally shows intense uptake, but it is not advantageous over MRI or transvaginal ultrasound for tumor staging. PET/CT may be advantageous for nodal staging, but its role is not clear. Studies have shown standardized uptake value $(SUV)_{max}$ to be an independent predictor of both disease free and overall survival. Cervical cancer will also generally show intense F-18 FDG avidity. Uptake in cervical cancer has no correlation with International Federation of Gynecology and Obstetrics (FIGO) staging, but higher uptake does appear to be associated with higher risk of nodal metastatic disease.
- **Metastatic disease**: Uterine metastases can arise from direct extension from nearby primaries, such as bladder, rectum, cervix, ovary, and fallopian tubes; or from lymphatic or hematogenous spread from extrapelvic malignancies, most commonly from breast, gastrointestinal, kidney, lung, or melanoma primaries.

## ▪ Additional Diagnostic Consideration

- **Infection:** While there is limited literature available discussing F-18 FDG PET/CT findings in pelvic inflammatory disease, it is reasonable to expect increased activity. Pelvic actinomycosis, a rare complication of intrauterine devices, can be very difficult to differentiate from malignancy as it can appear as a hypermetabolic invasive mass.

## ▪ Diagnosis

Physiologic endometrial uptake.

## ✓ Pearls

- Physiologic uterine FDG uptake occurs in premenopausal women mostly in the first 3 days of the cycle.
- Leiomyosarcoma will generally show higher uptake than leiomyoma, but there is no definitive cutoff.
- Pelvic actinomycosis can mimic malignancy on both anatomic and metabolic imaging.

## Suggested Readings

Kitajima K, Murakami K, Kaji Y, Sugimura K. Spectrum of FDG PET/CT findings of uterine tumors. AJR Am J Roentgenol. 2010; 195(3):737–743

Musto A, Grassetto G, Marzola MC, et al. Role of 18F-FDG PET/CT in the carcinoma of the uterus: a review of literature. Yonsei Med J. 2014; 55(6):1467–1472

Nishizawa S, Inubushi M, Okada H. Physiological 18F-FDG uptake in the ovaries and uterus of healthy female volunteers. Eur J Nucl Med Mol Imaging. 2005; 32(5):549–556

Vriens D, de Geus-Oei LF, Flucke UE, et al. Benign uterine uptake of FDG: a case report and review of literature. Neth J Med. 2010; 68(9):379–380

# Case 124

*Ely A. Wolin*

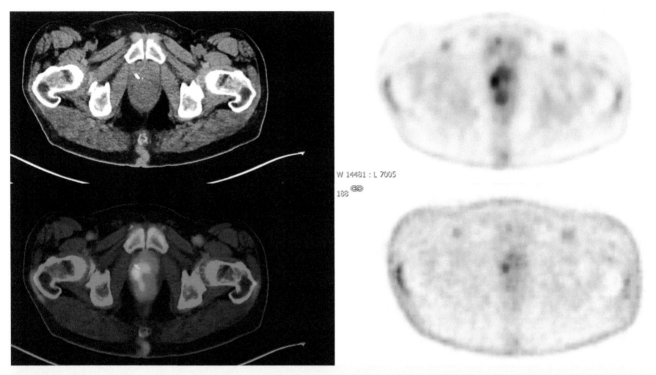

**Fig. 124.1** Axial CT, fused, attenuation corrected and non-attenuation corrected images from F-18 fluorodeoxyglucose positron emission tomography/computed tomography (PET/CT) show focal increased metabolic activity in the right posterolateral peripheral aspect of the prostate gland adjacent to coarse calcifications. The focal increased activity is also present on the non-attenuation corrected imaging excluding attenuation correction artifact.

W 14481 : L 7005
188

■ Clinical History

64-year-old male referred for follow up PET/CT for stage IV non-small-cell lung carcinoma on immunotherapy (▶ Fig. 124.1).

## ■ Key Finding

Increased prostate uptake on F-18 FDG PET/CT

## ■ Top 3 Differential Diagnoses

- **Prostate neoplasm.** The prostate gland normally exhibits very mild F-18 FDG uptake on PET/CT. Any increased uptake of the prostate raises suspicion for malignancy. Prostate adenocarcinoma represents the vast majority of primary prostate malignancies and shows variable, but often low, FDG avidity. This is likely due to the fact that well-differentiated prostate carcinoma uses less glucose than most other tumors. Increased FDG avidity often correlates with poorly differentiated neoplasms and high serum prostate-specific antigen (PSA) levels. Other prostate neoplasms can also demonstrate increased FDG avidity, including small cell, urothelial, squamous cell, and basal cell carcinoma, sarcoma (leiomyosarcoma and rhabdomyosarcoma), gastrointestinal stromal tumor (GIST), and lymphoma (most often diffuse large B-cell lymphoma). While focal increased FDG avidity in the peripheral zone is more concerning for malignancy, there is no accurate standardized uptake value (SUV) cutoff or uptake morphology for differentiating benign from malignant uptake. For this reason, any increased uptake in the prostate on PET/CT should likely lead to further evaluation with PSA levels and possible urology consultation for biopsy.

- **Benign prostatic hypertrophy.** The nodular fibromuscular and epithelial hyperplasia associated with benign prostatic hypertrophy (BPH) occurs within the transitional zone and periureteral area, versus the peripheral zone for prostate carcinoma. BPH can result in increased F-18 FDG uptake in the prostate.

- **Prostatitis.** Acute bacterial, chronic bacterial, asymptomatic inflammatory, autoimmune, and chronic prostatitis can all result in increased FDG uptake. Uptake can also be seen in granulomatous prostatitis, a known complication of bacillus Calmette–Guerin (BCG) instillation therapy for bladder cancer. Acute prostatitis will most often show diffuse increased uptake; chronic and granulomatous prostatitis may show more focal or multifocal uptake. As noted above, there are no uptake levels or patterns that have been shown to accurately differentiate benign from malignant uptake.

## ■ Diagnosis

Unknown, concerning for prostate adenocarcinoma.

## ✓ Pearls

- F-18 FDG PET/CT has low sensitivity for prostate carcinoma as many have lower glucose metabolism.
- Increased FDG uptake in prostate cancer suggests dedifferentiation and correlates with higher PSA levels.
- No uptake patterns or levels have been shown to accurately differentiate benign from malignant uptake.
- Increased prostate FDG uptake should likely lead to follow up PSA level and urology consultation.

## Suggested Readings

Dong A, Bai Y, Wang Y, Zuo C, Lu J. Spectrum of the prostate lesions with increased FDG uptake on (18)F-FDG PET/CT. Abdom Imaging. 2014; 39(4):908–921

Kim CY, Lee SW, Choi SH, et al. Granulomatous prostatitis after intravesical bacillus Calmette-Guerin instillation therapy: a potential cause of incidental F-18 FDG uptake in the prodtate gland on F-18 FDG PET/CT in patients with bladder cancer. Nucl Med Mol Imaging. 2016; 50(1):31–37

Kwon T, Jeong IG, You D, Hong JH, Ahn H, Kim CS. Prevalence and clinical significance of incidental (18)F-fluoro-2-deoxyglucose uptake in prostate. Korean J Urol. 2015; 56(4):288–294

Reesink DJ, Fransen van de Putte EE, Vegt E, et al. Clinical relevance of incidental prostatic lesions on FDG-positron emission tomography/computerized tomography – should patients receive further evaluation? J Urol. 2016; 195(4 Pt 1):907–912

# Part 11

## Tumor (not PET)

11

# Case 125

*Brian J. Lewis*

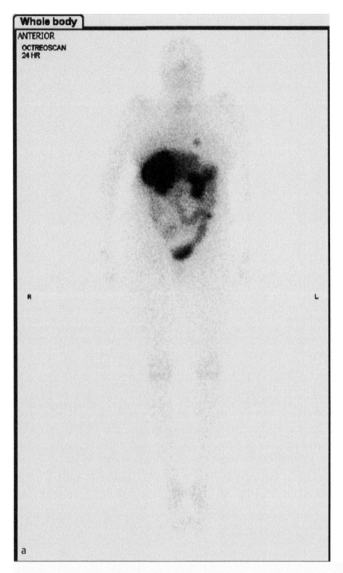 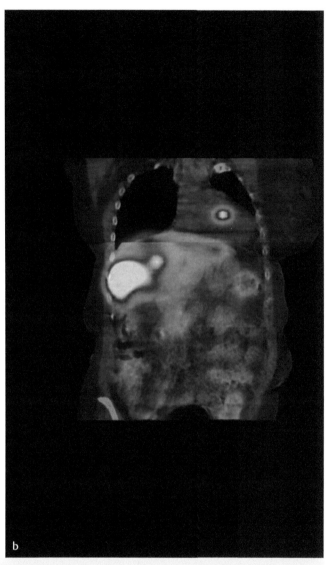

**Fig. 125.1** **(a)** Anterior whole-body planar and **(b)** coronal fused images from indium (In)-111 pentetreotide SPECT/CT are most notable for a large area of abnormal uptake in the liver as well as a focal area of activity in the heart.

## ■ Clinical History

69-year-old female with history of metastatic carcinoid and a cardiac mass initially noted on echocardiogram (▶ Fig. 125.1).

■ Key Finding

Abnormal uptake on In-111 pentetreotide scan (octreoscan)

■ Top 3 Differential Diagnoses

- **Neuroendocrine tumor.** In-111 has a physical half-life of 67.3 hours and gamma emission peaks of 173 and 247 keV. When coupled with pentetreotide, a somatostatin analogue, it is used in the evaluation of neuroendocrine tumors. Normal biodistribution includes spleen uptake, followed by the kidneys, bladder, and liver. Physiologic uptake is also normally seen in the blood pool, thyroid gland, gallbladder, and, on delayed images, the bowel. Imaging is performed at 4, 24, and possibly 48 hours, if needed. Whole-body planar imaging is performed with single-photon emission computed tomography (SPECT) or SPECT/CT added to improve sensitivity, especially in the chest and abdomen. Neuroendocrine tumors are derived from amine precursor uptake and decarboxylation (APUD) system cells. Carcinoid and pancreatic islet cell tumors are the most common indications for In-111 pentetreotide scanning. Other neuroendocrine tumors include medullary carcinoma of the thyroid, pheochromocytoma, neuroblastoma, paraganglioma, and small cell lung carcinoma. Octreoscan uptake varies by tumor and its subtypes. For islet cell tumors, octreoscan is most sensitive for gastrinomas and least sensitive for insulinomas.

- **Non-neuroendocrine tumor.** These tumors can also contain somatostatin receptors and, therefore, demonstrate radiotracer uptake on In-111 pentetreotide scan. These most commonly include lymphoma, breast carcinoma, non-small cell lung carcinoma, renal cell carcinoma, meningioma, and gliomas. Radiotracer uptake in these tumors tends to be highly variable. In-111 pentetreotide uptake can also be seen in thymoma and thymic carcinoma, helping to differentiate from thymic hyperplasia. In-111 pentetreotide scan may be ordered to evaluate known thymoma to determine if somatostatin therapy might be effective.

- **Inflammation.** Radiotracer uptake may also be demonstrated with inflammation, typically with chronic inflammatory conditions. This is classically described in granulomatous diseases such as sarcoidosis and tuberculosis. Other chronic inflammatory diseases include rheumatoid arthritis and inflammatory bowel disease. Uptake is secondary to lymphocyte somatostatin receptor expression. It is important to be aware of the patient's medical history, as these conditions can result in false-positive results.

■ Diagnosis

Carcinoid metastases in the liver and heart.

✓ Pearls

- Physiologic octreoscan uptake: spleen, kidneys/bladder, liver, gallbladder, bowel, and thyroid.
- Carcinoid and islet cell tumors are the most common indications for In-111 pentetreotide scan.

- Several non-neuroendocrine tumors contain somatostatin receptors and demonstrate uptake.
- Uptake can be seen in chronic inflammatory conditions, classically with granulomatous diseases.

Suggested Readings

Intenzo CM, Jabbour S, Lin HC, et al. Scintigraphic imaging of body neuroendocrine tumors. Radiographics. 2007; 27(5):1355–1369

Kvols LK, Brown ML, O'Connor MK, et al. Evaluation of a radiolabeled somatostatin analog (I-123 octreotide) in the detection and localization of carcinoid and islet cell tumors. Radiology. 1993; 187(1):129–133

Tan EH, Tan CH. Imaging of gastroenteropancreatic neuroendocrine tumors. World J Clin Oncol. 2011; 2(1):28–43

# Case 126

*Brian J. Lewis*

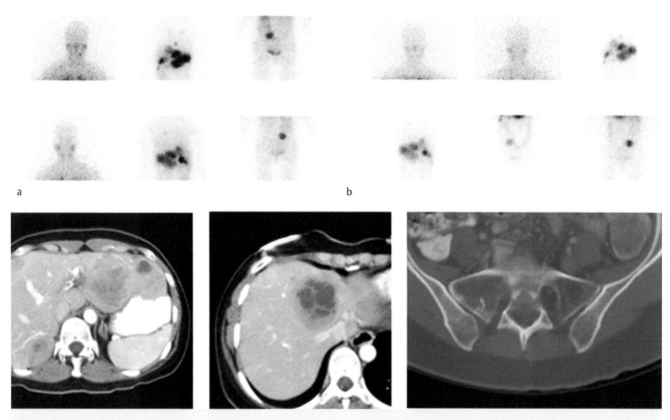

**Fig. 126.1** **(a)** Immediate and **(b)** 48-hour delayed whole-body imaging following administration of I-123 metaiodobenzylguanidine (MIBG) demonstrates heterogeneous and multifocal uptake within the region of the liver, as well as a focus of uptake within the right pelvis, suspicious for metastases. Axial contrast-enhanced CT images of the abdomen and pelvis demonstrate multifocal metastatic disease within the liver and right sacral ala.

## ■ Clinical History

43-year-old male with previous diagnosis of pheochromo-cytoma, status post resection of the primary lesion and chemotherapy (▶Fig. 126.1). (Case courtesy of Joseph S. Fotos, M.D., Penn State Hershey Medical Center.)

## Key Finding

Abnormal uptake on iodine-123 (I-123) metaiodobenzylguanidine (MIBG) scan in an adult

## Top 3 Differential Diagnoses

- **Pheochromocytoma/paraganglioma.** I-123 has a half-life of 13 hours and a photopeak of 159 keV. When coupled to MIBG, a norepinephrine analogue, it is useful for imaging sympathetic adrenergic tissue. Normal distribution includes the salivary glands, heart, liver, bladder, and faint kidney uptake. Thyroid uptake is blocked by preadministration of a potassium iodine (Lugol's) solution. Pheochromocytoma is a catecholamine-producing tumor that arises from the chromaffin cells of the adrenal medulla. The same tumor in an extra-adrenal location is known as a paraganglioma. Pheochromocytomas are classically solid hypervascular masses with high T2 signal intensity on magnetic resonance imaging (MRI). MIBG is most often used to identify clinically suspected tumors, for confirmation of suspected tumor found on anatomic imaging, or to evaluate for metastases. Diagnosis is critical, as catecholamine release may result in life-threatening hypertension or cardiac arrhythmia.
- **Carcinoid tumor.** These tumors arise from endocrine amine precursor uptake and decarboxylation (APUD) cells with about two-thirds of cases originating in the gastrointestinal (GI) tract, with the distal ileum being the most common location, and a quarter of cases arising from the tracheobronchial tree. GI carcinoids may produce 5-hydroxyindoleacetic acid (5-HIAA). They are usually sporadic but are also associated with multiple endocrine neoplasia (MEN) type 1, Zollinger–Ellison syndrome, and neurofibromatosis type I. Lesions may be found incidentally, or may present with bowel obstruction or GI bleeding. Carcinoid syndrome is typically seen when liver metastases are present. Desmoplastic reaction with calcification is classically present with mesenteric involvement, on anatomic imaging. Carcinoid tumors demonstrate variable uptake of MIBG, with the variability not completely understood. However, MIBG appears to be more sensitive for carcinoid tumor in the setting of elevated serum serotonin levels. Octreoscan is more frequently used for carcinoid imaging.
- **Medullary thyroid cancer.** It is a rare neuroendocrine tumor that arises from the parafollicular C cells of the thyroid gland and has a poorer prognosis than papillary and follicular subtypes. The average age of diagnosis is in the sixth decade of life, earlier if associated with MEN type 2 syndrome. Around a quarter of tumors less than 1 cm demonstrate nodal metastases, which jumps to 90% at greater than 4 cm. Typical thyroid imaging radiotracers are of little value, as these tumors poorly concentrate iodine. Fluorine-18 fluorodeoxyglucose positron emission tomography (F-18 FDG PET) is a more useful imaging radiotracer with a sensitivity around 60 to 95%. I-123 MIBG has a reported sensitivity of around 30%. Calcitonin and carcinoembryonic antigen (CEA) are useful biomarkers that aid in diagnosis and follow-up.

## Diagnosis

Metastatic pheochromocytoma.

## Pearls

- I-123 MIBG is favored over octreoscan for pheochromocytoma as there is less physiologic renal uptake.
- The distal ilium is the most common location for carcinoid tumor.
- Poor iodine concentration in medullary thyroid cancer renders I-123/I-131 imaging of little value.

## Suggested Readings

Ganeshan D, Bhosale P, Yang T, Kundra V. Imaging features of carcinoid tumors of the gastrointestinal tract. AJR Am J Roentgenol. 2013; 201(4):773–786

Ganeshan D, Paulson E, Duran C, Cabanillas ME, Busaidy NL, Charnsangavej C. Current update on medullary thyroid carcinoma. AJR Am J Roentgenol. 2013; 201(6):W867–76

Wiseman GA, Pacak K, O'Dorisio MS, et al. Usefulness of 123I-MIBG scintigraphy in the evaluation of patients with known or suspected primary or metastatic pheochromocytoma or paraganglioma: results from a prospective multicenter trial. J Nucl Med. 2009; 50(9):1448–1454

# Case 127

*Ely A. Wolin*

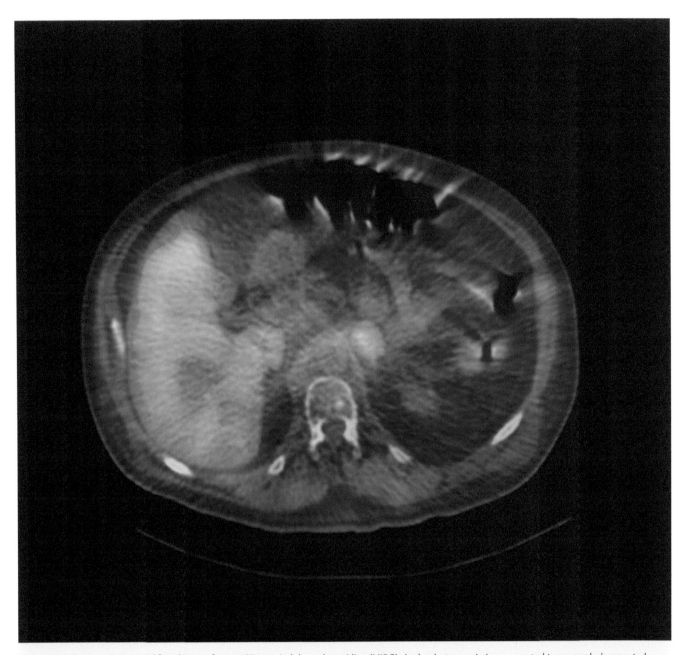

**Fig. 127.1** Representative axial fused image from I-123 metaiodobenzylguanidine (MIBG) single-photon emission computed tomography/computed tomography (SPECT/CT) shows mild uptake localizing to the body of the left adrenal gland. There was no anatomic correlate. The known left supraclavicular mass and pulmonary nodules did not demonstrate radiotracer uptake (not shown).

■ **Clinical History**

69-year-old male with metastatic paraganglioma referred for evaluation due to an enlarging left supraclavicular nodal mass and increasing pulmonary nodules (▶ Fig. 127.1).

■ **Key Finding**

I-123 metaiodobenzylguanidine (MIBG) adrenal gland uptake

■ **Top 3 Differential Diagnoses**

• **Normal.** MIBG is a norepinephrine analogue that is taken up by norepinephrine transporters and then stored intracellularly in neurosecretory granules. I-123 MIBG is used primarily for evaluation for pheochromocytoma due to less renal uptake than indium-111 (In-111) pentetreotide (which is also highly sensitive for paragangliomas). While norepinephrine transporter is predominantly present in neurons and sympathetic nerves, it is also present in chromaffin cells in the adrenal medulla. This means there is low level normal physiologic uptake of I-123 MIBG in the adrenal medulla, which may either mimic pathologic uptake or hide a small lesion. In general, physiologic adrenal uptake should be homogeneous and less intense than the liver. Physiologic uptake can be asymmetric around half of the time.

• **Pheochromocytoma.** A paraganglioma located within the adrenal gland is known as a pheochromocytoma. This is a usually benign tumor that can episodically secrete catecholamines resulting in symptoms of increased autonomic nervous system stimulation: paroxysmal hypertension, headache, sweating, palpitations, weight loss, etc. I-123 MIBG scintigraphy is used to verify the presence of a paraganglioma in the setting of suspicious clinical symptoms, or to confirm the diagnosis with a known mass and concerning biochemical features. The "rule of 10" has been used for paragangliomas: 10% are extra-adrenal, 10% are familial, 10% are malignant, 10% in pediatric patients, although this may no longer be accurate. Pheochromocytoma is associated with neurofibromatosis type I, von Hippel–Lindau syndrome, multiple endocrine neoplasia (MEN) type IIa and IIb, and Carney syndrome. I-123 MIBG scintigraphy has very high sensitivity for pheochromocytoma, higher than for extra-adrenal paraganglioma, with small lesions being the main cause for a false negative due to low level normal adrenal medullary uptake, as discussed above. Most pheochromocytomas will show focal increased I-123 MIBG activity with intensity exceeding the liver.

• **Medullary hyperplasia.** The amount of I-123 MIBG uptake seen with medullary hyperplasia is variable, but in general this will present with bilateral increased radiotracer uptake with preservation of an adreniform shape.

■ **Diagnosis**

Physiologic adrenal gland MIBG uptake. Multiple subsequent CT scans showed continued normal adrenal morphology.

✓ **Pearls**

• Adrenal scintigraphy with I-123 MIBG is useful in cases of suspected pheochromocytoma.
• Low-level physiologic adrenal medullary uptake of I-123 MIBG can mask small tumors.

• Symmetric homogeneous increased adrenal uptake with normal gland shape suggest hyperplasia.
• Pheochromocytoma usually show intense increased I-123 MIBG uptake, greater than liver.

**Suggested Readings**

Kurtaran A, Traub T, Shapiro B. Scintigraphic imaging of the adrenal glands. Eur J Radiol. 2002; 41(2):123–130

Wiseman GA, Pacak K, O'Dorisio MS, et al. Usefulness of 123I-MIBG scintigraphy in the evaluation of patients with known or suspected primary or metastatic pheochromocytoma or paraganglioma: results from a prospective multicenter trial. J Nucl Med. 2009; 50(9):1448–1454

# Case 128

*Ely A. Wolin*

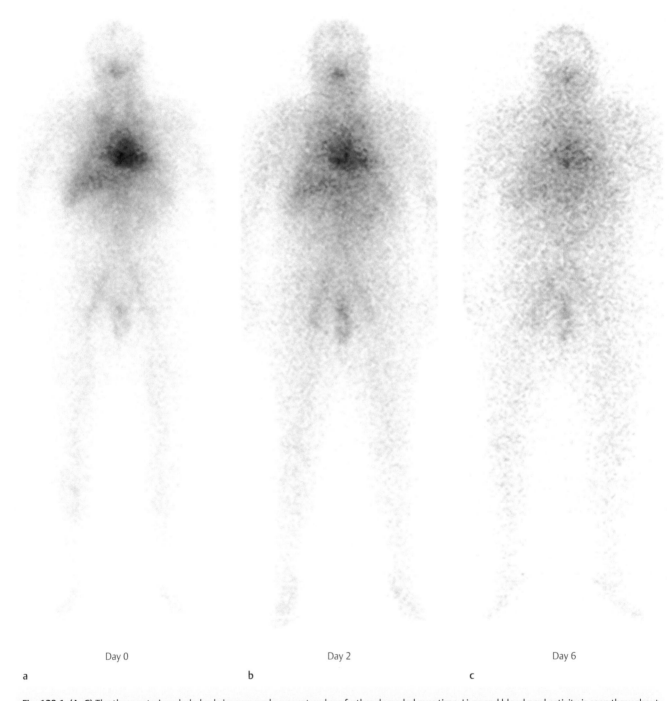

Day 0

Day 2

Day 6

a                  b                  c

**Fig. 128.1 (A–C)** The three anterior whole-body images are low count and are further degraded over time. Liver and blood pool activity is seen throughout the entire exam. Case reprinted with permission, originally published in: Appelbaum D, Miliziano J, eds. Rad Cases: Nuclear Medicine. Thieme 2011.

## ■ Clinical History

A 54-year-old woman with a relapsed low-grade lymphoma presents for therapy (▶Fig. 128.1).

## ■ Key Finding

Radionuclide therapy for lymphoma

## ■ Top 2 Differential Diagnoses

- **Yttrium-90 ibritumomab tiuxetan (Zevalin).** Lymphoma, a malignant lymphoid tissue tumor, is generally classified as either Hodgkin's disease (HD) or non-Hodgkin's lymphoma (NHL), based on histopathology. NHL can be either of B-cell or T-cell lineage. B cells have specific surface antigens, including CD20 which appears on maturing B cells prior to release from bone marrow. This antigen is the foundation for radionuclide lymphoma therapy. Monoclonal antibodies have been created which target CD20. In the case of Zevalin, the monoclonal antibody is ibritumomab. Standard nomenclature of monoclonal antibodies indicates that ibritumomab is a murine monoclonal antibody (mo = mouse, mab = monoclonal antibody) directed against a tumor (tu = tumor). Tiuxetan is used as a chelator to bind ibritumomab to In-111 for imaging, or Y-90 for therapy. Zevalin was initially approved for the treatment of refractory, relapsed, or transformed CD20 + NHL, but is now authorized as a first-line therapy. Zevalin protocol originally consisted of an initial dose of unlabeled rituximab, followed by 5 mCi of In-111 Zevalin for biodistribution scans obtained on day 1 and day 2, 3, or 4, then an additional dose of unlabeled rituximab prior to the Y-90 Zevalin therapy dose 7 to 9 days later. The biodistribution scan is no longer required. Dosing for the therapeutic infusion is based on weight and platelet count, 0.4 mCi/kg if platelets are over 150,000/mm$^3$, and 0.3 mCi/kg if platelet count is 100,000 to 150,000/mm$^3$. The radiotherapy is contraindicated if initial platelet count is below 100,000 mm$^3$, neutrophil count is below 1500/mm$^3$, and the patient has received external beam radiation to more than 25% of the marrow, or there is history of hypersensitivity to murine antibodies. The purpose of the unlabeled rituximab injections prior to either diagnostic or therapeutic Zevalin infusion is to block CD20 sites present on circulating B cells in the blood pool and spleen, allowing for more circulating time of labeled antibodies and thus more tumoral uptake. It is unclear why, but the unlabeled antibody does not seem to block the CD20 on tumor cells allowing pretreatment to result in increased target uptake. Since the monoclonal antibodies are murine, some patients will develop human antimurine antibody (HAMA). HAMA can make subsequent antibody infusions ineffective as well as initiate an immunologic response which can include fatal anaphylaxis. Because of this, patients must be monitored closely.
- **Iodine-131 tositumomab (Bexxar).** Similar to Zevalin, Bexxar was another approved radiolabeled monoclonal antibody for CD20 + NHL therapy, but is no longer available.

## ■ Diagnosis

Bexxar therapy for relapsed lymphoma with normal biodistribution (low count images due to I-131 label).

## ✓ Pearls

- Zevalin is a radiolabeled monoclonal antibody now approved for first-line therapy of CD20 + NHL.
- HAMA response can lead to fatal anaphylaxis; therefore, close monitoring of patients is required.
- Pretreatment with unlabeled monoclonal antibody, rituximab, allows for more tumor uptake of Zevalin.

## Suggested Readings

Goldsmith SJ. Radioimmunotherapy of lymphoma: Bexxar and Zevalin. Semin Nucl Med. 2010; 40(2):122–135

Hohloch K. Radioimmunotherapy of lymphoma: an underestimated therapy option. Lancet Haematol. 2017; 4(1):e6–e7

Rizzieri D. Zevalin(®) (ibritumomab tiuxetan): After more than a decade of treatment experience, what have we learned? Crit Rev Oncol Hematol. 2016; 105:5–17

Turner JH. Perspective: multimodality radionuclide therapy of progressive disseminated lymphoma and neuroendocrine tumors as a paradigm for cancer control. Cancer Biother Radiopharm. 2012; 27(9):525–529

# Case 129

*Ely A. Wolin*

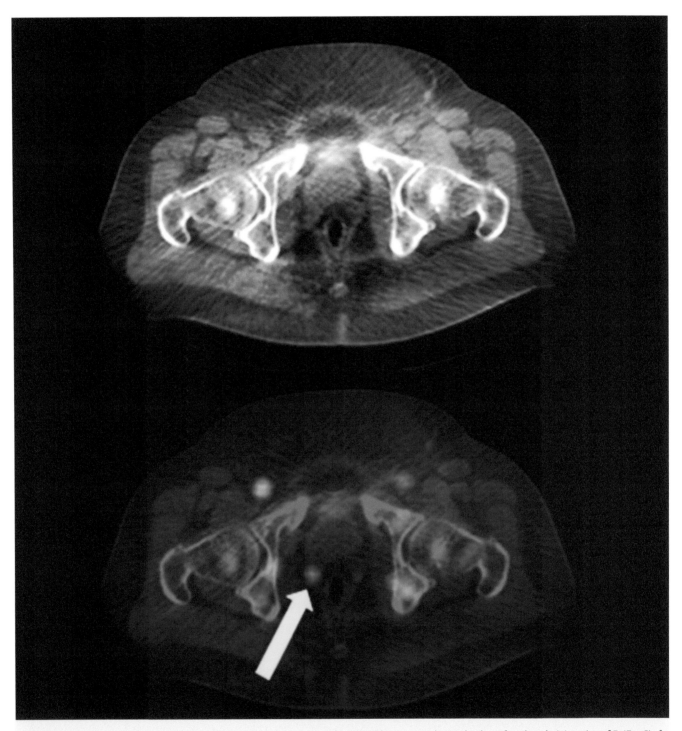

**Fig. 129.1** Axial CT and fused single-photon emission computed tomography (SPECT)/CT images obtained 4 days after the administration of 5.47 mCi of indium-111 (In-111) capromab pendetide show abnormal radiotracer uptake in the right seminal vesicle (*yellow arrow*).

■ Clinical History

67-year-old male with history of prostate cancer status post prostatectomy with new detectable prostate-specific antigen (PSA) over 2.0 (▶Fig. 129.1).

## Key Finding

Abnormal uptake on In-111 capromab pendetide (ProstaScint®; Cytogen Corporation, Princeton, NJ) scan

## Top 3 Differential Diagnoses

- **Prostate cancer.** Capromab is an IgG1 murine monoclonal antibody directed against prostate-specific membrane antigen (PSMA). Malignant prostate cells have a higher expression of PSMA, and expression appears to be upregulated in higher grade, androgen independent and metastatic prostate cancer. ProstaScint is capromab chelated to In-111 for imaging. It binds to an intracellular epitope of PSMA, meaning it will only localize in damaged or necrotic tumor cells. Care must be taken due to the possibility of human anti-mouse antibody (HAMA) response, particularly if the patient has previously received a murine antibody infusion. Physiologic distribution includes low-level uptake in the normal prostate, if present, liver, spleen, bone marrow, blood pool, genitourinary system, and bowel. Imaging typically involves whole-body planar imaging with single-photon emission computed tomography (SPECT)/CT of the pelvis 4 days after administration. Some may use a day 0 scan or alternatively use dual isotope imaging with Tc-99m red blood cell imaging, to map the blood pool. Blood pool imaging is not completely necessary with high-quality equipment allowing for accurate anatomic localization.

ProstaScint scan is indicated in patients with a diagnosis of prostate cancer who are thought to have localized disease after routine workup but are at high risk for nodal metastases. It is also indicated in the setting of a rising serum PSA post prostatectomy with a negative workup, concerning for occult metastatic disease. Bone scan remains more sensitive than ProstaScint for osseous metastases. PSMA PET imaging agents are now being used clinically which may allow for increased sensitivity and specificity.
- **Nonprostatic malignancy.** Uptake of In-111 capromab pendetide has been seen in several nonprostatic malignancies, including renal cell carcinoma (clear cell and chromophobe), bladder cancer (urothelial, adenocarcinoma, and small cell carcinoma), breast cancer, colon cancer, among others. The uptake in these malignancies is thought to be primarily due to PSMA expression associated with neovascularity. However, multiple malignancies have been shown to have tumoral expression of PSMA on histopathology.
- **Inflammation.** PSMA expression can exist within inflammatory lesions.

## Diagnosis

Recurrent metastatic prostate carcinoma in the right seminal vesicle.

## ✓ Pearls

- Prostate cancer PSMA expression is inversely related to the degree of cancer differentiation.
- PSMA imaging is indicated in patients believed to have localized high-risk prostate cancer.

- ProstaScint may help if PSA is increasing post prostatectomy with concern for occult metastatic disease.
- ProstaScint uptake is not specific and can be seen in nonprostatic malignancies and infection.

## Suggested Readings

Mhawech-Fauceglia P, Zhang S, Terracciano L, et al. Prostate-specific membrane antigen (PSMA) protein expression in normal and neoplastic tissues and its sensitivity and specificity in prostate adenocarcinoma: an immunohistochemical study using mutiple tumour tissue microarray technique. Histopathology. 2007; 50(4):472–483

Mohammed AA, Shergill IS, Vandal MT, Gujral SS. ProstaScint and its role in the diagnosis of prostate cancer. Expert Rev Mol Diagn. 2007; 7(4):345–349

Ristau BT, O'Keefe DS, Bacich DJ. The prostate-specific membrane antigen: lessons and current clinical implications from 20 years of research. Urol Oncol. 2014; 32(3):272–279

# Case 130

*Ely A. Wolin*

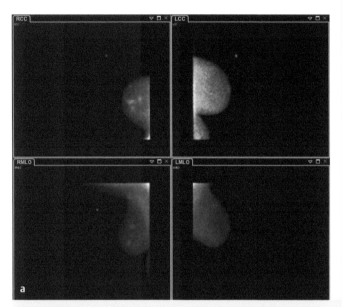
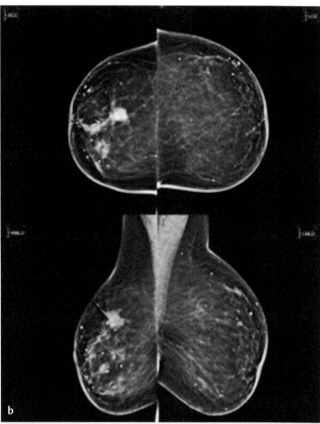

**Fig. 130.1** Images from breast-specific gamma imaging (BSGI) imaging performed after the administration of 20.5 mCi technetium-99m (Tc-99m) sestamibi **(a)** show three foci of abnormal uptake in the right breast with correlative mammographic abnormalities **(b)**.

## ■ Clinical History

75-year-old female with history of right breast cancer diagnosed 10 years prior and treated with lumpectomy and radiotherapy. Had biopsies 4, 5, and 8 years later for enlarging masses and asymmetry in the right lower inner breast, all of which showed stromal fibrosis and fat necrosis (▶ Fig. 130.1).

■ **Key Finding**

Focal breast uptake on BSGI

■ **Top 3 Differential Diagnoses**

- **Malignancy.** BSGI is a useful adjunct for the evaluation of breast cancer due to high resolution and small field of view Tc-99m sestamibi, a mitochondrial imaging agent, is injected followed by imaging of the breasts on dedicated high resolution, small field of view cameras after around a 10-minute delay. Imaging is based on the fact that malignant cells have increased vascularity and a higher concentration of mitochondria. Early attempts at scintimammography were limited by the relatively poor resolution of large field of view cameras, resulting in unacceptably low sensitivity for subcentimeter lesions. Dedicate high resolution, small field of view breast imaging cameras have corrected this issue, allowing for the breasts to be placed directly in contact with the detector and utilize standard mammographic projections. BSGI is not currently indicated for screening primarily due to the lack of data proving a mortality benefit like mammography, and increased radiation exposure (around 10 times the dose of mammography, and delivered to whole body not just breast tissue). There are several indications for BSGI to assist in both diagnosis and staging. In patients with a newly diagnosed breast malignancy, BSGI can evaluate for extent of disease, particularly useful in detecting multifocal, multicentric, and bilateral disease, as well as to assess response to neoadjuvant chemotherapy. BSGI can also be used when MRI is indicated but cannot be performed due to unavailability, presence of implanted devices that are not MRI compatible, decreased renal function preventing the use of gadolinium, or claustrophobia. BSGI has shown sensitivity similar to MRI with increased specificity. In screening of dense breasts, BSGI increases sensitivity over mammography from around 30 to over 90%. BSGI may also be particularly useful for invasive lobular carcinoma which can be more difficult to identify with mammography and ultrasound often leading to later stage disease with nodal metastases at diagnosis. The Society of Nuclear Medicine and Molecular Imaging procedure standards has defined interpretation criteria, merging scintigraphic findings with Breast Imaging Reporting and Data System (BIRADS) categories. BIRADS 1 is a normal scan that involves homogeneous uptake in the breast and axilla. BIRADS 5 has focal, moderate to intense uptake, with well-defined contours and is highly suggestive of malignancy. Diffuse or patchy, mild to moderately intense uptake with poorly delineated borders is more suggestive of benign disease.
- **High-risk lesions.** Focal increased uptake on BSGI has been seen in high-risk, but nonmalignant, lesions such as atypical ductal hyperplasia (ADH) and lobular carcinoma in-situ (LCIS).
- **Benign disease.** False-positive uptake on BSGI has been seen with multiple benign entities, including fibrocystic change, fibroadenoma, stromal fibrosis, and fat necrosis. Using a lesion to background ratio of 1.5 increases specificity.

■ **Diagnosis**

Stromal fibrosis and fat necrosis.

✓ **Pearls**

- BSGI, not for screening, is a useful adjunct in the evaluation of known or suspected breast malignancy.
- BSGI has shown sensitivity similar to MRI with increased specificity.
- Fibrocystic change, fibroadenoma, ADH, and LCIS, among others, can result in false-positive BSGI.

**Suggested Readings**

Fowler AM. A molecular approach to breast imaging. J Nucl Med. 2014; 55(2):177–180

Goldsmith SJ, Parsons W, Guiberteau MJ, et al. Society of Nuclear Medicine. SNM practice guideline for breast scintigraphy with breast-specific gamma-cameras 1.0. J Nucl Med Technol. 2010; 38(4):219–224

Holbrook A, Newel MS. Alternative screening for women with dense breasts: breast-specific gamma imaging (molecular breast imaging). AJR Am J Roentgenol. 2015; 204(2):252–256

# Case 131

*Vicki Nagano*

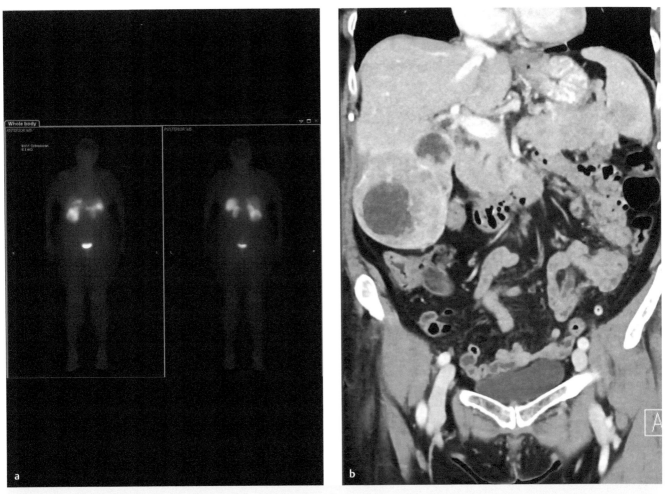

**Fig. 131.1** 24-hour delayed indium-111 pentetreotide images **(a)** show several regions of abnormal uptake within the liver and pancreatic tail with heterogeneous masses seen on corresponding CT **(b)**.

## ■ Clinical History

73-year-old female with right liver mass in the setting of pancreatic tail masses and smaller liver lesions (▶ Fig. 131.1).

## ■ Key Finding

Focal abdominal uptake on indium-111 (In-111) pentetreotide scan (octreoscan)

## ■ Top 3 Differential Diagnoses

- **Neuroendocrine tumor.** Somatostatin is a peptide that inhibits the release of anterior pituitary hormones and certain intestinal and pancreatic peptides, such as insulin, gastrin, glucagon, and cholecystokinin (CCK). In-111 pentetreotide (octreoscan) contains an amino acid analogue of somatostatin and is frequently used for the evaluation of neuroendocrine tumors. Normal radiopharmaceutical distribution includes intense splenic uptake with slightly less prominent uptake in the kidneys, followed by liver. Physiologic uptake is also seen within thyroid gland, gallbladder, bowel, and bladder. Planar imaging surveys the entire body; single-photon emission computed tomography (SPECT) imaging is essential in the chest and abdomen. Octreoscan is most commonly used for islet cell and carcinoid tumors. The sensitivity for islet cell tumors varies based upon the subtype: insulinoma (50%), gastrinoma (75–93%), glucagonoma (73%), and vipoma (88%). Sensitivity for various other neuroendocrine tumors is as follows: carcinoid (80–90%), neuroblastoma (over 85%), medullary thyroid carcinoma (54%), malignant pheochromocytoma (87%), paraganglioma (93%), and small cell carcinoma of the lung (100%). Neuroblastoma and pheochromocytoma are more com-monly imaged with I-123 metaiodobenzylguanidine (MIBG) as physiologic renal uptake with octreoscan may obscure an adrenal lesion.
- **Metastatic disease.** Non-neuroendocrine tumors which contain somatostatin receptors and can metastasize to the mesentery include non-small cell lung cancer, breast cancer, and lymphoma (sensitivity of 70% each). Lymphoma is the most common malignant neoplasm affecting the mesentery. Approximately 30 to 50% of patients with non-Hodgkin's lymphoma (NHL) will have disease in mesenteric lymph nodes.
- **Granulomatous disease.** Somatostatin receptors are also present in granulomatous diseases, such as sarcoidosis and tuberculosis (TB). Intra-abdominal TB lymphadenopathy has most commonly been reported in the lesser omental, mesenteric, and upper para-aortic regions. Contrast CT typically demonstrates rim enhancement in the peripheral inflammatory reaction and a low-attenuation center in the central caseous necrosis. In contrast, malignant and reactive lymph nodes generally demonstrate homogeneous enhancement on contrast CT. Enlarged mesenteric nodes can also be seen in some noninfectious, inflammatory conditions such as sarcoidosis.

## ■ Diagnosis

Metastatic pancreatic neuroendocrine tumor, likely gastrinoma.

## ✓ Pearls

- In-111 pentetreotide (octreoscan) is useful for imaging metastatic neuroendocrine tumors.
- Physiologic activity is seen within spleen, liver, gallbladder, kidneys, bowel, bladder, and faint thyroid.
- Uptake is also seen in granulomatous disease, lymphoma, meningioma, astrocytoma, and breast cancer.
- Neuroblastoma and pheochromocytoma are more commonly imaged with MIBG.

## Suggested Readings

Balon HR, Brown TLY, Goldsmith SJ, et al. Society of Nuclear Medicine. The SNM practice guideline for somatostatin receptor scintigraphy 2.0. J Nucl Med Technol. 2011; 39(4):317–324

Intenzo CM, Jabbour S, Lin HC, et al. Scintigraphic imaging of body neuroendocrine tumors. Radiographics. 2007; 27(5):1355–1369

Lucey BC, Stuhlfaut JW, Soto JA. Mesenteric lymph nodes seen at imaging: causes and significance. Radiographics. 2005; 25(2):351–365

Sheth S, Horton KM, Garland MR, Fishman EK. Mesenteric neoplasms: CT appearances of primary and secondary tumors and differential diagnosis. Radiographics. 2003; 23(2):457–473, quiz 535–536

# Case 132

*Britain A. Gailliot*

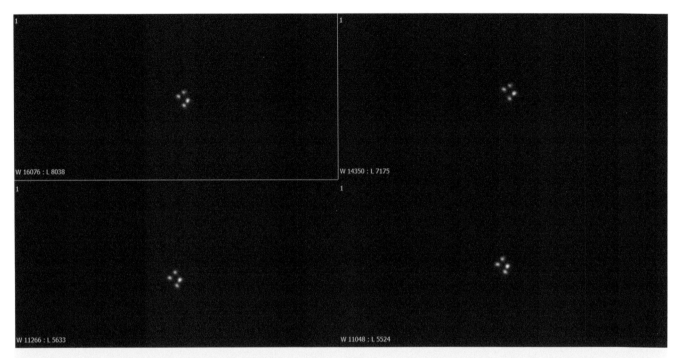

**Fig. 132.1** Representative images obtained over 2.5 hours after periareolar subdermal injection of 1 mCi technetium-99m (Tc-99m) filtered sulfur colloid injection divided in four equal doses show only the four injection sites.

## ■ Clinical History

62-year-old female referred for same day preoperative sentinel lymph node (SLN) localization prior to left breast cancer surgery (▶Fig. 132.1).

## ■ Key Finding

Lack of radiotracer migration on breast lymphoscintigraphy

## ■ Top 3 Differential Diagnoses

• **Lymphatic obstruction from cancer.** Preoperative breast lymphoscintigraphy is performed by superficial injection of filtered technetium-99m sulfur colloid (Tc-99m SC) allowing its progression through the lymphatic system to the SLN. When lymphatic architecture has been altered by a breast malignancy, in which it is typically very disorganized and ineffective, normal transit of the radiocolloid (RC) is prevented. This leads to retention of the RC within the mass and a delay in transit through the lymphatic chain, resulting in limited activity within the SLN. The highly disorganized lymphatic system within breast cancer is a reason intratumoral injection of RC is not performed. Failed migration of RC has also been shown to be more predictive of axillary node disease involvement.

• **Prior therapy.** As a result of lumpectomy, and often subsequent radiation therapy, lymphatic drainage pathways can be considerably damaged. The damaged lymphatic pathways lead to retention of the RC with significantly delayed clearance, resulting in an inability to detect activity within the SLN. Alternatively, in many cases of SLN remapping the results can be drastically different from the original procedure, resulting in SLN activity within the internal mammary nodes or contralateral axilla. This occurs as a result of alternative lymphatic drainage pathways being created by the initial therapies.

• **Poor technique/patient factors.** Various technical errors can occur in the performance of breast lymphoscintigraphy, for the most part involving injection and preparation of the RC. The amount of RC used for superficial injections is of very low volume, mostly for patient comfort. Failure to place a small amount of intervening air within the syringe can result in failure to adequately clear the RC from the needle. This results in too low a dose for SLN mapping. The RC is also contained in a suspension, and failure to gently agitate the suspension prior to injection can result in sedimentation of the RC within the syringe and inadequate administration. Technical errors in synthesis/preparation of the RC can also occur resulting in a high percentage of free Tc-99m. This presents as an elevated level of background and organ activity on imaging. If the RC is not appropriately filtered, migration failure may result as the particles will be too big for the lymphatic system. Some patient factors have also been shown to affect SLN visualization, such as large breasts and higher age.

## ■ Diagnosis

Lack of radiocolloid migration on preoperative breast lymphoscintigraphy, unknown cause.

## ✓ Pearls

• Breast lymphoscintigraphy is performed with filtered technetium-99m sulfur colloid (Tc-99m SC) (~100–200 nm).
• Lymphatic drainage may be disorganized with breast cancer and from prior surgery or radiation.

• Numerous technical errors can occur, most frequently with the preparation/injection of the radiotracer.
• Failed preoperative localization of an axillary SLN comes with a higher chance of axillary node disease.

## Suggested Readings

Brenot-Rossi I, Houvenaeghel G, Jacquemier J, et al. Nonvisualization of axillary sentinel node during lymphoscintigraphy: is there a pathologic significance in breast cancer? J Nucl Med. 2003; 44(8):1232–1237

Krynyckyi BR, Kim CK, Goyenechea MR, Chan PT, Zhang ZY, Machac J. Clinical breast lymphoscintigraphy: optimal techniques for performing studies, image atlas, and analysis of images. Radiographics. 2004; 24(1):121–145, discussion 139–145

Mariani G, Moresco L, Viale G, et al. Radioguided sentinel lymph node biopsy in breast cancer surgery. J Nucl Med. 2001; 42(8):1198–1215

# Case 133

*Cathy Zhou*

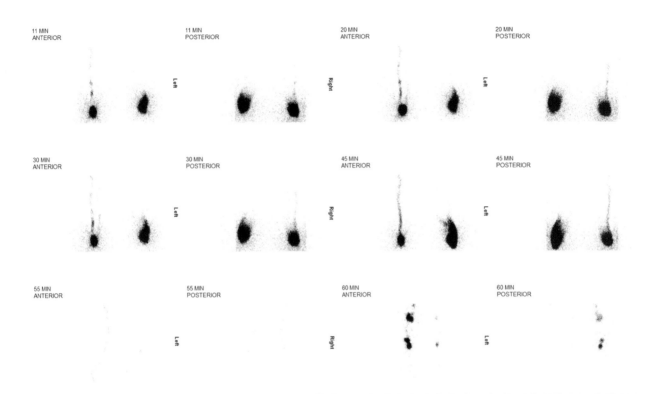

**Fig. 133.1** Following bilateral injections of technetium-99m-labeled microfiltered sulfur colloid between the first and second toes, anterior and posterior static images of the bilateral lower extremities at 11 minutes demonstrate prompt flow of radiotracer up the right lower extremity and no significant flow beyond the injection site on the left. Additional static images of the lower extremities at 20, 30, 45, and 55 minutes continue to reflect significantly delayed radiotracer flow on the left. At 60 minutes, images of the pelvis confirm significant asymmetry in amount of nodal radiotracer uptake, right greater than left.

## ■ Clinical History

14-year-old girl with a history of multiple bilateral lower extreity surgeries and left lower extremity edema (▶Fig. 133.1).

## ■ Key Finding

Delayed lower extremity radiotracer migration after subcutaneous injection of filtered technetium-99m sulfur colloid (Tc-99m SC)

## ■ Top 3 Differential Diagnoses

- **Primary lymphedema.** Lymphedema without an inciting cause is termed primary lymphedema, and is categorized on the basis of age of presentation. Congenital lymphedema presents before 2 years of age, and is usually attributed to a congenital or inherited condition such as Milroy's disease or Turner syndrome. Lymphedema precox, by far the most common type, arises around puberty, often in females. A small percentage of these are associated with Meige's disease. Lastly, lymphedema tarda presents after 35 years of age again mostly in females. The congenital type typically affects the bilateral lower extremity while lymphedema precox and tarda are limited to unilateral lower extremity below the knee. In a patient without a relevant clinical history, visualization of delayed/absent radiotracer movement, lymph vessels, and/or regional lymph nodes is considered diagnostic.

- **Malignancy-related lymphedema.** Impaired lymph flow primarily due to tumor infiltration or blockage/compression is rapid in onset and can be accompanied by paresthesias and weakness. Lymphedema can also arise more insidiously following lymphadenectomy, and the possibility is further increased with adjuvant radiation that destroys lymphatic channels. Unlike primary lymphedema, imaging is more likely to show prominent vessels or disrupted vessels with collaterals.
- **Postsurgical lymphedema.** Similar to lymphedema following cancer treatment, surgical interventions can also disrupt existing lymphatic channels. Factors that increase risk include increasing body mass index (BMI), extent of surgery, and postoperative delayed healing or infection. Findings are similar to that of malignancy-related lymphedema.

## ■ Additional Differential Diagnoses

- **Lymphatic filariasis:** This parasitic infection is the most common etiology for lymphedema worldwide, and is caused by three species, *Wuchereria bancrofti, Brugia malayi*, and *Brugia timori*, found in Africa and Asia. An estimated 120 million people are infected, but most are asymptomatic. Acutely, the

patient may endorse recurrent fever and painful lymphadenopathy, but severe lymphedema, sometimes referred to as elephantiasis, is a common late sequela. *Wuchereria bancrofti* often involves the lower extremities and genitals. Diagnosis is usually clinical, as lymphoscintigraphic correlation is poor.

## ■ Diagnosis

Postsurgical lymphedema.

## ✓ Pearls

- Primary lymphedema is suspected to be secondary to aplasia or hypoplasia of lymphatic vessels.
- Malignant lymphedema is most commonly attributed to sarcomas and lower extremity melanomas.

- Cancer treatment-related lymphedema is most often due to axillary lymph node dissection for breast cancer.

## Suggested Readings

Freedman DO, de Almeida Filho PJ, Besh S, Maia e Silva MC, Braga C, Maciel A. Lymphoscintigraphic analysis of lymphatic abnormalities in symptomatic and asymptomatic human filariasis. J Infect Dis. 1994; 170(4):927–933

Scarsbrook AF, Ganeshan A, Bradley KM. Pearls and pitfalls of radionuclide imaging of the lymphatic system. Part 2: evaluation of extremity lymphoedema. Br J Radiol. 2007; 80(951):219–226

Williams WH, Witte CL, Witte MH, McNeill GC. Radionuclide lymphangioscintigraphy in the evaluation of peripheral lymphedema. Clin Nucl Med. 2000; 25(6):451–464

# Case 134

*Ely A. Wolin*

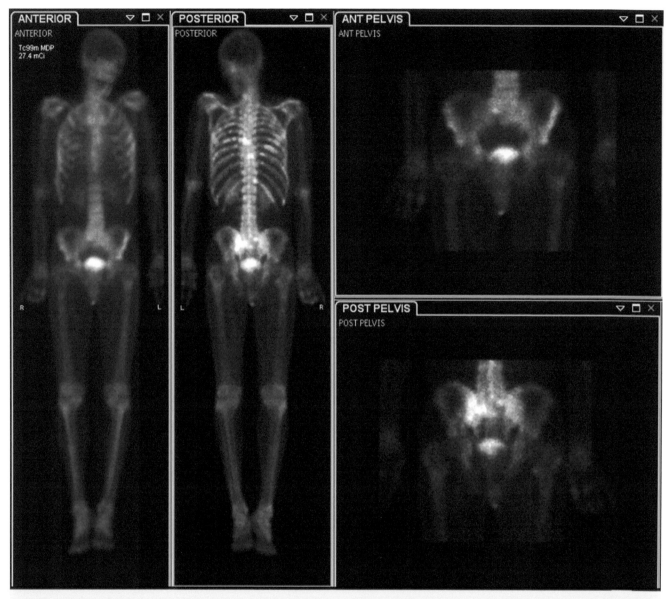

**Fig. 134.1** Anterior and posterior whole-body and spot images of the pelvis from Tc-99m methylene diphosphonate (MDP) bone scan show diffuse osteoblastic metastatic disease.

## ■ Clinical History

69-year-old male with castration-resistant metastatic prostate cancer referred for radionuclide therapy (▶Fig. 134.1).

## ■ Key Finding

Radiopharmaceutical therapy for painful bone metastases

## ■ Top 2 Differential Diagnoses

- **Disease-modifying therapy.** Recently added to the radiopharmaceutical therapy group, radium-223 (Ra-223) is the first to show disease-modifying capabilities. Ra-223 is primarily an alpha emitter with a physical half-life of 11.4 days. The alpha particles result in high energy transfer with a miniscule travel distance of 0.1 mm in soft tissue. The decay chain actually includes the release of four different alpha particles resulting in 282 MeV of energy deposition. Two beta particles and five gammas are also released, to a lesser extent, making biodistribution imaging possible if needed. Administered as the salt Ra-223 chloride, the radiopharmaceutical is incorporated into bone without the use of a chelator Ra-223 functions as a calcium analogue and is included in hydroxyapatite formation. Areas of increased bone metabolism will result in increased uptake. The majority of the radiopharmaceutical is deposited on the surface of the bone, and the high energy transfer prevents extensive radiation dose reaching the deeper marrow. The Alpharadin in Symptomatic Prostate Cancer (ALSYMPCA) trial was ended early after preliminary data showed Ra-223 therapy resulted in a 30% reduction in risk of death versus placebo in patients with castrate-resistant prostate cancer. Overall, Ra-223 was shown to increase survival, lengthen the time before alkaline phosphatase and PSA levels rose, increase the timespan before a symptomatic skeletal event, and show improved quality of life. This is without any significant difference in the frequency of hematologic or nonhematologic adverse events. Ra-233 chloride, sold by Bayer HealthCare Pharmaceuticals Inc. as Xofigo, is indicated in patients with castration-resistant prostate cancer with at least two sites of osseous metastases and no evidence of visceral metastatic disease. It is delivered as six intravenous doses spaced 4 to 8 weeks apart. Prior to receiving the first dose, the patient must have an absolute neutrophil count (ANC) of at least $1.5 \times 10^9$/L, platelet count (PLT) of at least $100 \times 10^9$/L, and hemoglobin of at least 10 g/dL, as myelosuppression remains the primary adverse concern. For subsequent dosing, the ANC must be at least 1 and PLT must be at least $50 \times 10^9$/L. If levels have not recovered after 6 weeks, a risk benefit analysis for continued therapy needs to be done. If a dose is delayed for more than 8 weeks, therapy is discontinued.
- **Pain palliation.** Several agents have previously been used for pain palliation with symptomatic bony metastatic disease with no proven survival benefit. These include strontium-89 (Sr-89), samarium-153 (Sm-153), phosphorus-32 (P-32), and rhenium-156 (Re-156). Sm-153 and Re-156 require a carrier to chelate to hydroxyapatite, such as ethylene diamine tetramethylene phosphonate (EDTMP) or hydroxyethylidene bisphosphonate (HDEP). These have shown good pain relief, with around 70% of patients experiencing some relief, but myelosuppression is the dose-limiting toxicity as the longer travel distance of the beta particles results in increased marrow suppression.

## ✓ Pearls

- Ra-223 provides pain palliation and disease modification in castration-resistant metastatic prostate cancer.
- Alpha particles have high energy transfer resulting in shorter travel distance, less marrow suppression.
- Myelosuppression is a dose-limiting toxicity for the beta-emitting pain palliation radiopharmaceuticals.
- Ra-223 therapy can be done as an outpatient with routine radiation protection precautions.

## Suggested Readings

Brady D, Parker CC, O'Sullivan JM. Bone-targeting radiopharmaceuticals including radium-223. Cancer J. 2013; 19(1):71–78

Florimonte L, Dellavedova L, Maffioli LS. Radium-223 dichloride in clinical practice: a review. Eur J Nucl Med Mol Imaging. 2016; 43(10):1896–1909

Nilsson S, Heinrich D, O'Sullivan JM, et al. Updated analysis of the phase III, double-blind, randomized, multinational study of radium-223 chloride in castration-resistant prostate cancer (CRPC) patients with bone metastases (ALSYMPCA). J Clin Oncol. 2012; 30(18_suppl)

# Part 12

## Quality Control

12

# Case 135

*Ely A. Wolin*

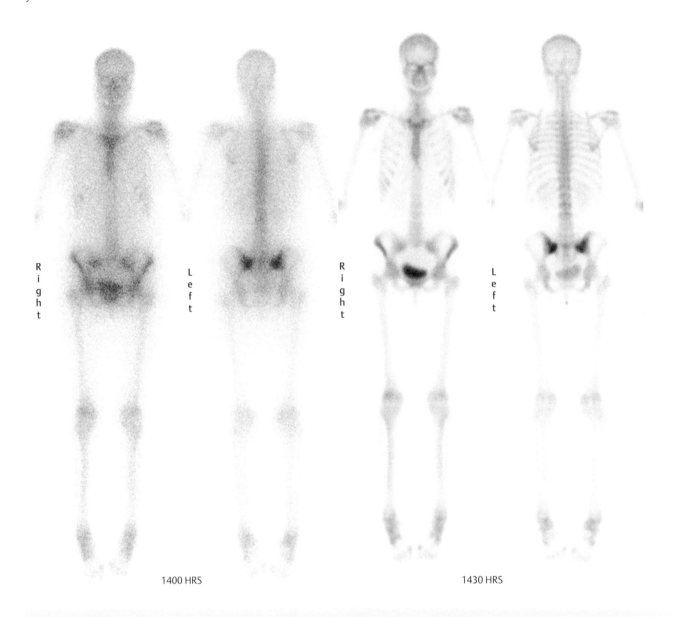

1400 HRS                    1430 HRS

**Fig. 135.1** Initial delayed whole-body bone scan (*left*) with technetium-99m (Tc-99m) hydroxy diphosphonate (HDP) demonstrates poor spatial resolution due to imaging acquisition at the wrong photopeak (122 keV for Co-57). Repeat imaging (*right*) at the correct photopeak setting (140 keV for Tc-99m) demonstrates improved spatial resolution. Incidentally, the patient had mild bilateral sacroiliitis which was seen on prior CT (not shown).

## ▪ Clinical History

24-year-old female with chronic hip pain. What is the difference between these two scans performed on the same day?
(▶Fig. 135.1)

## ■ Key Finding

Poor-quality bone scan

## ■ Top 3 Differential Diagnoses

- **Off-peak gamma camera.** For image acquisition, gamma cameras employ an energy window centered about the photopeak of the desired radioisotope in order to reject scatter radiation. In case of Tc-99m a 20% energy widow is centered about the 140 keV photopeak. Daily morning QC involves extrinsic field uniformity testing using a cobalt 57 (Co-57) sheet source prior to camera use for clinical studies. The extrinsic field uniformity test requires an energy window for Co-57 (122 keV) which is lower than Tc-99m. Failure to readjust the window setting for Tc-99m prior to clinical use results in a poor resolution scan due to downscatter from 140 keV photons into the 122-keV window. This is referred to as "off-peak" imaging.
- **Poor camera positioning.** Best image acquisition requires the gamma camera to be as close to the patient as possible. Minimizing the distance between source and detector allows for optimum performance of the external collimator, the largest limitation to overall resolution. As the detector is moved away from the target, photons with a greater angle of incidence will be allowed through the collimator because of the altered geometry. This leads to a blurry appearance of the obtained image. Using the wrong energy collimator could also similarly affect image quality.
- **Radiopharmaceutical preparation or administration error.** Administration of an incorrect radiopharmaceutical, incorrect dose of radiopharmaceutical (>20% difference from prescribed dose), or utilizing an unprescribed route of administration are classified as "misadministration" and may account for unexpected imaging results. Technical errors in radiopharmaceutical preparation can lead to chemical or radionuclidic impurities that may result in image degradation and, in some cases, increased patient dose. Infiltrated dose can lead to inadequate accumulation in the organ of interest resulting in a poor target-to-background and quantum mottle (image noise).

## ■ Additional Considerations

- **Medical event:** It is a subset of misadministration where the patient's whole-body dose exceeds 5 rem (0.05 Sv) or a single-organ dose exceeds 50 rem (0.5 Sv) requiring verbal and written notification of the Nuclear Regulatory Commission (NRC).
- **Radiopharmaceutical quality:** Regulations for radiopharmaceutical QC have been established by the NRC and the U.S. Pharmacopeia (USP). Examples for Tc-99m include less than 0.15 µCi of Mo-99 per 1 mCi of Tc-99m (at time of administration) and a maximum of 10 µg of aluminum break-through per 1 mL of Tc-99m eluate.

## ■ Diagnosis

Off-peak gamma camera.

## ✓ Pearls

- Off-peak imaging results in poor resolution imaging due to improper radiotracer photopeak selection.
- Poor resolution can also be seen with poor camera positioning and errors in radiotracer preparation/administration.
- "Medical event" is the misadministration of radiotracer exceeding the allowable limits of radiation dose.

## Suggested Readings

Cecchin D, Poggiali D, Riccardi L, Turco P, Bui F, De Marchi S. Analytical and experimental FWHM of a gamma camera: theoretical and practical issues. Peer J. 2015; 3:e722

Naddaf SY, Collier BD, Elgazzar AH, Khalil MM. Technical errors in planar bone scanning. J Nucl Med Technol. 2004; 32(3):148–153

Zanzonico P. Routine quality control of clinical nuclear medicine instrumentation: a brief review. J Nucl Med. 2008; 49(7):1114–1131

# Case 136

*Vicki Nagano*

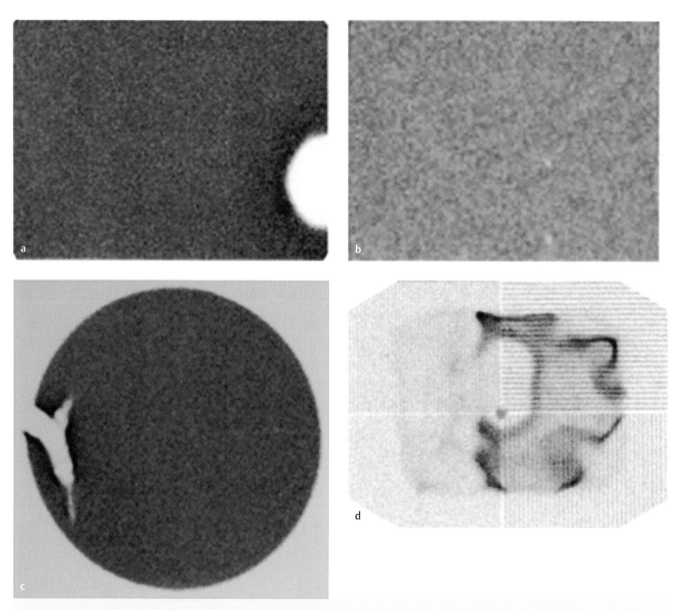

**Fig. 136.1** Multiple field uniformity flood images show a defective photomultiplier tube (PMT) **(a)**, two subtle photopenic defects due to dented lead in the collimator **(b)**, a crack in the sodium iodide crystal **(c)**, and an electronic problem affecting the main circuitry behind the PMTs **(d)**.

## ■ Clinical History

Technician presents flood field images for QC (▶ Fig. 136.1).

## Key Finding

Focal defect on QC images

## Top 3 Differential Diagnoses

- **PMT failure.** An array of PMTs behind the sodium iodide crystal converts the light pulse from the scintillation event into an electrical signal. Malfunction of the PMTs can be caused by a damaged tube, decoupling of the gel between the crystal and PMT, or a loose electrical connection. Scintillation events occurring due to defective PMT will not result in a measurable electrical signal. A round defect will be seen in the field uniformity image, corresponding to the position of the malfunctioning PMT. A similar focal defect can also be caused by an overlying attenuating structure on the camera head or by an air bubble in the liquid flood phantom.
- **Crystal defect.** Gamma ray photons produce a scintillation event within the sodium iodide crystal. A crack in the sodium iodide crystal on a flood-field image results in a branching white pattern due to lack of scintillations in this region. The surrounding dark edges are due to the edge-packing phenomenon.
- **Collimator defect.** The collimator helps to localize the radionuclide in the patient by allowing only those photons that travel in an appropriate direction to interact with the crystal. The soft lead in the collimators can be dented resulting in bending and distorting of the septa. The defect appears as a focal area of decreased activity on the flood-field image. Repeating the flood image with the collimator removed will show resolution of the defect.

## Additional Diagnostic Consideration

- **Electronic artifact:** Complex computer circuitry mounted along each PMT calculates the position and strength of the scintillation event. Electronic malfunctions can result in various artifacts, depending upon which electronic system is involved. The findings on flood imaging are less characteristic than those seen with other flood-field artifacts.

## Diagnosis

PMT failure (A); dented collimator (B); cracked crystal (C); electronic artifact (D).

## Pearls

- Daily QC includes extrinsic flood with Co-57 sheet source placed on the camera with collimator.
- Daily flood QC images should be reviewed if there is concern for external artifact on any diagnostic study.
- Weekly spatial resolution/linearity is tested with a bar phantom between the Co-57 sheet and collimator.
- Intrinsic flood (no collimator) and single-photon emission computed tomography (SPECT) QC are done monthly.

## Suggested Readings

Mettler FA, Guiberteau MJ. Essentials of nuclear medicine imaging, 6th ed. Philadelphia, PA: Elsevier, 2012

Zanzonico P. Routine quality control of clinical nuclear medicine instrumentation: a brief review. J Nucl Med. 2008; 49(7):1114–1131

Ziessman HA, O'Malley JP, Thrall JH. Nuclear medicine: the requisites, 4th ed. Philadelphia, PA: Elsevier, 2014

# Case 137

*David W. Erickson*

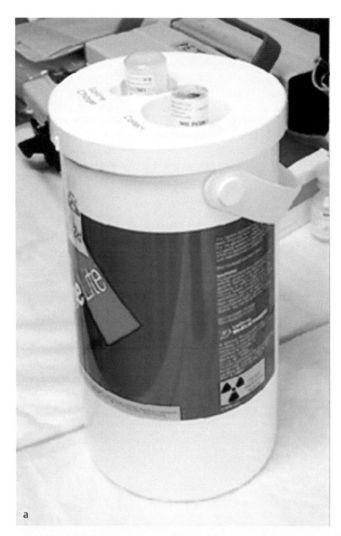
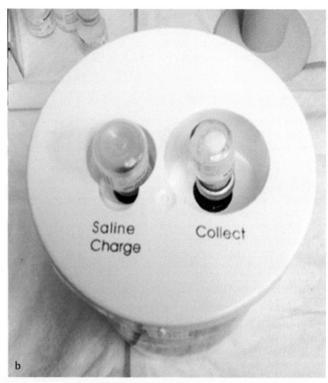

Fig. 137.1 Mo-99/technetium-99m (Tc-99m) elution generator **(a)**, top view of generator showing the saline charge vial and Tc-99m collection vial **(b)**.

## ▪ Clinical History

The nuclear medicine clinic has an Mo-99/Tc-99m generator shipped to the department on a weekly basis for providing readily available Tc-99m for imaging purposes. The technologist on shift elutes the generator each day to obtain a Tc-99m patient dose and administers it for a cardiac study. When the patient is placed on the scanner, the images acquired are not clinically usable (▶ Fig. 137.1).

## ■ Key Finding

No clinically usable image can be obtained

## ■ Top 3 Differential Diagnoses

- **Wrong energy window.** Before imaging a patient, the technologist can confirm that the energy window is centered on the correct photon energy with the correct energy window range. If the incorrect nuclide to be imaged is chosen on the scanner, it will be incorrectly throwing out counts from the Tc-99m 140 keV photons.
- **Wrong collimators.** Most gamma cameras have an option to change the collimators in order to optimize image acquisition for the injected radionuclide. For Tc-99m, low-energy collimators are used. The definition for low, medium, or high energy is decided by the manufacturer, but it is correlated to the height and thickness of the lead septa within the collimator. If the collimators on the gamma camera are intended for a higher

energy nuclide, it could take significantly longer time for an image to appear on the acquisition monitor and fully acquire.
- **Molybdenum-99 contamination.** In accordance with 10 coronary flow reserve (CFR) 35.204, the first eluate from a Tc-99m generator is required to be tested to ensure that the Mo-99 contamination is not more than 0.15 µCi per 1 mCi of Tc-99m. Mo-99 has a half-life of 66 hours, primarily decays through a 1.214 MeV beta transmission as well as high-level gamma photons, and will concentrate in the liver, mineral bone, and kidneys if internalized. In addition to its radiation hazards, the high-energy gamma photons from Mo-99 could be a disruption to the imaging of Tc-99m uptake. The technologist should check that Mo-99 contamination levels are compliant.

## ■ Additional Diagnostic Consideration

- **Aluminum contamination:** Generators should also be tested for any aluminum contamination in the eluate from the aluminum column contained in the generator.

## ■ Diagnosis

The technologist failed to check that the Mo-99 contamination level was within allowable limits. This failure to test and document the first eluate from a generator is a finding of noncompliance with 10 CFR 35.204 if identified by an inspector. At the time of writing this, the reporting of a generator that has failed the breakthrough test is not an Nuclear Regulatory Commission (NRC) reportable event but reporting requirements are being discussed. The unusable image from this patient was due to the Mo-99 contaminant level being beyond NRC thresholds with an activity of 2 to 3 mCi of Mo-99 for the

patient administered dose of approximately 20 mCi Tc-99m. With this large Mo-99 dose being administered to the patient, the collimators on the gamma camera were not able to attenuate its many high-energy gamma photons. Furthermore, the energy spectrum analyzer of the gamma camera has an autoranging display setting that scales to its largest signal, so the Tc-99m signal was dwarfed by the Mo-99 energy spectrum component. This unexpected energy spectrum was not verified by the technologist and the image acquired included the many scattered Mo-99 photons.

## ✓ Pearls

- The first eluate should not have Mo-99 levels above 0.15 µCi per 1 mCi of Tc-99m.
- Technologists should verify the energy spectrum, energy level, and energy window width on a per-patient basis.

- The Al³⁺ contamination test is no longer required by the NRC, but it is common practice to perform with each elution.

## Suggested Readings

Pappas, Virginia, Re: Nuclear Regulatory Commission: 10 CFR Part 35 [NRC-2008-0175]; Medical Use of Byproduct Material, SNMI 18 November 2014

Shearer DR, Pezzullo JC, Moore MM, Coleman P, Frater SI. Radiation dose from radiopharmaceuticals contaminated with molybdenum-99. J Nucl Med. 1988; 29(5):695–700

# Case 138

*Kathryn R. Wagner*

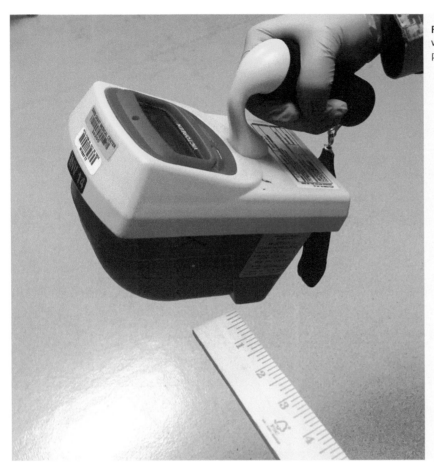

Fig. 138.1 Exposure rate measurement being taken with an ion chamber at one meter to determine if patient meets release criteria.

■ Clinical History

The radiation safety officer (RSO) takes surface and one-meter measurements from an inpatient who has received I-131 therapy. Based on calculations, the patient should be ready for release. The patient's one-meter measurement is 17 mR/hour (▶Fig. 138.1).

## ■ Key Finding

Patient with higher than expected one-meter measurement of 17 mR/hour

## ■ Top 3 Differential Diagnoses

- **Ionization chamber measurement error.** Prior to release from the facility, it must be determined that a patient who has been administered unsealed byproduct material will not overexpose a member of the public. In accordance with 10 coronary flow reserve (CFR) 35.75, which outlines patient release criteria, the total effective dose equivalent (TEDE) to a member of the public from a patient receiving unsealed byproduct material cannot exceed 500 mrem. Therefore, using calculations for I-131 taken from NUREG-1556 Volume 9 Revision 2, the dose rate at one meter at which a patient can be released is 7 mrem/hour (exposure rate of 7 mR/hour). Measurement occurs 1 m from the patient with an ionization chamber. In accordance with 10 CFR 35.61, survey instruments used for radiation surveys must be calibrated annually and "bump-checked" prior to use with a check source. If the indicated exposure rate differs from the anticipated exposure rate (determined during annual calibration) by more than 20%, then the survey meter must not be used.
- **Patient has compromised renal function.** Patients with thyroid disease who receive I-131 treatment and have compromised renal function pose a challenge when it comes to radiation safety. The excretion rate of I-131 in these patients is significantly slowed. This can cause a delay in release from the facility due to inaccurate calculations using the typical effective half-life of I-131. Excretion of I-131 from the body can significantly vary from patient to patient; any I-131 calculations should be verified with measurements.
- **Incorrect distance for measurement.** Due to the inverse square law, where intensity of the radiation beam decreases by $1/d^2$, where d is the distance from the source, the distance at which the measurement is taken can have a significant impact on the exposure rate measurement.

## ■ Additional Consideration

- **Public dose limits:** Two other public dose limits exist: 100 mrem per year and 2 mrem in any 1 hour (i.e., 2 mR/hour) in an unrestricted area (10 CFR 20.1301). These dose limits exclude background radiation and exposure from individuals released under 10 CFR 35.75 as described above. To show compliance, record of radiation surveys for any areas where radioactive materials are stored, used, or prepared should be kept on file. If a member of the public is likely to receive a dose in excess of 100 mrem from a patient who has been administered unsealed byproduct material, the patient must be given written instructions outlining proper precautions and restrictions.

## ■ Diagnosis

The ionization chamber used for the release survey was giving exposure measurements 10 times higher than the actual levels. The chamber was sent out for repair.

## ✓ Pearls

- Patients receiving unsealed byproduct material cannot give a member of the public a TEDE in excess of 500 mrem.
- Release instructions must be given if a member of the public is likely to receive a TEDE in excess of 100 mrem.
- Radiation intensity decreases by $1/d^2$, so the measurement distance is critical in showing that release criteria is met.

## Suggested Readings

Lee JH, Park SG. Estimation of the Release Time from Isolation for Patients with Differentiated Thyroid Cancer Treated with High-dose I-131. Nucl Med Mol Imaging. 2010; 44(4):241–245

Ravichandran R, Binukumar J, Saadi AA. Estimation of effective half life of clearance of radioactive Iodine (I) in patients treated for hyperthyroidism and carcinoma thyroid. Indian J Nucl Med. 2010; 25(2):49–52

# Case 139

*Kathryn R. Wagner*

Dose Cal Constancy Summary Report

Dose Calibrator: CRC - 25R          Manufacture :Capintec

| | | | Co-57 | Cs-137 | | | | | | |
|---|---|---|---|---|---|---|---|---|---|---|
| | Background | Voltage | Co - 57 | Cs -137 | F -18 | Ga-67 | I-123 | I-131 | In-111 | |
| | uCi | Volts | mCi | uCi | uCi | uCi | uCi | uCi | uCi | |
| 4/1/2016 7:35AM | 0.180 | 155.300 | 1.945 | 109.000 | 60.000 | 180.000 | 70.000 | 141.000 | 86.000 | |
| 4/2/2016 9:18AM | 0.160 | 155.300 | 1.955 | 108.000 | 59.000 | 178.000 | 69.000 | 139.000 | 85.000 | |
| 4/4/2016 6:32AM | 0.130 | 155.300 | 1.931 | 108.000 | 59.000 | 178.000 | 69.000 | 140.000 | 85.000 | |
| 4/5/2016 6:48AM | 0.260 | 155.300 | 1.927 | 109.000 | 59.000 | 179.000 | 69.000 | 140.000 | 85.000 | |
| 4/6/2016 6:49AM | 0.250 | 155.300 | 1.922 | 108.000 | 59.000 | 177.000 | 69.000 | 139.000 | 84.000 | |
| 4/7/2016 6:46AM | 0.170 | 155.300 | 1.915 | 108.000 | 59.000 | 178.000 | 69.000 | 139.000 | 85.000 | |
| 4/8/2016 6:40AM | 0.110 | 155.300 | 1.914 | 108.000 | 59.000 | 178.000 | 69.000 | 159.000 | 85.000 | |
| 4/11/2016 6:28AM | 0.200 | 155.300 | 1.897 | 108.000 | 59.000 | 178.000 | 69.000 | 139.000 | 85.000 | |
| 4/12/2016 6:53AM | 0.280 | 155.300 | 1.891 | 109.000 | 60.000 | 180.000 | 70.000 | 141.000 | 86.000 | |
| 4/13/2016 6:43AM | 0.270 | 155.300 | 1.887 | 107.000 | 59.000 | 177.000 | 69.000 | 139.000 | 85.000 | |
| 4/14/2016 6:41AM | 0.310 | 155.300 | 1.899 | 109.000 | 60.000 | 180.000 | 70.000 | 141.000 | 86.000 | |
| 4/15/2016 6:38AM | 0.230 | 155.300 | 1.894 | 108.000 | 59.000 | 177.000 | 69.000 | 140.000 | 84.000 | |
| 4/18/2016 6:18AM | 0.210 | 155.300 | 1.863 | 107.000 | 59.000 | 177.000 | 69.000 | 139.000 | 84.000 | |
| 4/19/2016 6:33AM | 0.200 | 155.300 | 1.878 | 107.000 | 59.000 | 177.000 | 69.000 | 139.000 | 84.000 | |

**Fig. 139.1** Dose calibrator daily constancy testing report.

## ■ Clinical History

The RSO reviews dose calibrator QC records for compliance with the Nuclear Regulatory Commission (NRC) (▶Fig. 139.1).

# ■ Key Finding

Errors with records of dose calibrator QC

# ■ Top 3 Differential Diagnoses

- **Constancy.** At installation and prior to daily use, the dose calibrator constancy test should be performed in order to determine that the precision of the instrument is within the permissible range (±10%), and that it is performing consistently from day to day. Constancy is typically performed with a Cs-137 check source, and the activity is measured on multiple radionuclide settings (gain settings) on the dose calibrator. One example would be checking the I-123 gain setting using a Cs-137 check source because Cs-137 is relatively long-lived and will provide constant measurement values each day in a properly functioning dose calibrator.
- **Linearity.** Linearity should be performed on the dose calibrator at installation and at every quarter to ensure that it is providing an accurate reading across a wide range of activities, from μCi to mCi. There are two ways to perform linearity: the decay method and the sleeve method. The decay method involves placing a vial of radiopharmaceutical in the dose calibrator and taking readings at various time intervals to plot the measured activity versus time on a semi-logarithmic graph, thus producing a linear representation of the decayed activity. The sleeve method uses cylindrical sleeves of increasing lead thickness to simulate the decay of the source. These values could also be plotted on a semi-log graph to produce a linear response but are more commonly corrected with calibration factors and compared. Measurements must be within ± 10% of the expected value.
- **Accuracy.** At installation and annually after, accuracy should be performed on the dose calibrator using a National Institute of Standards and Technology (NIST) source to determine that the dose calibrator is providing an accurate measurement of activity for a range of energies, within ±10% of the known activity value. Typically, Co-57, Ba-133, and Cs-137 are used to test low-, medium-, and high-energy ranges, respectively.

# ■ Additional Consideration

- **Geometry:** The dose calibrator geometry test should be performed at installation and after any move or repair. Geometry testing checks the dose calibrator's ability to give correct activity measurements across a variety of receptacles and volumes—vials, syringes, etc. Any receptacles used in the clinic should be tested to ensure that the dose calibrator is not dependent on the geometry of the object containing the dose.

# ■ Diagnosis

The dose calibrator QC records indicate that on April 8, 2016, constancy with the Cs-137 check source on the I-131 setting failed. Upon failure, this test should have been repeated to confirm a failure and the RSO notified to have the unit serviced immediately.

# ✓ Pearls

- Dose calibrator QC must be conducted per the manufacturer's instructions (per 10 coronary flow reserve (CFR) 35.60.)
- Required tests: constancy (daily), linearity (quarterly), accuracy (annually), geometry (after repair/move).
- Dose calibrator QC measurements must be within ± 10%, according to 10 CFR 35.61.

# Suggested Readings

American Association of Physicists in Medicine. AAPM Report 181 The Selection, Use, Calibration, and Quality Assurance of Radionuclide Calibrators Used in Nuclear Medicine. https://www.aapm.org/pubs/reports/RPT_181.pdf. Accessed June 27, 2016

Zanzonico P. Routine quality control of clinical nuclear medicine instrumentation: a brief review. J Nucl Med. 2008; 49(7):1114–1131

# Case 140

*Kathryn R. Wagner*

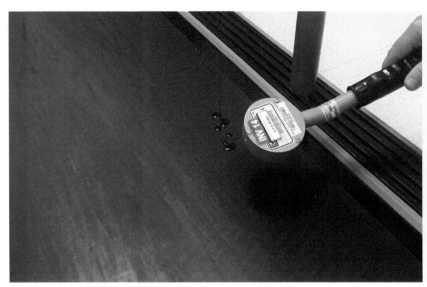

Fig. 140.1 Technologist surveys treadmill using a Geiger–Muller meter after patient IV leaks during a stress test. Technetium-99m (Tc-99m) is discovered on the treadmill.

## ■ Clinical History

During the stress portion of a myocardial perfusion study, the patient's IV leaks Tc-99m onto the treadmill (▶ Fig. 140.1).

■ **Key Finding**

An area of Tc-99m contamination is discovered

■ **Top 2 Differential Diagnoses**

• **Minor spill.** A minor spill consists of a small amount of radioactive material and poses less hazard in comparison to a major spill. During a response to a minor spill, individuals in the area of the spill should be notified, and the primary concern is prevention of further spread of contamination to other areas and among individuals. Individuals assisting in the clean-up should wear gloves, lab coats, and booties, and any other personal protective equipment available. The spill should be cleaned up using absorbent paper, and all contaminated items should be properly disposed of and labeled for decay in storage. The area and all personnel involved in the clean-up should be surveyed with a Geiger–Muller detector, which is sensitive enough to detect low levels of radiation. If any areas of contamination are unable to be cleaned up, they should be swiped for removable contamination. If removable contamination exits (above trigger limits), the area should be cordoned off until the spill has decayed to background. Finally, the incident should be reported to the RSO.

• **Major spill.** A major spill consists of larger amounts of radioactive material and requires more stringent clean-up and notification procedures. A spill is considered to be major if it involves Ci quantities of PET radionuclides, any amount of Ra-226, and amounts of radionuclides above the levels listed in the table below:

| Radionuclides | Threshold for major spill (mCi) |
|---|---|
| P-32, Fe-59, Co-60, Se-75, Sr-89, I-125, I-131 | 1 |
| Co-57, Co-58, Ga-67, Sr-85, In-111, I-123, Sm-153, Yb-169, Hg-197, Au-198 | 10 |
| Cr-51, Tc-99m, Tl-201 | 100 |

The important difference between procedures for major versus minor spills is the immediate notification to the RSO. In addition to the steps listed for minor spills, major spills may also require shielding of the source and securing the area to prevent other individuals from entering.

■ **Additional Consideration**

• **Reports to the Nuclear Regulatory Commission (NRC):** In accordance with 10 coronary flow reserve (CFR) 30.50, the NRC must be notified within 24 hours after the discovery of a contamination event that "requires access to the area to be restricted for more than 24 hours, and that involves a quantity of radioactive material greater than five times the annual limit on intake, and has access to the area restricted for a reason other than to allow isotopes with a half-life of less than 24 hours to decay prior to decontamination."

■ **Diagnosis**

Minor spill of Tc-99m (maximum around 30 mCi since stress dose). No notification to the NRC necessary.

✓ **Pearls**

• For both major and minor spills, the primary focus of clean-up is to prevent the spread of contamination.
• A major spill involves large quantities of radioactive material and requires immediate notification to the RSO.

• Contaminations meeting specific criteria outlined in 10 CFR 30.50 require notification to the NRC within 24 hours.

**Suggested Readings**

U.S. Nuclear Regulatory Commission. NUREG-1556 Vol. 9, Rev. 2. Program-Specific Guidance About Medical Use Licenses. http://www.nrc.gov/docs/ML0734/ML073400289.pdf. Accessed June 27, 2016

# Case 141

*Kathryn R. Wagner*

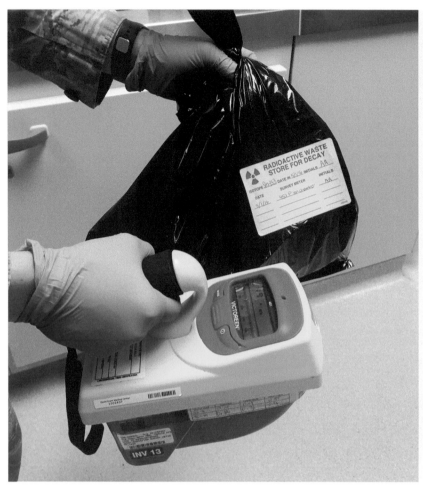

**Fig. 141.1** Technologist surveys radioactive waste using an ion chamber to determine if it has reached background for disposal as ordinary waste.

## ■ Clinical History

Technologist performs survey of samarium-153 (Sm-153) waste prior to disposal (▶ Fig. 141.1).

## ■ Key Finding

Waste receptacle survey measurements show the waste is still radioactive

## ■ Top 3 Differential Diagnoses

- **Clinic is in violation of regulations regarding decay-in-storage.** In accordance with 10 coronary flow reserve (CFR) 35.92, radiopharmaceutical waste and sharps can be held in decay-in-storage if the half-life is less than or equal to 120 days. The amount of activity that can be stored is not regulated.
- **Not enough half-lives have passed for disposal.** Before disposing of radioactive waste, it should be stored for approximately 10 half-lives and surveyed at the surface level (after removing any shielding) to ensure radiation levels are indistinguishable from background radiation levels. Once it has been determined that the radioactive waste has decayed to background levels, all radioactive labeling should be ablated,

and it can be disposed of with ordinary waste. Records containing the nature of disposal must be kept on file for 3 years.
- **Radiopharmaceutical contaminants.** During the production of radionuclides, specifically when using neutron activation, impurities in the target material will cause the production of other radionuclides also. To limit the contamination and maximize specific activity, radionuclides are produced by nuclear fission, rather than neutron activation, if possible. While contaminants are typically found in low percentages (e.g., 0.1%), they are often still detected and distinguishable from background levels.

## ■ Additional Considerations

- **Calibration of survey instruments:** In accordance with 10 CFR 35.61, survey instruments used for radiation surveys must be calibrated annually and "bump-checked" prior to use. If the indicated exposure rate differs from the calculated exposure rate (determined during annual calibration) by more than 20%, then the survey meter must not be used.
- **Daily and weekly area surveys:** Areas where radioactive materials are prepared, used, or stored should be surveyed

at the end of each day for contamination. In addition, surveys for removable contamination should be performed weekly (as recommended by NUREG-1556 Volume 9 Revision 2) by swiping commonly used surfaces and measuring the swipe with a counting instrument, such as a gamma counter or scintillation detector.

## ■ Diagnosis

Radioactive waste from an Sm-153 ethylene diamine tetramethylene phosphonate (EDTMP) metastatic bone pain palliation treatment was surveyed prior to disposal. Sm-153

contains a long-lived contaminant, Eu-154, with a half-life of 8.6 years that was detected in the waste.

## ✓ Pearls

- Radioactive waste should be held for approximately 10 half-lives and surveyed prior to disposing.
- Radiopharmaceuticals with half-lives less than 120 days can be kept in decay-in-storage.
- Some radiopharmaceuticals contain long-lived contaminants which could cause elevated survey levels.
- Areas where radiopharmaceuticals are prepared or stored should be surveyed at the end of each day.

## Suggested Readings

Kalef-Ezra JA, Valakis ST, Pallada S. Samarium-153 EDTMP for metastatic bone pain palliation: the impact of europium impurities. Phys Med. 2015; 31(1):104–107
Metyko J, Williford JM, Erwin W, Poston J, Jr, Jimenez S. Long-lived impurities of 90Y-labeled microspheres, TheraSphere and SIR-spheres, and the impact on patient dose and waste management. Health Phys. 2012; 103(5, Suppl 3): S204–S208

# Case 142

*Kathryn R. Wagner*

| Personal data | | | (All results in rem) External totals this monitoring period | | | | | | | |
|---|---|---|---|---|---|---|---|---|---|---|
| Name Last, First, MI | Monitoring period | | Eye Dose Equiv | Mead dose Equir (Deep) | Extressity Dose Equir | CD | Shallow Dose Equiv | Deep dose equiv whole body | | All Source TEDE |
| | From | To | | | | | | B/G/ | Neutron | |
| | 20150601 | 20150630 | 0.030 | 0.030 | 1.487 | NA | 0.028 | 0.030 | — | 0.030 |
| | 20150605 | 20150630 | 0.016 | 0.016 | 0.000 | NA | 0.015 | 0.016 | — | 0.016 |
| | 20150605 | 20150630 | 0.011 | 0.011 | 0.333 | NA | 0.010 | 0.011 | — | 0.011 |
| | 20150601 | 20150630 | 0.024 | 0.024 | 0.516 | NA | 0.023 | 0.024 | — | 0.024 |
| | 20150601 | 20150630 | 0.000 | 0.000 | 0.000 | NA | 0.000 | 0.000 | — | 0.000 |
| | 20150601 | 20150630 | 0.005 | 0.005 | 0.000 | NA | 0.005 | 0.005 | — | 0.005 |
| | 20150601 | 20150630 | 0.005 | 0.005 | 0.051 | NA | 0.005 | 0.005 | — | 0.005 |
| | 20150601 | 20150630 | 0.043 | 0.043 | 0.039 | NA | 0.041 | 0.043 | — | 0.043 |
| | 20150601 | 20150630 | 0.000 | 0.000 | 0.000 | NA | 0.000 | 0.000 | — | 0.000 |
| | 20150601 | 20150630 | 0.017 | 0.017 | 0.210 | NA | 0.016 | 0.017 | — | 0.017 |

Investigation Action Level (LAL):

| | | ***** | ***** |
|---|---|---|---|
| | Qty | 50 | 100 |
| | ***** | 200 | 500 |
| | ***** | 900**50 others | 1400 next, 100 others |
| | ***** | 20 deep,***** | 30 deep ******* |

**Fig. 142.1** Monthly dosimetry report for radiation workers shows totals for the monthly monitoring period. The extremity dose of 1.487 rem exceeds the monthly ALARA limits.

## ■ Clinical History

The RSO reviews the monthly dose reports for the nuclear medicine technologists (▶ Fig. 142.1).

## ■ Key Finding

Monthly dose reports for nuclear medicine technologists

## ■ Top 3 Differential Diagnoses

• **Individual has reached the annual occupational dose limit.** 10 coronary flow reserve (CFR) 20.1201 states that the annual occupational dose limit is 5 rem total effective dose equivalent or 50 rem committed dose equivalent to any individual organ or tissue, 15 rem to the lens of the eye, or 50 rem to the skin of the whole body or of any extremity. If an individual reaches any of these limits, he/she must be removed from duties as a radiation worker. Records of exposures must be kept until termination of the radioactive materials permit.

• **Individual is not required to be monitored for occupational radiation exposure.** At a minimum, a radiation dosimetry program must monitor individuals who are likely to receive 10% of the annual occupational dose limits in accordance with 10 CFR 20.1502. In addition, declared pregnant workers who are likely to receive a deep dose equivalent greater than 100 mrem must also be monitored. Monitoring determination should not be made from a single monitoring period alone. Time period of from 6 months to 1 year should be taken into account to consider changes in workload.

• **High dose limits.** Dosimetry reports for radiation workers should be reviewed after each monitoring period to ensure that individuals are on track to remain below the annual occupational dose limit. As directed by NUREG-1556 Volume 9 Revision 2, facilities should establish internal limits that trigger an investigation as to why the worker received a higher than usual dose during the monitoring period and to ensure workplace practices align with radiation safety ALARA (as low as reasonably achievable) principles. It is common for nuclear medicine students or new technologists to hit internal trigger limits often, specifically for ring badge doses, due to lack of experience and slower handling of materials. As experience level increases, occupational doses should decrease.

## ■ Additional Considerations

• **Additional employment records cause the individual to reach annual occupational dose limits:** Annual occupational dose limits are cumulative in nature and include any exposures to radiation in the workplace, regardless of what facility they occur. Therefore, the annual dose limits should be reduced by the amount of occupational dose received while employed by another facility in the same year.

• **Planned special exposures:** Planned special exposures, accidents, or emergences must be subtracted from annual occupational dose limits.

## ■ Diagnosis

The individual listed above shows an abnormal ring badge dose; if the worker continues to receive an equal or greater dose each monitoring period, he/she will be on track to meet or exceed the annual occupational dose limit and must be removed from duties as a radiation worker.

## ✓ Pearls

• Annual occupational dose limits are 5 rem TEDE, 15 rem to the eye lens, 50 rem to skin or an extremity.
• Workers must be on a dosimetry program if likely to receive 10% of the annual occupational dose limit.

• Annual dose limits are cumulative; records must include occupational exposures from all locations.

## Suggested Readings

Bayram T, Yilmaz AH, Demir M, Sonmez B. Radiation dose to technologists per nuclear medicine examination and estimation of annual dose. J Nucl Med Technol. 2011; 39(1):55–59

Kaljevic J, Stankovic K, Stankovic J, et al. Hand Dose Evaluation of Occupationally Exposed Staff in Nuclear Medicine. Radiat Prot Dosimetry. 2015

Leide-Svegborn S. External radiation exposure of personnel in nuclear medicine from 18F, 99 mTC and 131I with special reference to fingers, eyes and thyroid. Radiat Prot Dosimetry. 2012; 149(2):196–206

# Case 143

*Kathryn R. Wagner*

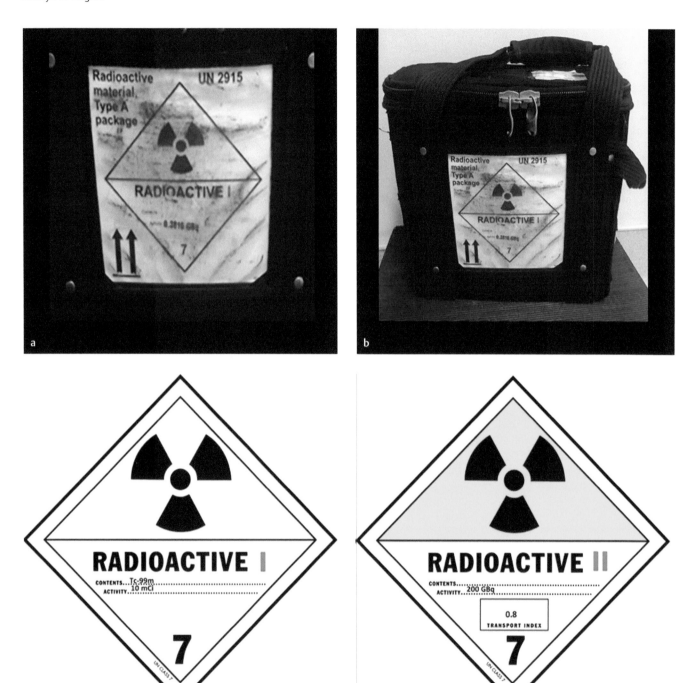

**Fig. 143.1** Package with 0.7 mR/hour surface reading labeled as White I package **(a)**; package with missing security seal **(b)**; label with incorrect activity units **(c)**; and label missing contents of package **(d)**.

## ■ Clinical History

Technician checks in radioactive package to the nuclear medicine clinic (▶Fig. 143.1).

## ■ Key Finding

Improper labeling/packaging for radioactive material shipments

## ■ Top 3 Differential Diagnoses

- **Missing security seal.** Normal Form (most radiopharmaceutical shipments) packages must have a security seal to verify that the integrity of the package has not been tampered with by the time it reaches its destination. A security seal can be nylon or paper tape, or a wire seal. Limited quantity packages (i.e., spent generators) do not require a security seal.
- **Improper labeling on radioactive package.** Category labeling for Normal Form radioactive packages is based on the radiation hazard as measured from the outside of the package. Measurements at the surface and at 1 m from the package are used to determine the proper label based on the chart below, per 49 coronary flow reserve (CFR) 172.403, Department of Transportation regulations:

| Label category | Surface reading (mR/hour) | Transport index (TI) (Based on measurement taken at 1 m in mR/hour, rounded up to the nearest tenth and unitless) |
|---|---|---|
| WHITE-I | <0.5 | 0 (considered to be 0 if measurement is < 0.05 mR/hour) |
| YELLOW-II | 0.5–50 | ≤1.0 |
| YELLOW-III | 50–200 | ≤10.0 |

In addition, Normal Form packages must be affixed with a "UN 2915, Radioactive Material, Type A package, non-special form, non-fissile, or fissile excepted" label.
- **Missing information on category label.** Normal Form packages must contain other information in addition to the label category. The contents and activity of the shipment must also be denoted on the label. The contents should include all radioactive materials contained in the package, and the activity must be listed in SI units (Becquerels). Traditional units for activity (mCi) may also be used in parentheses following SI units.

## ■ Additional Considerations

- **Missing category label:** Two category labels must be affixed to opposite sides of Normal Form packages.
- **Package measurements and swipes:** In accordance with 10 CFR 20.1906, all packages containing radioactive materials

(with the exception of Special Form shipment and gases) must be swiped over an area of 300 cm$^2$ for external contamination. The removable contamination limit is 6600 dpm/300 cm$^2$.

## ■ Diagnosis

Incorrect category label (A); missing security seal (B); missing information on category label (C and D).

## ✓ Pearls

- Normal Form packages should not be accepted if the mandatory security seal is missing or tampered.
- Category labels are based on surface and one-meter measurements, affixed to opposite sides of the package.
- The category label must include the radioisotopes included in the package and activity in Bq.
- The removable contamination limit for radioactive packages is 6600 dpm/300 cm$^2$ swipe.

## Suggested Readings

Transportation of Radioactive Materials "Nuclear Reactor Concepts" Workshop Manual, U.S. NRC

# Case 144

*Kathryn R. Wagner*

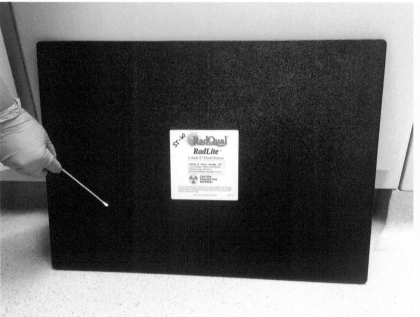

**Fig. 144.1** Technologist performs leak test on Co-57 flood source.

## ■ Clinical History

A flood source was shipped to your facility to be used for QC testing of gamma cameras (▶ Fig. 144.1).

## ■ Key Finding

Sealed source was received with accompanied leak test report

## ■ Top 3 Differential Diagnoses

- **Perform a leak test to meet frequency requirements.** In accordance with 10 coronary flow reserve (CFR) 35.67, a sealed source must be leak tested before use (unless the supplier provides proof of a leak test within 6 months before transfer) and at least every 6 months thereafter. To perform a leak test, a 100 cm² surface of the source is wiped with a swab or filter paper, focusing on areas like corners and edges that have a higher probability of leakage. The wipe is then counted in an instrument that must be capable of detecting levels of removable contamination as low as 0.005 µCi.
- **Source specifications do not meet requirements for performing leak tests.** Leak tests are not required to be performed on sealed sources with a half-life of less than 30 days and sources containing less than 100 µCi (if the material is a beta or gamma emitter) or less than 10 µCi (if the material is an α emitter). Additionally, sources that are being stored and not used are not required to be leak tested; however, a leak test must be performed before being put into use again or before transferring/shipping.
- **Leak test results require disposal of the source.** If a leak test detects the presence of removable contamination in excess of 0.005 µCi, a report must be made to the Nuclear Regulatory Commission (NRC) within 5 days, and the source should be removed from use and either disposed of or repaired.

## ■ Additional Consideration

- **Add sealed source to inventory:** A semiannual physical inventory of sealed sources must be conducted; therefore, sealed sources should be added to the inventory upon receipt. Records of semiannual inventories and leak tests must be kept for 3 years.

## ■ Diagnosis

The sealed source should be added to the inventory. Leak test results are current and below action limits; therefore, no leak test will be required for 6 months.

## ✓ Pearls

- Sealed sources with half-life < 30 days or containing < 100 µCi β/γ emitter or < 10 µCi α emitter do not require a leak test.
- Leak tests must be performed at intervals not to exceed 6 months.
- Leak tests detecting contamination > 0.005 µCi require a report and immediate removal from use.

## Suggested Readings

United States Nuclear Regulatory Commission. Requirements for Possession of Sealed Sources and Brachytherapy Sources. 10 CFR 35.67. 2015

# Case 145

*David W. Erickson*

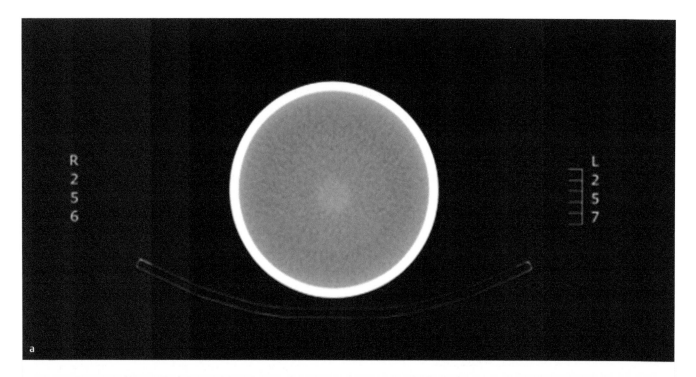

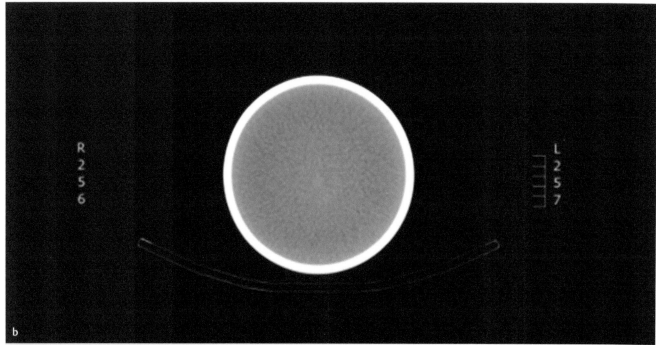

**Fig. 145.1** Image **(a)** shows a failed daily QC phantom image. Image **(b)** shows the same phantom image, with same acquisition settings after system calibrations were completed by field service technician.

## ■ Clinical History

Technologist performs daily QC for CT portion of single-photon emission computed tomography (SPECT)/CT system to ensure accurate attenuation correction (▶Fig. 145.1).

## ■ Key Finding

System failed Hounsfield unit (HU) standard deviation daily QC criteria

## ■ Top 3 Differential Diagnoses

- **CT detector gains drifting.** Most SPECT/CT hybrid imaging systems are not equipped with lower quality CT scanners to provide an attenuation correction map and basic anatomic localization. The system used here utilizes a cone-beam geometry with a single flat panel detector that utilizes thin-film transistor technology to create discrete detectors. Each individual pixel is provided a bias voltage supply after an exposure for a "readout" of the signal. These gains can drift over time producing an incorrect signal in the image. If left uncorrected, it can yield an artifact (most often a ring artifact) in the reconstructed image.
- **Phantom used.** The CT phantom used for routine QC is often provided by the manufacturer. Just like the imaging system, the phantom ages and can degrade with time. It is important to ensure the phantom is intact. Handling of the phantom could result in feature inserts being knocked loose.
- **QC technique.** Technique factors (kVp, mAs) used during routine QC are often preset in the imaging system to minimize any deviations from protocol. However, any facility with a high turnover of technologists should be especially mindful of protocols that allow technique factor adjustments. Technique factors used for QC protocols are important because CT systems used for attenuation correction need to operate at a higher kVp (120–140 kVp) to give an accurate attenuation correction map. Routine QC is most effective when the same protocol is followed. Any protocol deviations can yield unreliable QC values for trending system performance.

## ■ Additional Considerations

- **Attenuation correction:** Quick and simple daily QCs are the first line of defense for detecting a problem with the camera. Any minor issues found during a routine QC can typically be corrected at a later time that is convenient to the clinic. However, issues that produce artifacts that could be deemed clinically significant should be corrected immediately.
- **Uniformity:** Because this system utilizes the CT for attenuation correction and anatomic localization, it is important that uniform phantom areas appear uniform in the reconstructed image. A system out of calibration can incorrectly compute the attenuation correction, affect quantitative studies, and misrepresent the true anatomy of a patient.
- **Incorrect region of interest (ROI) placement:** It is clear in the first image that a center nonuniformity is present. Qualitatively the uniformity performance of this camera is poor. However, QC instructions are to obtain a center ROI and compare with correct performance criteria. While this nonuniformity issue is visible, marginal movement of the analysis ROI may obtain values that pass the vendor-specified threshold.

## ■ Diagnosis

Check positioning of CT phantom being imaged, look for any beam path obstructions, and rescan the phantom. If not better, the system should be serviced to perform CT calibrations.

## ✓ Pearls

- Routine QC and technologist experiences are the first identifiers for detecting a system problem early on.
- Nonuniformities/artifacts in the CT images also affect the nuclear medicine images.
- Both quantitative and qualitative analysis should be performed on QC images.

## Suggested Readings

Floyd CE, Jr, Warp RJ, Dobbins JT, III, et al. Imaging characteristics of an amorphous silicon flat-panel detector for digital chest radiography. Radiology. 2001; 218(3):683–688

Zanzonico P. Routine quality control of clinical nuclear medicine instrumentation: a brief review. J Nucl Med. 2008; 49(7):1114–1131

# Case 146

*David W. Erickson*

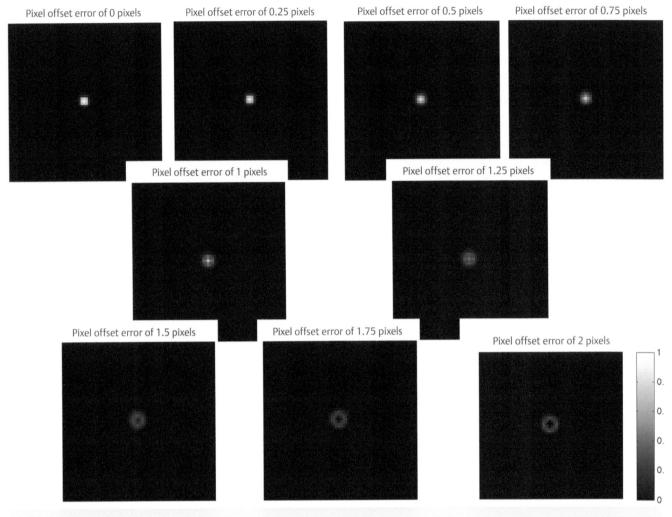

**Fig. 146.1** Simulated reconstruction of a point source with different center of rotation errors using MATLAB R2013a 64-bit (maci64). 64 × 64 matrix, 360 degree total angle of rotation, 360-degree projection angles, circular orbit. Point source is a 3 × 3 reconstruction into transverse slices using a ramp filter and filtered back projection.

## ▪ Clinical History

Center of rotation (COR) single-photon emission computed tomography (SPECT) performance (▶ Fig. 146.1).

## ■ Key Finding

Poor COR yields degraded tomographic resolution

## ■ Top 3 Differential Diagnoses

- **Routine COR QC.** Technologists should perform COR QC on SPECT systems monthly (or per the manufacturer's specifications) to ensure proper image reconstruction after acquisition. Degraded resolution or a ring artifact could be caused by a drift in alignment of the gamma camera heads. If routine QC is not an integral part of the clinic's operation, system errors will most likely be found when clinically usable images are no longer being produced and the system must be shut down until a service technician can repair.
- **QC performed but not reviewed.** All QC testing data should be routinely reviewed by a medical physicist to anticipate failures by trending system performance, and to ensure recorded values are within manufacturer specifications. For a typical system, both X and Y direction camera head alignment performance values should be within 2 mm. However, the frequency of testing and action level criteria are typically manufacturer driven. Moreover, loss of resolution and artifacts are likely to occur if a camera head is unstable during tomographic imaging.
- **System modifications.** It is especially important to ensure that a system is operating properly after any modifications, new installations, renovations, or adverse events take place. While most gamma camera systems have the capability to self-correct based on the COR QC data, this correction is dependent on the QC being completed. For example, if the gamma camera heads are inadvertently bumped with enough force from a patient bed, tomographic misalignment could occur.

## ■ Additional Diagnostic Considerations

- **Phantom mixing:** The typical method for visualizing a ring artifact due to misalignment is by the tomographic imaging of a 20-cm cylindrical phantom. This phantom is filled with Tc-99m and must be properly mixed before acquisition. Poor mixing can yield nonuniform, reconstructed, tomographic images.
- **Alignment checks:** Most systems have a method of viewing the sinogram data of an acquisition. This sinogram can be inspected for rough discontinuities which would indicate poor head alignment.

## ■ Diagnosis

Dual-headed gamma camera misalignment yields poor tomographic resolution.

## ✓ Pearls

- Cardiac imaging clinics must be especially conscious of camera alignment to avoid artifacts.
- COR QC should be performed and assessed weekly for maintaining adequate camera alignment.
- Minor COR offsets can significantly affect tomographic performance.

## Suggested Readings

Halama, James R. QC Protocols Gamma Camera & SPECT Systems, AAPM Meetings <http://www.aapm.org/meetings/amos2/pdf/35-9798-70158-156.pdf>. Accessed September 13, 2016

Zanzonico P. Routine quality control of clinical nuclear medicine instrumentation: a brief review. J Nucl Med. 2008; 49(7):1114-1131

# Case 147

*David W. Erickson*

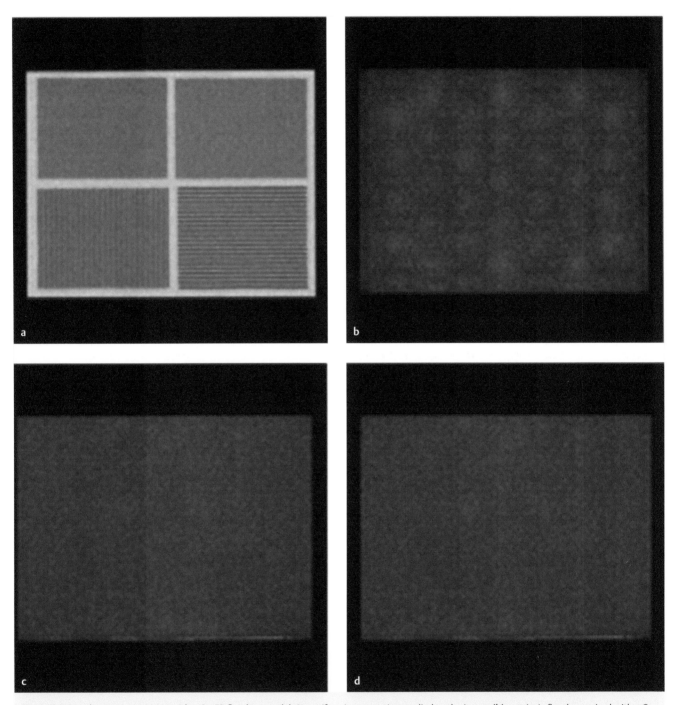

**Fig. 147.1** Bar phantom acquisition with a Co-57 flood source **(a)**. No uniformity correction applied to the image **(b)**, extrinsic floods acquired with a Co-57 sheet source having a Co-57 uniformity correction map applied to the image **(c)**, Tc-99m correction matrix applied to the image **(d)**.

■ **Clinical History**

Gamma camera linearity (▶ Fig. 147.1).

## ■ Key Finding

Technologist runs extrinsic uniformity QC with Co-57 sheet source and analysis shows degraded performance

## ■ Top 3 Differential Diagnoses

- **No correction map chosen.** Daily, before imaging patients, extrinsic uniformity QC should be accomplished to look for gross nonuniformities and ensure consistent performance. The technologist will place a sheet source (typically Co-57) on top of an upward-facing camera head with collimator (hence extrinsic) attached, and select an acquisition protocol to collect a 1 to 3 million count flood images, as defined by the manufacturer. This test should be performed with a consistent setup each day using the same collimator (typically the most heavily used). For all imaging protocols, there is an option to select a uniformity correction map. This correction map normalizes the high and low values within the image matrix to produce a uniform image. If the uniformity correction map is not chosen, the PMT arrangement will be visible in the acquired image resulting in poor uniformity.
- **Wrong correction map chosen.** The uniformity of a gamma camera is energy dependent. The two main contributors to a nonuniform detection efficiency are different and imperfect response characteristics of each PMT in the detector head and the position dependency on the scintillation event location (i.e., directly above a PMT vs in between two PMTs). Due to the imperfect response, gamma camera uniformity corrections are specific to the incident gamma ray energy and to the location where this gamma ray strikes the crystal face. For example, if a Tc-99m (140 keV) correction map is accidentally chosen but the camera is actually flooded with a Co-57 (122 keV) sheet source, the corrections applied will be incorrect for the actual incident gamma ray energy. The result will be a poorer uniformity response.
- **Resolution/linearity test.** Another extrinsic QC that is routinely performed implements a multiquadrant lead bar phantom. Commonly referred to as an extrinsic resolution test, the bar phantom is placed on an upward-facing camera head and then a sheet source is placed above the bar phantom. Each quadrant of the phantom has lead bars of varying line-pair thicknesses. The number of quadrants visible in the image (i.e., the smallest size lead bars that are resolvable) is the metric used to watch for any resolution degradation. A commonly forgotten application of this same phantom is its ability to test the linearity of the camera. By visually assessing the straightness of the lead bars in each quadrant, the X and Y position signals can be assessed for a linear response across the face of the detector (e.g., as a radiation source moves from the edge of a PMT to directly center of the PMT, the collection efficiency of that PMT increases in a nonlinear fashion). The bar phantom should be rotated each time QC is performed to check the directional performance of different areas of the crystal.

## ■ Additional Diagnostic Considerations

- **Co-57 sheet source:** The manufacturing process of Co-57 sheet sources is also imperfect and there is always a uniformity tolerance within the source itself. Sometimes image nonuniformities can be due to the sheet source itself.
- **Crystal thickness:** A higher energy gamma ray will have a scintillation event at a deeper depth within the detector crystal, thus having a smaller light-spread distribution. This typically results in worse uniformity but better resolution.

## ■ Diagnosis

Acceptable performance lines appear straight and three of four quadrants can be seen (A); poor uniformity due to no correction map (B); acceptable uniformity with correct energy uniformity map (C); acceptable uniformity with incorrect energy map (D).

## ✓ Pearls

- Gamma cameras implement energy, linearity, and uniformity corrections from calibration images.
- Gamma camera uniformity is energy and spatially dependent.
- Co-57 and Tc-99m energies are similar and thus have similar uniformity correction maps.

## Suggested Readings

Halama, James R. QC Protocols Gamma Camera & SPECT Systems, AAPM Meetings <http://www.aapm.org/meetings/amos2/pdf/35-9798-70158-156.pdf>. Accessed September 13, 2016

Zanzonico P. Routine quality control of clinical nuclear medicine instrumentation: a brief review. J Nucl Med. 2008; 49(7):1114-1131

# Index of Differential Diagnoses

# Index of Key Findings

*Note: The index is ordered by case number within each part*